Anticoagulation Therapy

A Point-of-Care Guide

William E. Dager, PharmD, BCPS (AQ Cardiology), FCSHP, FCCP, FCCM, FASHP

Pharmacist Specialist, UC Davis Medical Center
Clinical Professor of Medicine, UC Davis School of Medicine
Sacramento, California
Clinical Professor of Pharmacy
UC San Francisco School of Pharmacy
San Francisco, California
Clinical Professor of Pharmacy, Touro School of Pharmacy
Vallejo, California

Michael P. Gulseth, PharmD, BCPS

Program Director for Anticoagulation Services
Department of Pharmaceutical Services
Sanford USD Medical Center
Sioux Falls, South Dakota
Adjunct Assistant Professor of Pharmacy
South Dakota State University
Brookings, South Dakota

Edith A. Nutescu, PharmD, FCCP

Clinical Professor, Department of Pharmacy Practice & Center for Pharmacoeconomic Research
Director, Antithrombosis Center
College of Pharmacy and Medical Center
The University of Illinois at Chicago
Chicago, Illinois

American Society of Health-System Pharmacists®

Bethesda, Maryland

Any correspondence regarding this publication should be sent to the publisher, American Society of Health-System Pharmacists, 7272 Wisconsin Avenue, Bethesda, MD 20814, attention: Special Publishing.

The information presented herein reflects the opinions of the contributors and advisors. It should not be interpreted as an official policy of ASHP or as an endorsement of any product.

Because of ongoing research and improvements in technology, the information and its applications contained in this text are constantly evolving and are subject to the professional judgment and interpretation of the practitioner due to the uniqueness of a clinical situation. The editors, contributors, and ASHP have made reasonable efforts to ensure the accuracy and appropriateness of the information presented in this document. However, any user of this information is advised that the editors, contributors, advisors, and ASHP are not responsible for the continued currency of the information, for any errors or omissions, and/or for any consequences arising from the use of the information in the document in any and all practice settings. Any reader of this document is cautioned that ASHP makes no representation, guarantee, or warranty, express or implied, as to the accuracy and appropriateness of the information contained in this document and specifically disclaims any liability to any party for the accuracy and/or completeness of the material or for any damages arising out of the use or non-use of any of the information contained in this document.

Director, Special Publishing: Jack Bruggeman
Acquisitions Editor: Jack Bruggeman
Senior Editorial Project Manager: Dana Battaglia
Production Editor: Kristin Eckles
Cover and Page Design: David Wade

Library of Congress Cataloging-in-Publication Data

Anticoagulation therapy: a point-of-care guide / [edited by] William E. Dager, Michael P. Gulseth, Edith A. Nutescu.
   p.; cm.
  Includes bibliographical references and index.
  ISBN 978-1-58528-240-1
1. Anticoagulants (Medicine) 2. Anticoagulants (Medicine)—Therapeutic use.   I. Dager, William E.
II. Gulseth, Michael.   III. Nutescu, Edith A.   IV. American Society of Health-System Pharmacists.
  [DNLM: 1. Anticoagulants—therapeutic use. 2 Thromboembolism—drug therapy. QV 193]
  RM340.A536 2011
  615'.718—dc22

                    2011004926

ISBN 978-1-58528-240-1

DEDICATION

Without the continuous support of family, friends, students/
residents, and colleagues (including all the anticoagulation
practitioners that have inspired and helped me), projects,
such as this book, could never have occurred. To all the
patients who had a need for our services, stimulating a desire
to learn to improve their care. To my parents and the path
they lived and guided to serve the needs of others. For my
wife Karen and children William R., Jessica, and Laura for
their constant encouragement and understanding throughout
the years, I am forever grateful.

Bill

To my children Olivia, Luke, and Dominic, thank you for the
unconditional love and support you give to me every day.

Michael

To Michelle and Gabriel. Without your love, support, and
patience this would not have been possible.

Edith

ACKNOWLEDGMENTS

The editors and chapter authors would like to acknowledge the assistance provided by the individuals listed below during the preparation of this handbook. Your contribution is greatly appreciated.

Mikala Kanae, PharmD

Mahvish Ghufran, PharmD

Sok Lim, PharmD

Jacqueline Robichaud, PharmD

Lynnette Seyer, PharmD

Ashley Hansen, PharmD

William R. Dager

CONTENTS

PART III: Practical Monitoring and Coagulation Laboratory Insights

FOREWORD

Anticoagulation therapy can be dangerous and complicated. There are numerous indications for anticoagulant therapy, several agents that can be used, and many clinical risk factors that interplay with anticoagulant management. The complexity of issues that can affect anticoagulant therapy makes access to key information needed by clinicians a challenge. Where can the clinicians find all this essential information together in such a way that they can hone in on the information they need quickly and easily? There has been no easy answer.

Anticoagulation Therapy: A Point-of-Care Guide focuses on the clinical use of anticoagulant drugs. Emphasizing tabular presentation of information, the editors have organized the information in several valuable ways based on how clinicians typically frame or organize their thinking, particularly the nature of the underlying specific clinical problem. Determining the appropriate selection and dose of an anticoagulant drug in the patient who has unique clinical features is the continuing challenge of every clinician involved in managing anticoagulation therapy. What is the risk of stroke in a patient who has specified CHADS2 risk factors? What is the recommended perioperative treatment? What are the recommended screening criteria for a woman with recurrent fetal loss or the woman who had a prior major complication in pregnancy? What dose of a direct thrombin inhibitor should be used in a patient with HIT who has concomitant liver or renal disease? Answers to these and numerous other challenging anticoagulation questions can be found quickly in *Anticoagulation Therapy: A Point-of-Care Guide.*

In the ongoing clinical challenge to provide safe and effective anticoagulation therapy the editors have performed a great service for clinicians. *Anticoagulation Therapy: A Point-of-Care-Guide* should be an important component of your anticoagulation knowledge base. All clinicians are reminded that in addition to reviewing primary literature when necessary it is equally important to gather the insights and experience that local clinicians possess, based on hands-on management of complex patients.

Richard H. White, MD
Professor of Medicine, UC Davis School of Medicine
Chief of General Medicine and Director, UC Davis Anticoagulation Service
Sacramento, California

David A. Garcia, MD
Associate Professor
Division of Hematology/Oncology, University of New Mexico
    Health Sciences Center, Albuquerque, New Mexico
President, Anticoagulation Forum, Newton, Massachusetts

PREFACE

Despite their well-documented benefits in thrombosis prevention and treatment, anticoagulants continue to be associated with significant morbidity and mortality. Decades of experience, countless clinical trials, and numerous writings have explored ways to improve the safety of their use; however, anticoagulants are still among the top drugs causing patient harm. Since their first introduction in the 1940s, the number of agents in clinical use has expanded. Even though anticoagulants have long been considered as "high risk medications" by organizations such as the Institute for Safe Medication Practices, a recent analysis found that 8.2% of hospitalized patients on warfarin and 13.6% exposed to heparin experience an adverse drug event.[1] To compound the challenges in preventing anticoagulant-related adverse drug events, anticoagulation therapy is utilized by a broad spectrum of clinical specialties often faced with the challenge of caring for multiple patients and complex medical conditions both in the inpatient and outpatient settings. As clinicians, we (the editors) have also faced this challenge and wondered if an updated clinical reference could improve the safe and effective use of anticoagulants. We set out to create a unique, pocket-sized, point-of-care practice guide, which would give the clinician quick access to evidence-based and/or expert opinion information for the challenging clinical situations they may face.

To accomplish this aim, this point-of-care guide was designed to be the following:

- Light on text—The amount of "book style text" is intentionally minimized so a clinician will not have to read a whole chapter to find the "one nugget" they are seeking.

- Heavy on tables/figures—Our hope is that this allows the clinician to rapidly find the answers they are seeking.

- Easy to digest—The use of bullets and clinical pearl examples both present the information in a succinct fashion and highlight how the information applies to real life care.

- Comprehensive—While no book can cover every foreseeable topic, this book covers a lot of the potential challenges clinicians face.

- Expertly written—All of the authors are experts in the areas in which they write about and all chapters were carefully reviewed by all of the editors including the chapters written by other editors.

- Applicable to patients across the continuum of care—This book covers topics as diverse as how to care for the ambulatory patient in need of anticoagulation bridging for an invasive procedure to the pediatric patient on extracorporeal membrane oxygenation.

- Useful to a broad scope of disciplines—This handbook is intentionally designed to be a useful guide for clinicians in any discipline caring for patients on anticoagulation therapy.

The editors are deeply indebted to the authors who were willing to take on yet one more project and provided their expertise to improve the care of patients receiving anticoagulation therapy. We can never repay them for the time they took away from family and other professional commitments.

Finally, thank you to all clinicians who appreciate the challenges posed by these medications on a daily basis. There is no such thing as a "safe" anticoagulant, yet your efforts are what assure that these agents are used "safely" and in an evidence-based fashion. For that, we wish to thank you on behalf of your patients.

The Editors
December 2010

Note: you can find updates and additional information for *Anticoagulation Therapy: A Point-of-Care Guide* at www.ashp.org/anticoag.

REFERENCE

1. Classen DC, Jaser L, Budnitz DS. Adverse drug events among hospitalized Medicare patients: epidemiology and national estimates from a new approach to surveillance. *Jt Comm J Qual Patient Saf.* 2010;36(1):12–21.

EDITORS

William E. Dager, PharmD, BCPS
(AQ Cardiology), FCSHP, FCCP,
FCCM, FASHP
Pharmacist Specialist, UC Davis
    Medical Center
Clinical Professor of Medicine,
    UC Davis School of Medicine
Sacramento, California
Clinical Professor of Pharmacy,
    UC San Francisco School of Pharmacy
San Francisco, California
Clinical Professor of Pharmacy,
    Touro School of Pharmacy
Vallejo, California

Michael P. Gulseth, PharmD, BCPS
Program Director for Anticoagulation Services
Department of Pharmaceutical Services
Sanford USD Medical Center
Sioux Falls, South Dakota
Adjunct Assistant Professor of Pharmacy
South Dakota State University
Brookings, South Dakota

Edith A. Nutescu, PharmD, FCCP
Clinical Professor, Department of
    Pharmacy Practice & Center for
    Pharmacoeconomic Research
Director, Antithrombosis Center
College of Pharmacy and Medical Center
The University of Illinois at Chicago
Chicago, Illinois

CONTRIBUTORS

Douglas C. Anderson, Jr., BSPharm,
    PharmD, CACP
Professor and Chair
Department of Pharmacy Practice
Cedarville University School of Pharmacy
Cedarville, Ohio

William E. Dager, PharmD, BCPS
    (AQ Cardiology), FCSHP, FCCP,
    FCCM, FASHP
Pharmacist Specialist, UC Davis Medical
    Center
Clinical Professor of Medicine, UC Davis
    School of Medicine
Sacramento, California
Clinical Professor of Pharmacy, UC
    San Francisco School of Pharmacy
San Francisco, California
Clinical Professor of Pharmacy, Touro
    School of Pharmacy
Vallejo, California

Paul P. Dobesh, PharmD, FCCP,
    BCPS (AQ Cardiology)
Associate Professor of Pharmacy
    Practice
College of Pharmacy
University of Nebraska Medical Center
Omaha, Nebraska

John A. Dougherty, MBA, PharmD,
    BCPS
Director of Pharmacy
Nemours Children Hospital
Clinical Assistant Professor
University of Florida College of Pharmacy
Orlando, Florida

John Fanikos, RPh, MBA
Director of Pharmacy Business
Department of Pharmacy Services
Brigham and Women's Hospital
Boston, Massachusetts

Robert Gosselin, CLS
Coagulation Specialist, Department of
    Medical Pathology & Laboratory
    Medicine
Specialty Testing Center
The University of California, Davis Health
    System
Sacramento, California

Michael P. Gulseth, PharmD, BCPS
Program Director for Anticoagulation Services
Department of Pharmaceutical Services
Sanford USD Medical Center
Sioux Falls, South Dakota
Adjunct Assistant Professor of Pharmacy
South Dakota State University
Brookings, South Dakota

Jessica B. Michaud, PharmD, BCPS
Clinical Assistant Professor
The University of Illinois at Chicago
    College of Pharmacy
Clinical Pharmacist
The University of Illinois Medical Center at
    Chicago
Chicago, Illinois

Edith A. Nutescu, PharmD, FCCP
Clinical Professor, Department of
    Pharmacy Practice & Center for
    Pharmacoeconomic Research
Director, Antithrombosis Center
College of Pharmacy and Medical Center
The University of Illinois at Chicago
Chicago, Illinois

Kirsten H. Ohler, PharmD, BCPS
Neonatal/Pediatric Clinical Pharmacist
Clinical Assistant Professor in
    Pharmacy Practice
College of Pharmacy and Medical Center
The University of Illinois at Chicago
Chicago, Illinois

Lance J. Oyen, PharmD, BCPS, FCCP,
    FCCM
Assistant Director, Clinical Services,
    Pharmacy Department
Associate Professor, Mayo College of
    Medicine
Clinical Pharmacist, Surgical/Trauma ICU
Mayo Clinic
Rochester, Minnesota

Gregory J. Peitz, PharmD, BCPS
Clinical Pharmacist, Adult Intensive
    Care/Cardiology
Department of Pharmaceutical and
    Nutrition Care
Adjunct Assistant Professor, Pharmacy
    Practice
University of Nebraska Medical
    Center
Omaha, Nebraska

Nancy L. Shapiro, PharmD, BCPS,
    FCCP
Clinical Associate Professor
Operations Manager, Antithrombosis
    Clinic
The University of Illinois at
    Chicago
Chicago, Illinois

Maureen A. Smythe, PharmD, FCCP
Coordinator of Student and Resident
    Education
Department of Pharmaceutical
    Services
Beaumont Hospital
Royal Oak, Michigan
Professor (Clinical) of Pharmacy
    Practice
Wayne State University
Detroit, Michigan

Sarah A. Spinler, PharmD, FCCP, FAHA,
    FASHP, BCPS (AQ Cardiology)
Professor of Clinical Pharmacy
Residency Programs Coordinator
Philadelphia College of Pharmacy
University of the Sciences in Philadelphia
Philadelphia, Pennsylvania

Zachary A. Stacy, PharmD, BCPS
Clinical Pharmacy Specialist, Cardiology
St. Luke's Hospital
Associate Professor of Pharmacy Practice
St. Louis College of Pharmacy
Saint Louis, Missouri

Toby C. Trujillo, PharmD, BCPS
    (AQ Cardiology)
Associate Professor
University of Colorado Denver School of
    Pharmacy
Clinical Specialist, Anticoagulation/
    Cardiology
University of Colorado Hospital
Aurora, Colorado

Daniel M. Witt, PharmD, FCCP, BCPS,
    CACP
Senior Manager, Clinical
    Pharmacy Research & Applied
    Pharmacogenomics
Kaiser Permanente Colorado
Aurora, Colorado

Ann K. Wittkowsky, PharmD, CACP,
    FASHP, FCCP
Clinical Professor
University of Washington School of
    Pharmacy
Director, Anticoagulation Services
University of Washington Medical Center
Seattle, Washington

ABBREVIATIONS

A	apixaban
AAOS	American Association of Orthopedic Surgery
AAP	American Academy of Pediatrics
ACA	anticardiolipin antibody (also often abbreviated as aCL)
ACC	American College of Cardiology
ACC/AHA	American College of Cardiologists/American Heart Association
ACCP	American College of Chest Physicians
ACS	acute coronary syndrome
ACT	activated clotting time
AF	atrial fibrillation
AFFIRM	Atrial Fibrillation Follow-up Investigation of Rhythm Management
AHA	American Heart Association
AHA/ASA	American Heart Association/American Stroke Association
AIS	arterial ischemic stroke
ALL	acute lymphoblastic leukemia
ALT	alanine aminotransferase
AMI	acute myocardial infarction
AP	antiplatelet
APC	activated protein C
APLA syndrome	antiphospholipid antibody syndrome (also often abbreviated APS and APLS)
APLAs	antiphospholipid antibodies
aPTT	activated partial thromboplastin time
ASA	aspirin
ASSENT	Assessment of the Safety and Efficacy of a New Thrombolytic
AST	aspartate aminotransferase

AT	antithrombin
AUC	area under the serum concentration versus time curve
AVR	aortic valve replacement
BID	twice daily dosing
BMI	body mass index
BP	blood pressure
CABG	coronary artery bypass graft
CAD	coronary artery disease
CAP	College of American Pathologists
CBC	complete blood count (including platelets)
CBS	cystathionine β synthase
CHD	coronary heart disease
CI	confidence interval
CLIA	Clinical Laboratory Improvement Amendments
CLSI	Clinical Laboratory Standards Institute (formerly NCCLS or National Committee on Clinical Laboratory Standards)
Cmax	maximum serum concentration
CPK	creatinine phosphokinase
CPR	cardiopulmonary resuscitation
CrCL	creatinine clearance
CRRT	continuous renal replacement technique
CRUSADE	**C**an **R**apid risk stratification of **U**nstable angina patients **S**uppress **AD**verse outcomes with **E**arly implementation of the ACC/AHA guidelines
CSCT	colloidal-silica clotting time
CT	computed tomographic
CVA	cerebrovascular accident
CVAD	central venous access device
CVL	central venous line
D	dabigatran

D5W	5% dextrose in water
DBP	diastolic blood pressure
Dec	decrease
DIC	disseminated intravascular coagulation
dL	deciliter
dPT	dilute prothrombin time
dRVVT	dilute Russell's viper-venom time
DTI	direct thrombin inhibitor
DVT	deep vein thrombosis
ECG	electrocardiogram
ECLS	extracorporeal life support
ECMO	extracorporeal membrane oxygenation
ELISA	enzyme-linked-immunosorbent assay
Enox	enoxaparin
EU	European Union
FDA	Food and Drug Administration
FFP	fresh frozen plasma
FVL	factor V Leiden mutation
GAGs	glycosaminoglycans
GCS	Glasgow Coma Scale
GCS	graduated compression stockings
GI	gastrointestinal
Gp llb/lll	glycoprotein llb/llla receptor
GUSTO	global use of strategies to open occluded coronary arteries
HAT	heparin-associated thrombocytopenia (nonimmune mediated)
Hct	hematocrit
Hgb	hemoglobin
HIT	heparin-induced thrombocytopenia (immune mediated)

HITTS	heparin-induced thrombocytopenia thrombosis syndrome (immune mediated)
hr	hour
HR-ACT	high response activated clotting time
HR	heart rate
HTN	hypertension
IBD	inflammatory bowel disease
ICD	implantable cardioverter defibrillator
ICH	intracranial hemorrhage
IgG (IgA, etc.)	immune globulin G, etc.
IM	intramuscular
Inc	increase
INR	international normalized ratio
IPC	intermittent pneumatic compression
ISI	International Sensitivity Index
ISTH	International Society of Thrombosis and Haemostasis
IUGR	intrauterine growth restriction
IV	intravenous
IVC	inferior vena cava
KCT	kaolin clotting time
kD	kilodalton
Kg	kilogram
Kg/m^2	kilogram/meter squared
LA	lupus anticoagulant
LIA	latex immunoassay
LMWH	low molecular weight heparin
LR ACT	low range activated clotting time
LV	left ventricular
mg	milligrams

Mg	magnesium
MI	myocardial infarction
Min	minutes
mL/min	milliliter/minute
MODS	multiple organ dysfunction syndrome
MRI	magnetic resonance imaging
MTHFR	methylene-tetrahydrofolate reductase
MVP	mechanical valve prosthesis
MVR	mitral valve replacement
NA	not available
NHP	normal human plasma
NIBSC	National Institute of Biological Standards and Controls
NINDS	National Institute of Neurological Disorders and Stroke
NPSG	National Patient Safety Goal
NS	normal saline
NSAIDs	nonsteroidal anti-inflammatory drugs
NSR	normal sinus rhythm
NSTE	non-ST-segment elevation
NSTEMI	non-ST-segment elevation myocardial infarction
OR	operation room
PAD	peripheral arterial disease
PCC	prothrombin complex concentrate
PCI	percutaneous coronary intervention
PE	pulmonary embolism
PF-4	platelet factor 4
PICC	peripherally inserted central catheter
Plt	platelet
POC	point of care

PPH	primary pulmonary hypertension
PRBCs	packed red blood cells
PT	prothrombin time
Pt yr	patient-year
R	rivaroxaban
RACE	RAte Control vs. Electrical cardioversion for persistent atrial fibrillation study
RCT	randomized clinical trial
rFVIIa	recombinant factor VII activated
RRR	relative risk reduction
rt-PA	recombinant tissue plasminogen activator
RVT	renal vein thrombosis
SBP	systolic blood pressure
SC	subcutaneous
SCAI	Society for Cardiac Angiography and Interventions
SCD	sickle cell disease
SCr	serum creatinine
SOB	shortness of breath
SQ	subcutaneous
SRA	serotonin release assay
SSC	Scientific Subcommittee (part of ISTH)
SSRI	selective serotonin reuptake inhibitors
STEMI	ST-segment elevation myocardial infarction
T1/2	elimination half life
TBW	total body weight
TE	thromboembolism
TEE	transesophageal echocardiography
THR	total hip replacement
TIA	transient ischemic attack

TIA	transient ischemic attack
TIMI	thrombolysis in myocardial infarction
TKR	total knee replacement
TMA	thrombotic microangiopathy
Tmax	time to maximum serum concentration
TNK	tenecteplase
tPA	tissue plasminogen activator
TPN	total parenteral nutrition
TT	thrombin time
TTE	transthoracic echocardiography
UFH	unfractionated heparin
Vit K	vitamin K or phytonadione
VKA	vitamin K antagonist
VKOR	vitamin K epoxide reductase
VTE	venous thromboembolism
vWF	von Willebrand's factor
WARSS/APASS	Warfarin vs. Aspirin Recurrent Stroke Study/ Antiphospholipid Antibodies in Stroke Study
WHO	World Health Organization

PART I: Anticoagulant Medication Management

Introduction to Anticoagulation Management

1

William E. Dager, Michael P. Gulseth, Edith A. Nutescu

INTRODUCTION

In the setting where anticoagulation therapy is necessary, clinicians are faced with the challenge of utilizing agents that inherently have a small therapeutic window and the ability for medication mishaps when not used appropriately. However, this risk is balanced against the need to prevent against or treat thrombosis, which can also have life altering consequences. Therefore, clinicians utilizing anticoagulants must not only have a firm grasp of the pharmacology and pharmacokinetics of the agents they are utilizing, but they must also be current with the evidence regarding their use and understand how an individual patient's situation can influence management decisions.

This reference book was developed with these challenges in mind in order to seed thoughts and provide information that assists the clinician in assuring the safe and optimal use of anticoagulants. The information in the chapters is intended to provide key concepts based on the literature and experiences of the authors when evidence is more limited. Evidence-based recommendations by expert panels are included when available. This handbook is intended to provide insights that can assist in decision process and not to replace the clinician's judgment.

JOINT COMMISSION NATIONAL PATIENT SAFETY GOALS (NPSGS) FOR ANTICOAGULATION, 2010 VERSION (NPSG 03.05.01, FORMALLY NPSG 3E)[1]

- Because of the high incidence of reported adverse event rates associated with anticoagulation therapy or suboptimal approaches to prevention of VTE, several regulatory agencies have initiated processes to address their concerns. One example is the NPSGs issued by the Joint Commission. The primary goal of the anticoagulation NPSGs is to reduce the likelihood of patient harm associated with the use of anticoagulant therapy.

- The full text and requirements of the NPSGs can be found at http://www .jointcommission.org/standards_information/npsgs.aspx.

- Of note is that the NPSGs are driven by the frequency of reported adverse events associated with anticoagulation therapy. Thus, newer agents, or infrequently used agents may not receive as much attention or regulatory oversight. This does not necessarily make their use any less challenging.

TABLE OF USEFUL RESOURCES

Table 1-1: Resources Involving Anticoagulation Therapy

Reference	Website	Comment
ACCP guidelines	http://chestjournal .chestpubs.org/ content/133/6_suppl	The oldest and most established evidence-based guideline involving antithrombotic therapy
AHA guidelines	http://my.americanheart .org/professional/ guidelines.jsp	The American Heart Association regularly published guidelines that cover different arterial disease states, often in conjunction with other societies
FDA	http://www.fda.gov/	The FDA regularly posts any alerts concerning marketed medications and materials that are reviewed by advisory committees
Clinical Trials.gov	http://www.clinicaltrials .gov/	Describes current clinical trials being conducted
PubMed	http://www.ncbi.nlm.nih .gov/pubmed/	Excellent free site available for searching Medline from the United States National Library of Medicine

(*continued*)

Table 1-1: (Continued)

Reference	Website	Comment
Anticoagulation Forum	http://www.acforum.org/	Multidisciplinary professional organization for those who manage anticoagulation therapy; helpful clinical resources are posted on the site
ClotCare	http://www.clotcare .com/clotcare/index .aspx	Regularly updated site mainly focused on keeping professionals abreast of cutting edge information involving antithrombotic therapy; site also does contain helpful information for patients

TOOLS FOR SUCCESS

Considerations in applying professional organizations' expert evidence-based guidelines to patient care:

- Expert panels representing the American College of Chest Physicians (ACCP) and American Heart Association (AHA) (published in conjunction with the American College of Cardiology (ACC)) have provided evidence-based recommendations to aid clinicians in selecting appropriate patient care. Often, these guidelines are considered the final word. Adherence to these guidelines by nature ignores how an individual patient situation may cause variance from the guidelines. It should be kept in mind that such guidelines are established based on the strength of the evidence available. In many cases, evidence or trials may have not included selected situations or populations, or negative experiences were not published. Clinicians need to view and use these guidelines as they are intended; evidence-based tools designed (or developed) to aid in patient care.

- The following tables explain the evidence ranking system of the both ACCP and AHA guidelines. These evidence grades are extensively mentioned in subsequent chapters.

Table 1-2: Interpreting the ACCP Antithrombotic and Thrombolytic Therapy Evidence-Based Clinical Practice Guidelines Evidence Grades[2,a]

Grade of Recommendation (recommendation strength/evidence grade)	Quality of Evidence	Implications
1A	Consistent findings from randomized clinical trials (RCTs) or extremely strong evidence from observational studies	Recommendation applies to most patients in most situations
1B	RCTs that have important limitations or strong evidence from observational studies	Recommendation applies to most patients in most situations
1C	At least one important outcome has been assessed in case series, observational studies, or from a seriously flawed RCTs; indirect evidence also can be used	Recommendation applies to most patients in many situations
2A	Consistent findings from randomized clinical trials (RCTs) or extremely strong evidence from observational studies	The appropriate treatment may vary based on patient/society values
2B	RCTs have important limitations or strong evidence from observational studies	The appropriate treatment may vary based on patient/society values
2C	At least one important outcome has been assessed in case series, observational studies, or from a seriously flawed RCTs; indirect evidence also can be used	Other treatment options may be equally desirable

[a]Grade 1 recommendations are considered "strong" recommendations and grade 2 are considered "weak" recommendations. Grade A evidence comes from RCTs or observational studies with very large effects. Grade B evidence comes from RCTs with limitations or strong evidence from observational trials. Grade C evidence comes from observational trials or RCTs with major limitations.

Table 1-3: Interpreting the ACC/AHA Evidence Grades Used in Scientific Statements[3]

Grade of Recommendation (class/evidence grade)	Quality of Evidence
1 (A)	Strong recommendation that a treatment or procedure is helpful; robust supporting data
1 (B)	Strong recommendation that a treatment or procedure is helpful; more limited supporting data
1 (C)	Strong recommendation that a treatment or procedure is helpful; largely based on expert opinion, standard of care, or case studies
IIa (A)	Recommendation that a treatment or procedure is helpful; data available contains some conflicting evidence
IIa (B)	Recommendation that a treatment or procedure is helpful; data available contains some conflicting evidence
IIa (C)	Recommendation that a treatment or procedure is helpful; largely based on expert opinion, standard of care, or case studies
IIb (A)	Recommendation that a treatment or procedure may be considered; supporting data contains significant conflicting evidence
IIb (B)	Recommendation that a treatment or procedure may be considered; available data contains significant conflicting evidence
IIb (C)	Recommendation that a treatment or procedure may be considered; largely based on expert opinion, standard of care, or case studies
III (A)	Recommendation that a treatment or procedure should *not* be considered; robust supporting data
III (B)	Recommendation that a treatment or procedure should *not* be considered; more limited supporting data
III (C)	Recommendation that a treatment or procedure should *not* be considered; largely based on expert opinion, standard of care, or case studies

Considerations when evaluating clinical trials involving anticoagulants

- Clinical trials frequently have preselected inclusion and exclusion criteria that create a focus for the concept being studied. In many cases with anticoagulation therapy, patient groups (advanced age, bleeding history, organ dysfunction, critically ill, hypercoagulable condition) initially excluded from the clinical trials may receive the therapy. Clinicians should consider that trials serve as a foundation to managing thrombosis, but that excluded populations may respond differently to a given therapy.

- Anticoagulants or reversal therapies may frequently be used in conditions where the agent has not been adequately explored. The limited evidence with such "off-label" use should be used with caution, with consideration that the optimal dose, duration or approach to their use in such settings has not been determined.

- In many situations, current approaches to anticoagulation regimens have evolved based on postmarketing experiences. Populations originally excluded in the clinical trials may provide signals on how therapies may need to be adapted. In some settings, limited single center case reports where no additional information exists may drive practice. In others, concepts based in theory but not yet validated (e.g., overlapping parenteral anticoagulants for two additional days after the INR on warfarin is over 2) are utilized.

- When reviewing data derived from observations collected from registries, the reviewer should consider the voluntary structure and potential cleaning of data prior to submission to eliminate any perception of poor management. The coding of the information prior to being extrapolated may also create certain bias, or limitations on the quality of the research.

Table 1-4: Additional Considerations When Evaluating Clinical Trials

Concept	Comment
Population studied	• The inclusion and exclusion criteria describe who was or was not studied in the analysis. Be sure the patients you are considering for therapy based on the trial would have been included.
	• The number of eligible subjects vs. those actually studied can also describe potential challenges in repeating the observations in the general population.

(*continued*)

Table 1-4: (Continued)

Concept	Comment
Methods	• The methods should be cross compared to the setting of the study. For example, ethnic differences in a region or the assay used may create results that may have some limitations when being implemented in a different setting.
Results	• Many of the new trials involving anticoagulants are "noninferiority" in design. If the medication is found to be "noninferior" to the comparator, be sure to carefully review the noninferiority criteria to assure it is appropriate. Also, when compared to warfarin, how well controlled was the warfarin?
	• Carefully consider the clinical significance of the primary endpoint of the trials. For example, many orthopedic trials commonly include venographically derived asymptomatic DVT, which many would argue is not as clinically significant as symptomatic DVT/PE. These results may be "statistically significant," but that is very different than "clinically significant."
	• Data should be carefully assessed for "robustness." Were any signals present suggesting different outcomes within the study population? Who was excluded? Where additional analysis done to confirm the primary endpoint findings or conclusions made?
	• Was any subgroup analysis included in the initial study design, or was it derived posthoc to create a positive spin on the study. Caution should be exercised if considering applying post hoc analysis to patient care.
	• When assessing a clinical observation or reported result, consider the potential error in the data. Single, unexpected, or atypical observations should be confirmed with additional analysis.
	• Trends in data that support a result create a higher level of confidence than the single outlier.
Limitations	Be sure the study clearly identifies the limitations of the analysis. The study should attempt to describe how the limitations affect interpretation/application of the results. It is also helpful if they have done additional data analysis to assess the impact of the limitations.
Summary/ conclusion	Be sure the conclusion is appropriate considering the data and its limitations. Often, conclusions overreach the observed result, ignoring important limitations, which could potentially harm patients if applied without this consideration.

Meta-analysis interpretation cautions

- Guidelines strive to incorporate the best evidence available when developing recommendations. This frequently can be influenced by meta-analysis that explores similar trials. It should be kept in mind that trials may not be published, particularly small negative trials. This can create a literature base that is influenced by positive outcomes. In some cases, single large trials may dominate the observations. Such data basis should utilize concepts such a funnel plots to describe any potential bias in the data base. (See reference 4 for an example of how this can help detect publication bias.)[4]

- Differences in the approach to the study and the patients actually studied may have influenced the variable results reported in the meta-analysis. These trials, while having enough power to detect small treatment effects, often include a diverse population of patients by their nature.

- Medical advances in both technology and management approaches over time can independently influence outcomes. Since trials included in a meta-analysis are usually conducted during different time periods, this can create challenges in interpreting the results.

Treat the patient and consider all of the patient's potential needs

- Each patient is unique, and clinicians will combine their knowledge and experience along with resources, such as this handbook, to derive and adapt anticoagulation therapy. In many cases, deficiencies in the information used limit its application. Lab results or other surrogate markers may not be validated to hard outcomes of bleeding, thrombosis, morbidity, or death. Quality of life or limitations such as the ability to be adherent to the management plan, affordability of the therapy, or monitoring can influence management plans.

  - Observations away from the bedside may not always agree with the patient presentation. For example, increasing the level of anticoagulation based on laboratory results may not be optimal if the patient is bleeding. The lab test is intended to lend assistance in determining appropriate patient management and must not be interpreted apart from the individual patient situation. Caution should be considered with the management of anticoagulation therapy by assessing information solely from a computer screen, even in facilities with the most advanced electronic medical record systems. Critical information (bleeding, consideration for an LP, potential invasive procedures) may be missed, due to delay in availability or ommission of information. This can limit the level of care provided.

- Just because something is ordered does not mean the intended therapy is carried out. Handing out a prescription or order where hurdles to fulfill the prescription exist may delay or prevent therapy. (Classic example is the patient never filling the prescription when he or she leaves the hospital.)

- Even when a patient is handed a dose, this does not always equate to the patient taking it. In time, this may be discovered by a lack of INR response to warfarin. One consideration is to assure the therapy is administered is by requesting nurse/family to witness swallowing of the medication.

- When arranging ambulatory anticoagulation patient care followup, has the treatment team determined if the patient can get the prescribed followup laboratory monitoring? Are they capable of utilizing the medication prescribed, including injectables? Is the patient able to afford the prescribed medication regimen?

- The level of patient acuity should be considered. Clinical trials may not have explored critically ill patients, yet the therapy may be regularly used in such a population. Management plans may at times be short-term and should be adapted as changes occur. In many cases, therapy involves multiple agents or changing settings. A management plan should consider both short- and long-term goals, and what options are available. Sometimes, the agent chosen in a management plan may not be the one that is "best" based on evidence, but instead the agent that is most likely to succeed considering the patient's individual situation.

  - Often, newer agents may be preferable, but if financially unreasonable for the patient, could lead to suboptimal results.

  - Patients are often moving in or out of different care settings during therapy. This can influence the choice of agents utilized in the management plan.

  - Management should consider how the patient is clinically changing in interfering factors such as interacting drugs or disease states and adapt as necessary.

- Practitioners who also have practice management responsibilities should strive to break down transitional care barriers that lead to unsafe care. When patients are admitted, it is important to obtain an accurate medication history. This is particularly critical regarding their antithrombotic drug therapy, which is often taken from electronic records and may not be current with the patients' actual regimen. Patients being discharged should be promptly handed off to the responsible managing clinician, with critical information relayed. The clinician needs to understand how the inpatient care experience may have influenced the patients' antithrombotic therapy needs. This is a particularly high-risk time period in the patients' therapy, and too often, patients do not understand their individual management plan, which leads to adverse drug events. Further, it also common for the medication reconciliation process to not be completed correctly at discharge. For example, patients can be put back on their home warfarin dosing (assuming it was correctly identified at admission!), which is no longer clinically appropriate considering their condition at discharge. Others may revise the regimen based on an altered response during an acute illness (elevated INR during acute decompensated heart failure or an infection), and not re-adjust the dose back once the patients baseline has been reestablished (heart failure or infection resolved). In this situation, a period of catch up may occur after discharge.

- Each patient is unique and hence a special population. However, generalizations of certain clinical situations create a "special management population." Examples include the elderly patients, pediatric patients, critically ill patients, patients with certain concurrent disease states, patients with a hypercoagulable condition, patients with multiple indications for anticoagulation, impaired organ function, etc. These patient populations are frequently discussed in this text.

REFERENCES

1.   Unknown. The Joint Commission National Patient Safety Goals. July 1, 2010; http://www.jointcommission.org/NR/rdonlyres/868C9E07-037F-433D-8858-0D5FAA4322F2/0/July2010NPSGs_Scoring_HAP2.pdf. Accessed August 7, 2010.

2.   Guyatt GH, Cook DJ, Jaeschke R, et al. Grades of recommendation for antithrombotic agents: American College of Chest Physicians Evidence-Based Clinical Practice Guidelines (8th Edition). *Chest.* 2008;133(6 Suppl):123S–131S.

3.   Kushner FG, Hand M, Smith SC Jr., et al. 2009 Focused Updates: ACC/AHA Guidelines for the Management of Patients With ST-Elevation Myocardial Infarction (updating the 2004 Guideline and 2007 Focused Update) and ACC/AHA/SCAI Guidelines on Percutaneous Coronary Intervention (updating the 2005 Guideline and 2007 Focused Update): a report of the American College of Cardiology Foundation/American Heart Association Task Force on Practice Guidelines. *Circulation.* 2009;120(22):2271–2306.

4.   Wein L, Wein S, Haas SJ, et al. Pharmacological venous thromboembolism prophylaxis in hospitalized medical patients: a meta-analysis of randomized controlled trials. *Arch Intern Med.* 2007;167(14):1476–1486.

TWO

Chapter

2

Warfarin

Ann K. Wittkowsky

INTRODUCTION

Vitamin K antagonists (VKAs), including warfarin, have been the core of oral anti-coagulation for decades. Warfarin is used for stroke prevention in atrial fibrillation, prevention of valvular thrombosis in biologic and mechanical valve replacement, and prevention and treatment of deep vein thrombosis, pulmonary embolism, and other manifestations of venous and arterial thromboembolism. Due to a narrow therapeutic index, highly variable dose response and the significant impact of diet, disease, and drugs on warfarin pharmacokinetics and pharmacodynamics, it is an agent that requires frequent monitoring and dosage adjustment to maintain its efficacy and safety.

PHARMACOLOGY[1]

Warfarin and other VKAs act by inhibition of the hepatic synthesis of vitamin K dependent clotting factors II, VII, IX, and X. These clotting factors (and the anticoagulant substances protein C and protein S) become biologically active by gamma-carboxylation involving vitamin KH2. In a vitamin K hepatic recycling process that maintains a continuous supply of vitamin KH2 for clotting factor synthesis, vitamin KH2 is oxidized to vitamin KO and subsequently converted to vitamin K by vitamin K epoxide reductase (VKOR) and then back to vitamin KH2 by vitamin K1 reductase. Warfarin inhibits VKOR and vitamin K1 reductase, resulting in accumulation of biologically inactive vitamin KO and a reduction in vitamin K dependent clotting factor synthesis. The full anticoagulant effect of warfarin occurs when previously activated clotting factors are depleted at rates consistent with their biologic half-lives (Table 2-1).

Table 2-1: Proteins and Half-life

Vitamin K Dependent Proteins	Elimination Half-life
Factor II	42–72 hr
Factor VII	4–6 hr
Factor IX	21–30 hr
Factor X	27–48 hr
Protein C	8 hr
Protein S	60 hr

PHARMACOKINETICS/PHARMACODYNAMICS[2]

Warfarin is a racemic mixture of R and S enantiomers that differ with respect to elimination half-life, metabolism, pathways of oxidative metabolism, and potency (Table 2-2).

Table 2-2: Differences in R and S Enantiomers

	R-Warfarin	S-Warfarin
Elimination half-life	45 hr (20–70 hr)	29 hr (18–52 hr)
Metabolism	40% reduction 60% oxidation	10% reduction 90% oxidation
Oxidative metabolism	1A2>3A4>2C19	2C9>3A4
Potency	1.0 (reference)	2.7–3.8 × R-warfarin

The pharmacokinetic and pharmacodynamic properties of other VKAs available outside the US are quite different from those of warfarin (Table 2-3).

Pictured are Jantoven brand warfarin tablets with permission by Upsher-Smith Laboratories, Inc., Maple Grove, MN. This color scheme is also used for other brands of warfarin and can be used to determine a patient's tablet strength and dose.

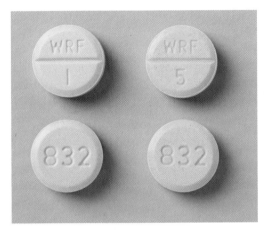

1 mg   Pink   5 mg   Peach

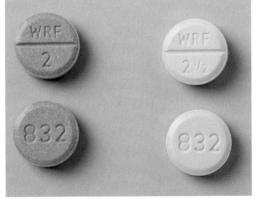

2 mg   Lavender   2.5 mg   Green

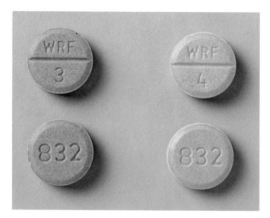

3 mg   Tan   4 mg   Blue

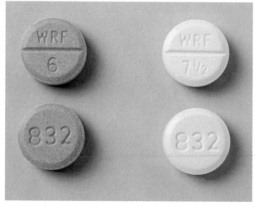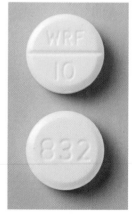

6 mg   Teal   7.5 mg   Yellow   10 mg   White

Table 2-3: Other K Antagonists

	Acenocoumarol	**Phenprocoumon**
Elimination half-life	R: 9 hr S: 0.5 hr	R: 5.5 days S: 5.5 days
Oxidative metabolism	R: 2C9 > 2C19 S: 2C9	R: 2C9 S: 2C9 ⅓ eliminated unchanged
Potency	R more active due to faster clearance of S	S 1.5–2.5 × more potent than R

Genetic variations in CYP2C9 genotype can influence the clearance of warfarin, leading to lower-than-average warfarin dosing requirements in patients in patients who are CYP2C*1/*2, CYP*1/*3, and CYP*2/*3 heterozygotes, and even lower dosing requirements in CYP*2/*2 and CYP*3/*3 homozygotes. In addition, VKORC1 haplotype influences warfarin responsiveness. A number of dosing algorithms that incorporate CYP2C9 genotype and VKORC1 haplotype are currently being investigated, but genetic testing to guide warfarin dose determination is not yet a routine component of clinical care.

Clinical Pearls

- Clinicians managing warfarin therapy will encounter patients who cannot take warfarin enterally. If the International Normalized Ratio (INR) is in range or close to being in range, using IV warfarin can prevent disruption of stabilized patients. This avoids use of other injectable anticoagulants and re-titration of warfarin. These patients often require lower IV doses from baseline despite equal bioavailability of oral warfarin secondary to acute illnesses, medication used to treat the illness, and/or decreased nutritional intake of vitamin K.

- Due to the long half-life of warfarin, every dose taken within the last 7 days must be considered when making dosing decisions. However, doses taken 2–3 days ago will have the most prominent effect on current day's INR, and these require careful consideration when making further dosage adjustments.

Vitamin K interactions[3]

Changes in dietary vitamin K intake can alter response to warfarin therapy. Accordingly, patients should be instructed to recognize foods high in vitamin K and to maintain a stable and consistent intake of high vitamin K-containing foods. Examples of foods high in vitamin K are listed below (Table 2-4). A thorough list of vitamin K content of various foods is from the USDA at www.nal.usda.gov/fnic/foodcomp/data/SR17/wtrank/sr17w430.pdf.

Table 2-4: Sample Foods High in Vitamin K

Broccoli	Lettuce
Brussels sprouts	Kale
Cabbage	Mustard greens
Chard	Parsley
Chives	Scallions
Collard greens	Spinach
Endive	Turnip greens

Clinical Pearl

- Hospitalized patients often have changes in diet causing fluctuating warfarin requirements and dosing that is distinctly different from their outpatient requirements. Further, enteral and parenteral nutritional supplements containing vitamin K further complicate matters. It is important for clinicians to follow changes in feeding rates and diets as these influence warfarin dosing.

Disease state interactions

Numerous disease states influence the pharmacokinetics and pharmacodynamics of warfarin (Table 2-5). Progression and improvement in these factors can influence warfarin dosing requirements and should be considered when evaluating INR response to warfarin therapy.

Table 2-5: Drug-Disease State Interactions[2]

Clinical Condition	Effect on Warfarin Therapy
Advanced age	Increased sensitivity to warfarin due to reduced vitamin K stores and/or lower plasma concentrations of vitamin K dependent clotting factors
Pregnancy	Teratogenic; avoid exposure during pregnancy
Lactation	Not excreted in breast milk; can be used postpartum by nursing mothers
Alcoholism	• <u>Acute ingestion:</u> inhibits warfarin metabolism, with acute elevation in INR • <u>Chronic ingestion:</u> induces warfarin metabolism, with higher dose requirements
Liver disease	• May induce coagulopathy by decreased production of clotting factors, with baseline elevation in INR • May reduce clearance of warfarin
Renal disease	Reduced activity of CYP2C9, with lower warfarin dose requirements
Heart failure	Reduced warfarin metabolism due to hepatic congestion
Cardiac valve replacement	Enhanced sensitivity to warfarin postoperatively due to hypoalbuminemia, lower oral intake, decreased physical activity, and reduced clotting factor concentrations after cardiopulmonary bypass
Nutritional status	Changes in dietary vitamin K intake (intentional or as the result of disease, surgery etc) alter response to warfarin
Use of tube feedings	Decreased sensitivity to warfarin, possibly caused by changes in absorption or vitamin K content of nutritional supplements

(continued)

Table 2-5: (Continued)

Clinical Condition	Effect on Warfarin Therapy
Thyroid disease	• <u>Hypothyroidism:</u> decreased catabolism of clotting factors requiring increased dosing requirements • <u>Hyperthyroidism:</u> increased catabolism of clotting factors causing increased sensitivity to warfarin
Smoking and tobacco use	• <u>Smoking:</u> may induce CYP1A2, increasing warfarin dosing requirements. • <u>Chewing tobacco:</u> may contain vitamin K, increasing warfarin dosing requirements
Fever	Increased catabolism of clotting factors, causing acute increase in INR
Diarrhea	Reduction in secretion of vitamin K by gut flora, causing acute increase in INR
Acute infection/inflammation	Increased sensitivity to warfarin
Malignancy	Increased sensitivity to warfarin by multiple factors

Clinical Pearls

- Patients who experience acute liver dysfunction (hypotensive episodes, liver metastasis, etc.) while in the hospital will be extremely sensitive to warfarin. Vigilance is necessary when managing warfarin in these patients (daily INRs and warfarin adjustments) and sometimes holding warfarin until liver function recovers is required. Close consultation with the attending physician is advised in these situations.

- Thyroid status is often not a clinical concern unless thyroid status is changing. In other words, stable levothyroxine patients in euthyroid status should be treated like patients without thyroid issues. Hypothyroid patients initiated on levothyroxine or having levothyroxine dose increases may require warfarin dose reduction. Patients undergoing hyperthyroid treatment will likely require warfarin dose increases.

- Previously stabilized warfarin patients often have elevated INRs when admitted with decompensated heart failure. This often requires holding or reducing their warfarin dose by about 50% for 1–2 days after admission, but as they diurese and improve, they often require their previous warfarin dose. Clinicians are often reluctant to resume previous dosing thinking "the dose made them go high" overlooking the acute illness as the cause rather than the dose. As with all warfarin patients, it is important for the clinician to understand the patient's complete clinical status and not just "treat the numbers."

Drug-drug interactions[4]

Numerous prescription and nonprescription drugs as well as natural/herbal products interfere with the pharmacokinetics and/or pharmacodynamics of warfarin. The addition or discontinuation of interacting agents can profoundly impact warfarin dose-response and requires that current medication use be evaluated routinely in patients taking warfarin so that appropriate monitoring and dosage adjustments may occur. Timely management can avoid significant interactions, and allow for interacting drugs to be used concurrently with warfarin. There is considerable variability in the time of onset, extent of influence, and time of offset of drug interactions with warfarin, requiring individualization of dosing and monitoring any time a potentially interacting medication is started, stopped or used on an as-needed basis (Tables 2-6 and 2-7).

Clinical Pearls

- Patient and medical staff education on warfarin interactions reduces hospital admissions by improving warfarin management and preventing warfarin misadventures. Hospital admissions secondary to warfarin drug interactions provide an opportunity to educate the prescriber, patient's outpatient pharmacy, and patient on interaction screening.

- Interactions involving inhibition of S-warfarin metabolism are more severe and may require preemptive warfarin dose

Table 2-6: Warfarin Drug Interactions

Target	Effect	Response	Examples (Noninclusive)		
Clotting factors	Increased synthesis	Decreased INR	Vitamin K		
	Decreased synthesis	Increased INR	Broad spectrum antibiotics		
	Increased catabolism	Increased INR	Thyroid hormones		
	Decreased catabolism	Decreased INR	Methimazole	Propylthiouracil	
Warfarin metabolism	Inhibition	Increased INR	Acetaminophen	Allopurinol	Amiodarone	Azole antifungals
			Cimetidine	Fluroquinolones	Macrolides	Metronidazole
			Propafenone	SSRIs	Statins	Sulfa antibiotics
	Induction	Decreased INR	Barbiturates	Carbamazepine	Doxycycline	Griseofulvin
			Nafcillin	Phenytoin	Primidone	Rifampin

(continued)

Table 2-6: (Continued)

Target	Effect	Response	Examples (Noninclusive)			
Hemostasis	Additive antithrombotic effects	Increased bleeding risk	Aspirin	NSAIDs	Salicylates	GPIIb/IIIa inhibitors
	Additive anticoagulant response	Increased bleeding risk	Heparin	LMWH	Direct thrombin inhibitors	Thrombolytics
Absorption	Reduced	Decreased INR	Cholestyramine	Colestipol	Sucralfate	
Unknown		Decreased INR	Ascorbic acid	Azathioprine	Corticosteroids	Cyclosporin
		Increased INR	Androgens	Clofibrate	Cyclophosphamide	Gemfibrozil

adjustments or interchange to safer alternatives. Interactions involving the less potent R-isomer can often be managed by daily INR monitoring and usually cause less dramatic INR elevations.

- Clearly determining if a medication, even those known to interact, caused an INR elevation in hospitalized patients is difficult because acute illnesses may also elevate the INR. A good example is a patient receiving metronidazole for *Clostridium difficile* colitis. When an INR bump occurs, is it from the metronidazole, the severe diarrhea, poor vitamin K intake, or all of the above? Often, it is a combination of factors and the presumed "drug interaction" may become less pronounced as the patient recovers from illness.

Table 2-7: Indications and Goal INR[1]

Indication	Target INR (range)
Atrial fibrillation	2.5 (2–3)
Atrial flutter	2.5 (2–3)
Cardioembolic stroke	2.5 (2–3)
Left ventricular dysfunction	2.5 (2–3)
Myocardial infarction	2.5 (2–3)
Venous thromboembolism (treatment and prophylaxis)	2.5 (2–3)
Valvular heart disease	2.5 (2–3)
Valve replacement, bioprosthetic	2.5 (2–3)
Valve replacement, mechanical	
Aortic, bileaflet	2.5 (2–3)
Aortic, other	3 (2.5–3.5)
Mitral, all	3 (2.5–3.5)

DOSE MANAGEMENT

Dosage form availability

Warfarin is available in brand (Coumadin), branded generic (Jantoven) and various unbranded generic formulations that are 100% bioavailable. The tablets, which can be crushed, are color coded to identify strength. The 10-mg tablet contains no dyes and can be used for patients in whom dye allergies are suspected or confirmed. Warfarin is also available in an intravenous formulation that can be given IV push over 1–2 minutes and can be used in patients who are NPO, have actual or perceived difficulties with warfarin absorption, or in patients with suspected noncompliance with oral administration (Table 2-8).

Table 2-8: Tablet Strengths and Colors (see color insert page)

Tablet Strength	Color
1 mg	Pink
2 mg	Lavender
2.5 mg	Green
3 mg	Tan
4 mg	Blue
5 mg	Peach
6 mg	Teal
7.5 mg	Yellow
10 mg	White

Initiation dosing

After obtaining a baseline INR, which can be used to identify patients with underlying coagulopathy, warfarin therapy is initiated at a starting dose. Two general methods of warfarin initiation dosing are available.

Average daily dosing method[2,5]

Although dosing requirements vary considerably among patients, from as little as ≤1 mg/day to ≥20 mg/day to reach a therapeutic INR of 2.0–3.0, the average dosing requirement is approximately 5 mg daily. The "average daily dosing method" for warfarin initiation uses a starting dose of 5 mg daily, with subsequent dosing adjustments guided by INR response. A well-known algorithm uses two 5-mg doses and day 3 INR to guide doses on days 3 and 4, following by a day 5 INR to guide doses on days 5–7. An institutional hybrid using 5 mg daily for 3 days (2.5 mg daily for patients with factors known to increase sensitivity to warfarin) is described below. This type of initiation is useful for outpatients, in which daily INR monitoring is inconvenient and can also be a reasonable starting point for inpatients that are otherwise clinically stable (Table 2-9).

Table 2-9: Warfarin Initiation Nomogram

	Nonsensitive Patients	**Sensitive Patients**
Initial dose	5 mg every day x 3 days	2.5 mg every day x 3 days
First INR		
<1.5	7.5–10.0 mg every day x 2–3 days	5.0–7.5 mg every day x 2–3 days
1.5–1.9	5 mg every day x 2–3 days	2.5 mg every day x 2–3 days
2.0–3.0	2.5 mg every day x 2–3 days	1.25 mg every day x 2–3 days
3.1–4.0	1.25 mg every day x 2–3 days	0.5 mg every day x 2–3 days
>4.0	Hold until INR <3.0	Hold until INR <3.0
Subsequent dosing and monitoring	Continue dose escalation and frequent monitoring until lower limit of therapeutic range is reached	

Flexible initiation dosing nomograms[2,6-8]

For inpatients, in which daily INR monitoring is available, a flexible initiation nomogram can be helpful. Several algorithms have been developed that utilize daily INR results to guide warfarin dosing for the first 4–6 days of therapy. These algorithms may begin with either a 5-mg or 10-mg starting dose, but 10 mg initiation typically results in a higher likelihood of over-anticoagulation.

It is critical to appreciate that warfarin dosing nomograms/algorithms have most often been developed and validated in stable, healthy outpatients. Many of these studies have significant exclusion criteria such that a majority of hospitalized patients were not included and provide no information on whether or not changes in interacting drugs were included or considered. Dosing nomograms offer a reasonable starting point for warfarin dose adjustments but should never be used in an "absolute" manner. Thorough patient assessment and clinical judgment are imperative components of warfarin dose management.

Clinical Pearl

- Clinicians need to identify factors that may increase sensitivity to warfarin when initiating therapy, including interacting medications, elderly, race, malnutrition, and disease states like heart failure, acute infections, etc. For these reasons, acutely ill patients starting warfarin should be initiated on lower doses such as 2.5–3.0 mg of warfarin per day.

Maintenance dosing[2]

Once the therapeutic INR range has been reached and warfarin therapy is essentially at steady state, dosing adjustments are based on routine INR monitoring and assessment of factors that may have resulted in the INR being below, within or above the therapeutic range. Dosing adjustments are based on percent changes in the weekly (or in some cases, daily) dose, taking into consideration the tablet size available to the patient. As with initiation therapy algorithms, maintenance therapy algorithms must be used with considerable clinical judgment. When the INR test result is unexpected or does not fit the clinical context, laboratory error should be considered (Table 2-10).

Table 2-10: Warfarin Maintenance Dosing Nomogram

For Goal INR 2–3	Adjustment	For Goal INR 2.5–3.5
INR <1.5	• Increase maintenance dose by 10% to 20% • Consider a booster dose of 1.5–2 times daily maintenance dose • Consider resumption of prior maintenance dose if factor causing decreased INR is considered transient (e.g., missed warfarin dose/s)	INR <2.0

(continued)

Table 2-10: (Continued)

For Goal INR 2–3	Adjustment	For Goal INR 2.5–3.5
INR 1.5–1.8	• Increase maintenance dose by 5% to 15% • Consider a booster dose of 1.5–2 times daily maintenance dose • Consider resumption of prior maintenance dose if factor causing decreased INR is considered transient (e.g., missed warfarin dose/s)	INR 2.0–2.3
INR 1.8–1.9	• No dosage adjustment may be necessary if the last two INRs were in range; if there is no clear explanation for the INR to be out of range, and if in the judgment of the clinician, the INR does not represent an increased risk of thromboembolism for the patient • If dosage adjustment needed, increase by 5% to 10% • Consider a booster dose of 1.5–2 x daily maintenance dose • Consider resumption of prior maintenance dose if factor causing decreased INR is considered transient (e.g., missed warfarin dose/s)	INR 2.3–2.4
INR 2.0–3.0	Desired range	INR 2.5–3.5
INR 3.1–3.2	• No dosage adjustment may necessary if the last two INRs were in range; if there is no clear explanation for the INR to be out of range, and if in the judgment of the clinician, the INR does not represent an increased risk of hemorrhage for the patient • If dosage adjustment needed, decrease by 5%–10% • Consider resumption of prior maintenance dose if factor causing elevated INR is considered transient (e.g., acute EtOH ingestion)	INR 3.6–3.7
INR 3.3–3.4	• Decrease maintenance dose by 5% to 10% • Consider resumption of prior maintenance dose if factor causing elevated INR is considered transient (e.g., acute alcohol ingestion)	INR 3.8–3.9

(continued)

Table 2-10: (Continued)

For Goal INR 2–3	Adjustment	For Goal INR 2.5–3.5
INR 3.5–3.9	• Consider holding 1 dose • Decrease maintenance dose by 5% to 15% • Consider resumption of prior maintenance dose if factor causing elevated INR is considered transient (e.g., acute alcohol ingestion)	INR 4.0–4.4
INR ≥4.0	• Hold until INR <upper limit of therapeutic range • Consider use of minidose oral vitamin K • Decrease maintenance dose by 5% to 20% • Consider resumption of prior maintenance dose if factor causing elevated INR is considered transient (e.g., acute alcohol ingestion)	INR ≥4.5

Frequency of INR monitoring[1,2]

Frequency of monitoring should be guided by clinical considerations (initiation versus maintenance dosing; stable versus unstable therapy, etc.) as well as by practical issues (patient convenience, vacations, weekends, etc.). If followup intervals need to be extended for a particular circumstance, a more conservative dosing strategy may be warranted (Table 2-11).

Table 2-11: Frequency of Monitoring by Clinical Setting

Clinical Setting		Frequency of Monitoring
Initiation therapy	Inpatient initiation	Daily
	Outpatient flexible initiation	Daily through day 4, then within 3–5 days
	Outpatient average daily dosing method	Every 3–5 days until INR >lower limit of therapeutic range, then within 1 week

(*continued*)

Table 2-11: (Continued)

Clinical Setting		Frequency of Monitoring
	After hospital discharge	If stable, within 3–5 days If unstable, within 1–3 days
	First month of therapy	At least weekly
Maintenance therapy	Medically stable inpatients	Every 1–3 days
	Medically unstable inpatients	Daily
	After hospital discharge	If stable, within 3–5 days If unstable, within 1–3 days
	Routine followup in medically stable and reliable patients	Every 4–6 weeks
	Routine followup in medically unstable or unreliable patients	Every 1–2 weeks
	Dose held today for significant over-anticoagulation	In 1–2 days
	Dosage adjustment today	Within 1–2 weeks
	Dosage adjustment ≤ 2 weeks ago	Within 2–4 weeks

Clinical Pearls

- Data on how often INRs are required in the inpatient setting is scarce. Considering the instability of patients in high acuity settings, increased probability of medication interactions, and changes in dietary intake of vitamin K, many hospitals often have policies requiring daily INRs and daily warfarin dosing. This ensures patients, at least in theory, are reassessed daily.

- Many hospitals standardize their warfarin administration time to the evening so dose adjustments can be made the same day as an INR check and to match when most patients take warfarin at home.

Management of nontherapeutic INRs with or without complications[1,9]

While general guidelines are available for the management of patients with non-therapeutic INRs as well as bleeding or thromboembolic complications, some practical issues should be considered as well. For patients with limited access to healthcare or who live in remote areas, it may be advisable to prescribe several tablets of vitamin K 2.5 mg to have available on an "as needed" basis. Patient with a significant degree of variability in INR response may benefit from same-daily-dosing of warfarin (5 mg every day, 5.5 mg every day, etc.) rather than alternating dosing (e.g., 7.5 mg Mondays and Friday, and 5 mg all other days), as well as supplementation with minidose vitamin K (50–100 mcg orally using commercial products available in health food stores as dietary supplements). Most importantly, the clinical context of out-of-range INRs needs to be considered before any intervention is made (Table 2-12).

Table 2-12: INR Strategies

INR	Strategy
Thromboembolic recurrence	Treat with full intensity heparin/LMWH/fondaparinux for typical duration of treatment
INR <1.5	Increase maintenance dose if appropriate
	Consider bridge therapy until INR is greater than the lower limit of therapeutic range
<5	Lower maintenance dose if appropriate
	Consider omitting dose(s) until INR is less than the upper limit of therapeutic range
5.0–8.9	Omit one or two doses; or omit dose and give vitamin K (≤5 mg orally)
	Repeat vitamin K (1–2 mg orally) if INR is still elevated at 24 hr
≥9	Hold warfarin and give vitamin K (5–10 mg orally)
	Use additional vitamin K if necessary

(*continued*)

Table 2-12: (Continued)

INR	Strategy
Serious bleeding with high INR	Hold warfarin and give vitamin K (10 mg by slow IV infusion) supplemented with fresh frozen plasma, prothrombin complex concentrate, or recombinant factor VIIa; may repeat vitamin K q 12 hr if necessary
Life-threatening bleeding	Hold warfarin and give prothrombin complex concentrates or recombinant factor VIIa supplemented with vitamin K (10 mg by slow IV infusion); repeat as necessary

Clinical Pearl

- Injectable vitamin K can be given orally when doses less than 2.5 mg are desired.

HEMORRHAGIC RISK ASSESSMENT[10-12]

Bleeding is the most significant adverse effect associated with warfarin therapy. Two scoring systems have been developed to assess the risk of major bleeding in patients taking warfarin. These scoring systems can be helpful in determining risk versus benefit of oral anticoagulation and in guiding the management of overanticoagulation in individual patients (Table 2-13).

Table 2-13: Bleeding Risk Scoring Systems

Scoring System	Criteria	Point Scores	Risk of Major Bleeding	
Outpatient bleeding risk index	AGE >65	1 point	Score	Major bleeding
	History of GI bleed	1 point	0	0.8%/pt yr
	History of stroke	1 point	1–2	2.6%/pt yr
	One or more of diabetes, Hct<30, Scr >1.5 or recent MI	1 point	3–4	9.7%/pt yr

(continued)

Table 2-13: (Continued)

Scoring System	Criteria	Point Scores	Risk of Major Bleeding	
HEMMORRHAGES	Hepatic or renal disease	1 point	Score	Major bleeding
	Ethanol abuse	1 point	0	1.9%/pt yr
	Malignancy	1 point	1	2.5%/pt yr
	Older (age >75)	1 point	2	5.3%/pt yr
	Reduced platelet count or function	1 point	3	8.4%/pt yr
	Rebleeding risk	2 points	4	10.4%/pt yr
	Hypertension (uncontrolled)	1 point	≥5	12.3%/pt yr
	Anemia	1 point		
	Genetic factors (CYP2C9 polymorphism)	1 point		
	Excessive fall risk	1 point		
	Stroke	1 point		

Clinical Pearls

- Patient education on bleeding: minor nose bleeds, gum bleeding after brushing, and increased bruising are common for warfarin patients. However, they may also indicate an elevated INR in a patient not used to these experiences while therapeutic on warfarin. Patients require education on how to manage these symptoms and advice on specific symptoms requiring medical attention. Patients prone to minor nose bleeds should be informed of nasal moisturizers that reduce this occurrence. Patients tend to bruise easily on warfarin; however, bruises should not continue to grow after several days.

- Red or brown urine, or red or black tarry stools, are often symptoms of more serious bleeding. These require medical attention and INR check. Patients with hemorrhoids or frequent constipation may have blood on toilet paper. Stool softeners can be helpful in this situation. This, however, should also be evaluated by a physician in patients recently starting warfarin or for those not having this problem previously. Positive stool guaiacs and red or black tarry stools can be symptoms of a more serious condition such as malignancy or the result of excessive anticoagulation. Warfarin patients who develop occult GI bleeding have a 5% to 25% chance of finding a malignant source with further evaluation. Any bleeding regardless of source, that doesn't resolve quickly with minor attention, requires medical attention and check of the INR.

REFERENCES AND KEY ARTICLES

1. Ansell J, Hirsh H, Hylek E, et al. Pharmacology and management of the vitamin K antagonists: American College of Chest Physicians Evidence-based Clinical Practice Guidelines (8th ed.). *Chest.* 2008;133(suppl 6): 160s–198s.

2. Wittkowsky AK. Warfarin. In: Murphy JE, ed. *Clinical Pharmacokinetics.* 4th ed. Bethesda, MD: ASHP; 2008.

3. Booth SL, Centurelli MA. Vitamin K: a practical guide to the dietary management of patients on warfarin. *Nutr Rev.* 1999;57(9 pt 1):288–296.

4. Wittkowsky AK. Drug interactions with oral anticoagulants. In: Colman RW, Marder VJ, Clowes AW, et al. *Hemostasis and Thrombosis. Basic Principals and Clinical Practice.* (5th ed.). Philadelphia, PA: Lippincott Williams & Wilkins; 2006.

5. Kovacs MJ, Anderson DA, Wells PS. Prospective assessment of a nomogram for the initiation of oral anticoagulant therapy for outpatient treatment of venous thromboembolism. *Pathophysiol Haemost Thromb.* 2002;32:131–133.

6. Fennerty A, Dolben J, Thomas J, et al. Flexible induction dose regimen for warfarin and prediction of maintenance dose. *Br J Med.* 1984;288:1268–1270.

7. Roberts GW, Helboe T, Nielsen CBM, et al. Assessment of an age-adjusted warfarin initiation protocol. *Ann Pharmacotherapy.* 2003;37:799–803.

8. Crowther MA, Harrison L, Hirsh J. Warfarin: less may be better. *Ann Intern Med.* 1997;127:332–333.

9. Schulman S, Beyth RJ, Kearon C, et al. Hemorrhagic complications anticoagulant and thrombolic treatment: American College of Chest Physicians Evidence-Based Practice Guidelines (8th ed.). *Chest.* 2008;133(suppl 6): 275s–298s.

10. Beyth RJ, Quinn LM, Landefeld CS. Prospective evaluation of an index for predicting risk of major bleeding in outpatients treated with warfarin. *Am J Med.* 1998;105:91–99.

11. Aspinall SL, DeSanzo BE, Trilli LE, et al. Bleeding risk index in an anticoagulation clinic: assessment by indication and implications for care. *J Gen Intern Med.* 2005;20:1008.

12. Gage BF, Yan Y, Milligan PE, et al. Clinical classification schemes for predicting hemorrhage: results from the National Registry of Atrial Fibrillation (NRAF). *Am Heart J.* 2006;151:713–719.

THREE

Chapter 3

Unfractionated Heparin

William E. Dager

INTRODUCTION

Unfractionated heparin is one of the most commonly used parenteral anticoagulants. Heparin is used in a wide variety of settings to prevent or treat thromboembolism. It can be used systemically, instilled in catheters, or used to coat artificial surfaces and lines to prevent thrombotic complications. As one of the oldest anticoagulant agents in use, many of its applications developed over time, with limited assessment of efficacy from rigorous trials. Despite availability of newer anticoagulants, unfractionated heparin remains a commonly used anticoagulant due to its quick onset and offset and ease to reverse.

PHARMACOLOGY[1,2]

- Unfractionated heparin (UFH) is a highly sulfated mucopolysaccharide, heterogeneous compound of which one third contains the pentasaccharide unit responsible for anticoagulant activity.

- UFH is an indirect acting anticoagulant that forms a complex with antithrombin, increasing the affinity and anticoagulant activity of antithrombin against clotting factors IIa (18 saccharide sequence required) and Xa (5 saccharide sequence required). Factors IXa, XIa, and XIIa are also inactivated.

- At higher concentrations, heparin chains unrelated to the pentasaccharide sequence can catalyze thrombin by inhibiting thrombin via heparin cofactor II, or separately factor Xa generation through antithrombin and heparin cofactor II.

- UFH will not dissolve a formed clot but prevent its propagation and growth.

- No differences in antithrombotic activity have been demonstrated between the various UFH preparations.

INDICATIONS

Table 3-1: Approved Indications for UFH

Prophylaxis and treatment of venous thromboembolism

Prophylaxis and treatment of pulmonary embolism

Diagnosis and treatment of acute and chronic consumptive coagulopathies (DIC)

Atrial fibrillation with embolism

Prevention of clotting in arterial and cardiac surgeries

Prophylaxis and treatment of peripheral arterial embolism

Anticoagulant in blood transfusions, extracorporeal circulation, dialysis procedures

Anticoagulant in blood samples for laboratory purposes

PHARMACOKINETICS/PHARMACODYNAMICS

Table 3-2: Pharmacokinetic Properties of UFH[3-5]

UFH Properties	
Source	Extracted from porcine intestinal mucosa or beef lung (no longer available in the USA)
Molecular weight (daltons)	Mean 15,000 (range 3,000–30,000)
SC bioavailability	20% to 70% (dose dependent); see Table 3-3
Activated clotting factors inhibited	Factors IIa, IXa, Xa, XIa, XIIa
Binding to proteins other than target	Nonspecific binding to proteins and other cells; presence of heparin binding proteins including acute phase reactants can vary in concentration during acute illness and affect the aPTT
Ratio anti-Factor Xa activity: anti-IIa activity	1:1
Onset of action	Rapid if sufficient amounts administered; IV faster than SC

(*continued*)

Table 3-2: (Continued)

UFH Properties	
Primary route of elimination	Enzymatic degradation at low doses and renal at higher dose; both zero-order and first order process can be present
	Clearance (CL): 0.015–0.12 L/hr/kg
	Higher clearance can occur in the setting of pulmonary embolism
Half-life (SC route)	30–150 min (dose and administration site dependent with slower clearance at higher doses); may be slightly prolonged in liver disease and end stage renal disease
Volume of distribution	0.07 L/kg (range 0.04–0.14 L/kg; typically reflects blood volume; distribution into the tissues can occur with large doses (during bypass surgery)
Effects of protamine	Complete neutralization

- The pharmacokinetics of UFH can be altered by factors such as age, thromboembolism location, hepatic or renal impairment, and obesity.

Table 3-3: Bioavailability of Heparin[5]

Oral	• UFH administered orally is not absorbed by the gastrointestinal tract
IV	• 100%
	• Rapid onset of anticoagulation action can occur with an IV bolus followed by a continuous infusion; in some situations (e.g., during cardiac procedures), IV bolus doses may be repeated to maintain desired effects
SC	• ~30%; can be up to 70% with high doses
	• Because of the nonspecific binding of UFH to various cellular proteins and cells, and poor SC bioavailability, significant and intrapatient variability in anticoagulant dose-response can occur
	• Effects from SC injections typically last 8–12 hr; bioavailability may decrease when vasoconstrictors are in use, or in the critically ill in general

Clinical Pearls

- The aPTT/anti-Factor Xa activity from UFH can be checked to verify appropriateness of the dose for a particular treatment dosing interval. In addition, if the value is too low at 12 hours, an 8-hour interval may be considered. If the 8-hour value is in the upper portion of the target range or higher, a 12-hour dosing interval can be considered for ease of use. A repeat trough value can be considered to validate the regimen. Risk assessment for thrombosis, bleeding, and compliance should be considered when determining a SC dosing regimen.

- Intramuscular administration is not recommended due to erratic absorption and risk of hematoma formation.

Change in calibrators for UFH and potency

In 2009, the United States Pharmacopeia (USP) monograph for heparin was updated to be consistent with the World Health Organization (WHO) standards. This update resulted in up to a 10% reduction in heparin potency (potency per USP unit of heparin was up to 10% less than International Units). This conversion created a concern among clinicians for a potential under dosing of heparin. Consensus to date, however, suggests that impact of this change on clinical outcomes is unlikely although data is being accumulated and reviewed. Clinicians should be aware of this change and develop an alternative strategy if necessary.[6]

INITIATING THERAPY

UFH is usually administered parenterally by IV or SC injection. In some situations, heparin may be used by other means such as bath for instruments or coating of dialyzers prior to use. It can also be imbedded into catheter linings during their manufacture.

UFH for flushing catheters

- Saline and heparin are frequently instilled into catheters to keep them from clotting. Saline is the preferred agent in peripheral IV lines.
- The concentration and volume of heparin instilled will vary between catheters with suggestions provided by the manufacturer of the catheter. The lowest amount of heparin to maintain patency should be considered.

Table 3-4: Examples of Heparin Locking in Adults for Selected Devices

Device	Heparin	Volume
Midline	10 units/mL	3 mL
PICC, nontunneled and tunneled	10 units/mL	5 mL
Port	100 units/mL	3–5 mL

- When using an agent that is incompatible with heparin, consider flushing first with saline prior to instilling the heparin.

- In some cases, high amounts of heparin are used and the possibility of a sufficient amount reaching the circulation to cause systemic anticoagulant effects should be considered.

Clinical Pearl

- Line flushing during PCI: 200 units of IV heparin was used to flush catheters in individuals receiving fondaparinux undergoing PCI in the OASIS 5 trial to reduce thrombosis on the guidewire.[7]

ADMINISTRATION IV OR SC

Bolus dosing

- Is typically used when immediate anticoagulation is necessary. If immediate anticoagulation is not required, a bolus may not be necessary.

- Dosing guidelines may consider specifying a maximum bolus and infusion rate that triggers an additional assessment step for safety to prevent unintended excessive doses of heparin (see Dose capping section).

- Continuous IV infusion is preferred over intermittent IV boluses. Intermittent bolus injections result in high peak anticoagulant levels and have been associated in some observations with a higher risk of major bleeding.

- Dosing of UFH is generally based on patient's weight. (See Table 3-9.)

  - Weight-based UFH dosing regimens are more likely to exceed the therapeutic aPTT threshold in the first 24 hours after initiating treatment compared to more traditional dosing regimens such as a 5,000-unit bolus dose followed by an infusion administered at 1,000 units/hr.[9]

Table 3-5: Evidence Supporting Weight-Based Dosing Compared to a "Preset" Bolus and Infusion Rate and the Importance of Achieving Minimal aPTT Targets[9,a]

N = 115 (VTE = 80)

Time	Standard UFH Bolus: 5,000 Continuous Infusion started at 1,000 units/hr	Weight-based UFH 80 units/kg to 18 units/kg/hr (total body weight)	P value
24 hr aPTT			
Therapeutic	35%	57%	<0.001
Subtherapeutic	58%	15%	<0.001
Supratherapeutic	7%	27%	<0.001
48 hr aPTT			
Therapeutic	44%	65%	<0.001
Subtherapeutic	49%	18%	<0.001
Supertherapeutic	8%	18%	<0.001
Minor/major bleeding	2%/1%	2%/0	
Recurrent VTE (3 mo)	8/32 (25%)	2/41 (5%)	

[a]The key points of this analysis was that using a weight-based approach (total body weight was used) led to a higher incidence of aPTT values within or above the target rage in the first 24–48 hours without increasing bleeding instances but decreasing recurrent VTE events fivefold. Some observations have linked increased bleeding to frequent excessive aPTT values or higher doses during prolonged courses or therapy, suggesting some caution regarding frequent supratherapeutic values beyond 48 hours.[10,11]

Dose capping

- Adjusted and total body weight to a certain maximum dose should be considered to minimize potential excessive anticoagulation. The amount can vary between indications.

  - Bolus: outside of arterial disease or during surgical procedures, bolus doses beyond 4,000–5,000 units may not add any clinical benefit and should be avoided.

  - Large bolus doses may not be necessary to get an anticoagulation effect. In one analysis, 3,000 units of heparin prior to cardiac catheterization produced therapeutic aPTT values, with half >140 seconds. Low values were only seen if the dose was <32 units/kg (weight >92 kg).[8]

- Infusions: depending on the situation, infusions are typically initiated at 12–18 units/kg/hr, but may go up to 25 units/kg/hr.[12] Capping the initial allowed infusion rate unless otherwise specifically justified can avoid unintended excessive dosing. On occasion, higher infusion rates adjusted based on aPTT, etc., may be needed.

  - It has been suggested that the risk of bleeding may increase when daily doses exceed 31,000 units/day.[13]

  - In ACS, daily doses >1,667 units/hr (>40,000 units/day) may not need to be adjusted upwards when the aPTT remains low if the measured anti-Factor Xa activity is at least 0.35 units/mL.[14]

Clinical Pearl

- Setting a maximum "capped" bolus dose and separately infusion rate may avoid dosing errors that might occur from an incorrect weight (or units such as pounds for kg), or extra digit (800 intended but 8,000 ordered). Capped doses may be different based on the indicated use. Lower capped doses may be considered in the setting of ACS compared to PE. Higher doses may occur in the setting of PE secondary to enhanced elimination.

Table 3-6: Recommended Dosing for the Initiation of UFH[1,14-17]

	Indication	Bolus Dose	Maintenance Dose
IV	VTE treatment (DVT or PE)	80 units/kg (or 5,000 units)	18 units/kg/hr; aPTT range established by laboratory; calibrated to correspond to anti-Factor activity of 0.3–0.7 International Units/mL
IV	PCI (with GP IIb/IIIa inhibitor)	50–70 units/kg	Additional bolus doses (common target low response ACT 200–250 sec)
IV	PCI (without GP IIb/IIIa inhibitor)	60–100 units/kg	Additional bolus doses (target low response ACT 250–350 sec)
IV	Acute STEMI (patients receiving full-dose rt-PA)	60 units/kg Max: 4,000 units	12 units/kg/hr Max: 1,000 units/hr (common target aPTT 50–70 sec)[a]
IV	Acute STEMI (combination regimen with rt-PA)	40 units/kg Max: 3,000 units	7 units/kg/hr Max: 800 units/hr (target aPTT 50–70 sec)[a]
IV	Unstable angina or NSTEMI	60 units/kg Max: 4,000 units	12 units/kg/hr Max: 1,000 units/hr; some institutions use a higher threshold to achieve target ranges earlier
SC	DVT prophylaxis		5,000 units q 8–12 hr (Note: q 12 hr dosing intervals may be considered in low/moderate risk, elderly, low weight) See Chapter 10
SC	VTE treatment (DVT or PE, with monitoring)	250 units/kg (or 17,500 units)	250 units/kg q 12 hr
SC	VTE treatment (DVT or PE, without monitoring)	333 units/kg	250 units/kg q 12 hr
IM	IM administration should be avoided because of frequent hematomas		

[a] aPTT range will depend on the reagents sensitivity to heparin unique to each laboratory. aPTT target range selection of VTE treatment may consist of the middle to upper portion of the anti-Factor Xa activity calibration. Anti-Factor Xa activity targets with concurrent thrombolytic therapy or ACS are unclear. See Chapter 6 (Table 6-5) for heparin dosing recommendations when thrombolytic therapy is used.

Transitioning from IV to SC UFH

Table 3-7: Estimating a SC Heparin Regimen When Transitioning for an IV Infusion in Treatment of VTE

Dose SQ administered q 12 hr = [last IV infusion rate/hr x 24] [1.2]/2

"[1.2]" reflects the approximately 20% loss of bioavailability with the SC route

The common 250 units/kg q 12 dose for VTE treatment was determined by this approach; 20% over the common 18 units/kg IV infusion rate used in VTE

- Depending on dose, onset of effect occurs within 1–2 hours with peak effect achieved around 3 hours. Several days may be required to reach steady-state pharmacodynamic assessment values when SC UFH is given in full therapeutic doses.
- Due to its lower and variable bioavailability of the SC route of administration, higher doses of UFH should be initiated in order to attain therapeutic anticoagulation effect quickly.
- For VTE treatment, target aPTT values (or equivalent anti-Factor Xa activity of 0.3–0.7 units/mL) at 6 hours postadministration should be considered.[17]

Clinical Pearl

- In selected situations where an LMWH may not be an available option, UFH can be administered SC every 8–12 hours. The dose can be estimated from the IV infusion rate in Table 3-7. It may take several days for the aPTT to reach steady state. The risk for HIT with long-term SC UFH is not known. If bleeding at injection sites is observed, consider checking an aPTT and also the size of the needle used. Doses of 5,000 units in elderly, low-weight individuals may yield aPTT values in the therapeutic range.

Use of UFH in selected procedures

Table 3-8: Examples of UFH Dosing in Selected Invasive Procedures for Adults[18-20]

	Indication	Initial Bolus Dose	Maintenance Dose
IV Administration	CABG	80–350 units/kg	(Target HR-ACT 250 to >400 sec)
	On-pump CABG	400 units/kg	(Target HR-ACT ≥400 sec)
	Off-pump CABG (with aspirin 650 mg PR)	180 units/kg	3,000 units q 30 min (target HR-ACT ≥350 sec)
	Vascular reconstruction	100–150 units/kg	50 units/kg q 45–50 min
	Dialysis (normal bleeding risk)	50 units/kg	500–1,500 units/hr (target LR-ACT 80% above baseline)
	Dialysis (increased bleeding risk)	10–25 units/kg	250–500 units/hr (target LR-ACT 40% above baseline)
Other	Dialysis (very high bleeding risk or active bleeding)	Rinse dialyzer with 5,000–20,000 units and flush with 0.5–2 L saline	Rinse dialyzer intermittently with saline (target blood flow ≥250 mL/min)

- The amount of heparin required to maintain a hemodialysis circuit is variable depending on the approach (intermittent, extended duration, continuous, etc.), the properties of the dialysis circuit in addition to the patient

- Some hemodialysis machines are programmed to use preselected heparin concentrations (i.e., 1,000 units/mL) for continuous infusions

- Heparin requirement may be lower in extended daily dialysis (~650 units/hr) compared to continuous renal replacement therapy (~1,100 units/hr)

- Fewer patients on extended duration dialysis may require heparin compared to CRRT

Table 3-9: Weight Considerations for UFH Dosing in Obesity

Source	
Raschke R et al.[4]	Table 3-5 (actual body weight [ABW] used)
Yee W et al.[19]	ABW more likely to get aPTT in range by 24 hr
	Median infusion rate: 13 units/kg/hr
	Morbidly obese: potential for severe overdose at 18 units/kg/hr
	Max bolus 10,000 units max infusion 1,500 units/hr
	Max weight: 184 kg (this patient therapeutic at 1,700 units/hr)
Rosborough TK[20] anti-Factor Xa activity monitoring	Loading dose (units): 450 x estimated blood volume (liters)
	Initial infusion (units/hr): 344.335 x estimated blood volume (liters) x 257.962 − (age − years x 4.951)
	Estimated blood volume: (liters)
	Males: (0.3669 x height "m³") + (0.03219 x wt "kg") + 0.6041
	Females: (0.3561 x height "m³") + (0.03308 x wt "kg") + 0.1833
	Weight: median 77 kg (range 30 − 184 kg)
Myzienski AE et al.[21]	Literature review and case report in a 388-kg patient suggests a dosing weight of IBW + 0.4[ABW − IBW]
Riney JN et al.[22]	For aPTT similar to anti-Factor Xa activity 0.3−0.7 units/mL
	BMI ≥40 kg/m²: 11.5 units/kg/hr (mean wt 141 ± 32 kg)
	BMI 25−39.9 kg/m²: 12.5 units/kg/hr (mean wt 89 ± 16 kg)
	Normal: 13.5 units/kg/hr (mean wt 62 ± 11 kg)

- Consider using total body weight with a preselected maximum infusion rate "cap" (i.e., 2,000 units/hr) that triggers a additional assessment to limit unintended excessive dosing

Clinical Pearl

- As obesity is a risk factor for VTE, it is important to achieve adequate anticoagulation as soon as possible. The volume of distribution for heparin correlates to blood volume and thus creates a risk for overshooting targets in the very obese patient (BMI $\geq$40 kg/m^2 or >200 kg) if weight-based dosing is not capped or adjusted accordingly. Dosing caps can be considered to reduce the risk of excessive anticoagulation; however, aPTT (or anti-Factor Xa activity) should be carefully measured and infusions promptly adjusted to achieve targets as soon as possible in the setting of an acute thromboembolic event. Table 3-9 provides insights on how to approach heparin dosing in this setting.

MONITORING AND DOSING ADJUSTMENTS

Table 3-10: Laboratory Tests Used in the Monitoring of UFH (see Chapter 18)

	Monitoring
aPTT	Target range will vary between assays depending on the lot of each reagent used; the aPTT is typically used for lower intensity of heparin anticoagulation effects such as prophylaxis to VTE treatment; this assay can identify presence diminished response to UFH if antithrombin deficiency is present
Anti-Factor Xa activity	As with the aPTT, anti-Factor Xa activity is an alternative assay for measuring lower intensity of heparin anticoagulation effects such as prophylaxis to VTE treatment; this assay can identify presence of diminished response to UFH if high factor VIII concentrations are present
Low response ACT	Typically used in cardiac interventional procedures such as PCI; measures the intermediate range of heparin anticoagulation; ACT values may vary between tests (Hemochron values >MedTronic values in the upper part of the ACT range)
High response ACT	Used during high ranges of heparinization such as cardiothoracic surgery; may not detect presence of heparin at concentrations used to treat VTE
Protamine titration	See Chapter 18

Table 3-11: Target Anti-Factor Xa Activity Levels Considerations for Selected Indications Using UFH (these values have not been verified in clinical trials)[23]

Indication	Target Anti-Factor Xa Activity Level
VTE prophylaxis	0.1–0.3 units/mL
VTE treatment	0.3–0.7 units/mL
ACS	Target values of 0.35–0.7 units/mL have been proposed (not validated) and may depend on concurrent therapies (i.e., thrombolytics) used
Pregnancy	0.35–0.7 units/mL

Table 3-12: Trials Describing That Achieving a Therapeutic aPTT in the First 24–48 Hours After Initiating UFH Has Been Shown to Lower the Risk of Recurrent VTE[a]

	UFH Dose	VTE Recurrence
Raschke R 1992[9]	Weight-based vs. 5,000 unit-bolus and 24,000 units/24 hr	See Table 3-5 Weight-based had a fivefold lower incidence of recurrent VTE at 3 mo
Hull 1997[24]		aPTT <therapeutic range at 24 hr: 23.3% incidence VTE recurrence (p = 0.02) 4% to 6% with aPTT >therapeutic range at 24 hr Outlines importance of aPTT reaching target range early
Anand 1996 Five Trials[25]	30,000 units/ 24 hr	aPTT subtherapeutic 24 hr: 6.3% aPTT >lower therapeutic limit: 7% Outlines that if 30,000 units/day is provided, no evidence of improved efficacy observed with earlier aPTT in range
Anand 1999 Three Trials[26]	5,000 bolus + ≥1,250 units/hr	Low aPTT: odds 1.3 vs. therapeutic aPTT (at 24 and 48 hr) p = 0.56 Suggests the value of infusing at least 1,250 units/hr

[a]Controversy: it is unclear if an aPTT value within the target range at 24–48 hours or if doses 24,000–30,000 units are used lead to different outcomes. Lower daily doses and subtherapeutic aPTT values in the setting of acute thromboembolism may be associated with increased recurrent thromboembolism.

Clinical Pearl

- Most trials comparing UFH to LMWH for VTE treatment used aPTT ratios for heparin. Given the more sensitive heparin assays now in use, under dosing of UFH may have been present compared to current doses derived from aPTT ranges determined by anti-Factor Xa activity titration. This may have created a bias favoring LMWH in clinical trials compared LWMH to UFH targeting a predetermined aPTT (60–80 seconds) when more sensitive assays to heparin (e.g., aPTT target 80–110 for anti-Factor Xa activity of 0.3–0.7).[27]

Table 3-13: Example of an Adjusted Dosing Nomogram for Continuous Heparin Infusions Using the aPTT in VTE Treatment[a]

APTT (sec)	Dose Adjustment		Comments
	Weight-Based	**Nonweight[b]**	
<35	Bolus 40–80 units/kg Increase by 3 units/kg/hr	Bolus 2,500–5,000 units Increase by 200–250 units/hr	Consider bolus option if emergent anticoagulation is necessary
35–49	Bolus 20–40 units/kg Increase by 2 units/kg/hr	Bolus 2,500 units Increase by 100–200 units/hr	
50–59 (50–70); see Clinical Pearl below	Increase by 1 unit/kg/hr	Increase by 50–100 units/hr	Increase by 50–70 units/hr if target range the upper part of the anti-Factor Xa activity titration range
60–90[c] (70–90); see Clinical Pearl below	No change	No change	(70–90 units/hr) if upper end titration range targeted
91–105	Decrease by 1 unit/kg/hr	Decrease by 50–100 units/hr	

(*continued*)

Table 3-13: (Continued)

APTT (sec)	Dose Adjustment		Comments
	Weight-Based	**Nonweight[b]**	
105–125	Decrease by 2 units/kg/hr	Decrease by 100–200 units/hr	Option: hold 30–60 min
>124	Decrease by 3 units/kg/hr	Decrease by 200 units/hr	Option: hold 1–2 hr

[a]Each nomogram should consider the reagent range used in each lab. This sample nomogram assumes an aPTT treatment range of 60–90 seconds based on anti-Factor Xa activity titration of 0.3–0.7 International Units/mL for VTE treatment. The aPTT range has to be calibrated by each lab and will vary between lots of even the same reagent. See Chapter 18.

[b]Dose increase of 50–100 units/hr may depend on the patient weight.

[c]Institution-specific therapeutic aPTT range of 60–90 seconds is equivalent to a plasma heparin concentration of 0.3–0.7 anti-Factor Xa activity units/mL or 0.2–0.4 units/mL by protamine titration. Range may vary depending on the assay sensitivity to heparin for a particular reagent. Repeat aPTT 4–8 hours post-rate change; 4 hours if no bolus; 6–8 hours if a bolus is administered (see Figure 3-1).

Clinical Pearl

- The upper end of the titration curve may be selected for the aPTT range to assure adequate anticoagulation in acute VTE treatment (in this example, 70–90 seconds).

Table 3-14: Adjusted Dosing Nomograms (units/kg/hr) for Continuous Heparin Infusions Using the Anti-Factor Xa Activity in VTE Treatment[28,a]

Anti-Factor Xa Activity (units/mL)	Dose Adjustment	Comment
≤0.2	Bolus 26–30 units/kg Increase rate 3–4 units/kg/hr	Consider bolus option if emergent anticoagulation is necessary
0.21–0.29	Bolus 15 units/kg Increase rate 2 units/kg/hr	Consider bolus option if emergent anticoagulation is necessary; option 0.21–0.39
0.3–0.7	No change	Option: 0.4–0.7 for more aggressive activity (VTE treatment)
0.71–0.8	Decrease 1 unit/kg/hr	
0.81–0.99	Decrease 2 units/kg/hr	Option: hold 30–60 min if notable bleeding risks present
≥1.0	Hold infusion 1–2 hr Decrease 3 units/kg/hr	

[a]Repeat anti-Factor Xa activity 4–8 hours after infusion rate change. Earlier draw (4–6 hours) can be done if no bolus (see Figure 3-1). Once two consecutive anti-Factor Xa activity levels are 0.3–0.7 units/mL, draw every 24 hours.

Table 3-15: Sample Adjusted Dosing Nomogram for SC Heparin in VTE Treatment

aPTT	Dosing Adjustment	Next aPTT
<40	Increase by 36–48 units/kg q 12 hr	6 hr postdose
40–59	Increase by 24–36 units/kg q 12 hr	6 hr postdose

(*continued*)

Table 3-15: (Continued)

aPTT	Dosing Adjustment	Next aPTT
60–90	No change	Next morning, then daily (less frequent monitoring may be required with long-term use)
91–103	Decrease by 6–12 units/kg q 12 hr	6 hr postdose
104–124	Decrease by 12–24 units/kg q 12 hr	6 hr postdose
>124	Decrease by 24–36 units/kg q 12 hr	6 hr postdose

- Initial dose is 250 units/kg SC administered q 12 hr (or 17,500 units q 12 hr)
- Converting from IV infusion to SQ: multiply total 24-hour dose by 1.2 (assumes 20% loss in bioavailability, which can be greater then 20%), then divide total q 12 hr (see Table 3-7)
- aPTT should be drawn at 6 hr (mid-interval) after dose
- In pregnancy, an 8- or 12-hr aPTT can be considered to determine if the dosing interval needs to be changed to q 8 hr dosing is necessary; institution-specific therapeutic range of 60–90 sec is equivalent to anti-Factor Xa activity titration of 0.3–0.7 anti-Factor Xa activity units/mL or 0.2–0.4 units/mL by protamine titration; see comments in Table 3-13

- The bolus dose influences measured aPTT values up to 8 hours depending on the amount administered.
- aPTT assessments shortly after a bolus may suggest a higher degree of anti-coagulation than provided by the continuous infusion alone.
- Depending on the amount of a bolus (dashed line) administered, the aPTT will rise to a point higher than achieved by the continuous infusion (dotted line). The measured aPTT (solid line) in this situation will then drop over time to a value reflective of the infusion rate.

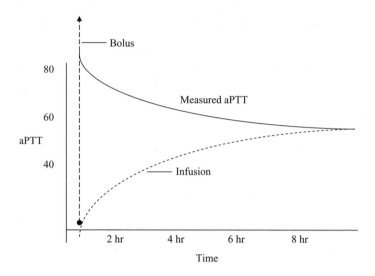

Figure 3-1: Bolus Dosing and Impact on Timing Laboratory Values for Adjusting a Continuous Infusion

Clinical Pearl

- Figure 3-1 describes the influence of the bolus dose on measured aPTT (or anti-Factor Xa activity) and subsequent dosing adjustments. Early aPTT measures after a bolus dose may be higher than observed should no bolus have been administered. This may lead to no dosing adjustment or a downward adjustment. The subsequent aPTT (or anti-Factor Xa activity) may then be below the target range creating a delay in reaching target values. Checking aPTT values earlier than 6 hours after initiating the UFH infusion may be requested in order to determine if an adequate infusion rate is present (aPTT value close to baseline.) UFH bolus doses of >5,000 International Units can also have an effect on aPTT values drawn up to 8 hours later.

Heparin resistance[1]

- Lack of a measurable heparin response can occur secondary to reduced antithrombin (benefit of the aPTT assay), excessive factor VIII (benefit of anti-Factor Xa activity assay), or excessive fibrinogen. Consider checking an alternative assay (anti-Xa), antithrombin, Factor VIII, and fibrinogen with infusion rates above 25 units/kg/hr and subtherapeutic assay measurements. If additional clarification is required, consider sending samples to an outside lab for validation.

- Patients with acute thrombosis may frequently need higher UFH dose requirements to attain therapeutic effect as these patients have been noted to eliminate UFH more rapidly, possibly because of increased binding to acute phase reactants.

- Lower aPTT values during awake periods compared to when asleep have been observed.[28]

Clinical Pearls

- aPTT or anti-Factor Xa activity values can vary during a 24-hour period secondary to a potential pharmacokinetic effect. Values can be higher during sleeping periods (early a.m.) compared to during awake hours.[29] Dosing increases and decreases may subsequently occur. For prolonged infusions and frequent daily dosing adjustments, the infusions ordered may be modified (i.e., measuring the aPTT or anti-Factor Xa activity at the same time each day) to simplify management.

- If resistance to UFH is suspected, check an aPTT value shortly after a bolus dose to see if a measure response occurs. If no response (Increase in aPTT or anti-Factor Xa activity) is noted for example 30 minutes after a 5,000-unit IV bolus, the assay may need to be checked (run anti-Factor Xa activity off the aPTT, ACT) or an alternative approach to anticoagulation considered.

CONSIDERATIONS IN STROKE PATIENTS

- Out of concerns for bleeding, bolus doses of UFH during initiation and during dosing adjustments are not typically administered.

- Usual starting doses are 12–15 units/kg/hr with maximum initial rates of 1,000–1,500 units/hr.

- The approach to heparin when combined with a GPIIb/IIIa agent for arterial stent placement will depend on the device and approach used.

Table 3-16: UFH Dosing in Continuous Renal Replacement Therapy[30,a]

APTT (sec)	Dose Adjustments
<35	Bolus 1,000–2,500 units Increase by 200 units/hr
35–49	Bolus 1,000 units Increase by 50–100 units/hr[b]
50–65[c]	No change
66–75	Decrease by 50–100 units/hr[b]
76–90	Decrease by 100–200 units/hr Option: hold 30–60 min
>90	Decrease by 200 units/hr Option: hold 1–2 hr

[a]Each nomogram should consider the reagent range used in each lab. The aPTT range has to be calibrated by each lab and will vary between lots of even the same reagent. See Chapter 18. Initial bolus doses of 25 units/kg (range 10–30 units/kg) followed by an infusion of 5–10 units/kg/hr (range 5–25 units/kg/hr) is one approach. Target aPTT should be a minimum of 1.5 times control or as established within the 0.3–0.7 units/mL anti-Factor Xa activity calibrations. Variations may exist between dialysis therapies.

[b]Dose increases or decreases of 50–100 units/hr may depend on the patient weight.

[c]Institution-specific therapeutic aPTT range of 45–75 seconds is equivalent to a plasma heparin concentration of 0.3–0.7 anti-Factor Xa activity units/mL or 0.2–0.4 units/mL by protamine titration. Range may vary depending on the assay sensitivity to heparin for a particular reagent.

- Repeat aPTT 4–8 hours post-rate change; 4 hours if no bolus; 6–8 hours if a bolus is administered.

- Survival of filter and heparin requirements may depend on the material (filter) used.

- Autoanticoagulated patients at high risk of bleeding may not undergo anticoagulation of the circuit.

- Regional heparin (patients with high bleeding risk and filter life span is too short to accept): continuous UFH (500 International Units/mL) into arterial line (i.e., 9 × blood flow [mL/min]). Continuous infusion protamine (5 mg/mL) into venous line starting at a 1:100 (protamine 1 mg/100 units UFH). Check circuit aPTT (arterial line post-UFH) and patient aPTT (arterial line preheparin). Target circuit aPTT is >55 seconds and patient aPTT <45 seconds.

Extracorporeal membranous oxygenation (ECMO) or extracorporeal life support (ECLS)

- Infusion rates may be center specific. Rates of 20 units/kg/hr have been used.
- Infusion rates over 60 units/kg/hr have been associated with diminished outcomes.
- Can lead to a drop in AT level. Impact of replacing AT or impact on heparin requirements unknown.
- Dosing adjustments may be done by bedside ACT (typically every 1–2 hours).
- Infusion rates and target goals may depend on the age of the patient, circuit, bleeding concerns, and cannulation site.

Clinical Pearl

- During ECLS/ECMO, the measured ACT or aPTT may vary without changes in the infusion rate. If one is not corresponding to dosing adjustments, consider adding the other for conformation. For pediatric patients, small peditubes can be used to minimize blood loss. Make sure the correct ACT test is used consistently.

Table 3-17: Drug Incompatibilities with Heparin

Alteplase	Droperidol	Levorphanol tartrate
Amikacin	Drotrecogin alfa	Methylprednisolone
Amobarbital	Ergonovine maleate	Mitoxantrone
Amphotericin B Deoxychoate	Erythromycin	Morphine sulfate
Atropine	Filgrastin	Nesiritide
Chlordiazepoxide	Gentamycin	Noripinephrine bitartrate
Ciprofloxacin	Haloperidol deconate	Orphenadrine citrate
Clarithromycin	Haloperidol lactate	Pentamidine
Codeine	Hyaluronidase	Phenytoin sodium
Cytarabine	Hydrocortisone sodium	Polymyxin B sulfate
Daunorubicin	Phosphate	Prochlorperazine
Diazepain	Hydroxyzine HCl	Promethazine
Doxorubicin	Idarubicin HCl	Quinupristin/dalfopristin
Doxycycline	Kanamycin sulfate	
	Levofloxacin	

SIDE EFFECTS, PRECAUTIONS, CONTRAINDICATIONS

Table 3-18: Side Effects, Precautions, and Contraindications to UFH

Side Effects	Precautions	Contraindications
<ul><li>Bleeding</li><li>Thrombocytopenia, HAT, HIT, HITT (see Chapter 15)</li><li>Local irritation</li><li>Hypersensitivity</li><li>Long-term use:<ul><li>– Alopecia</li><li>– Priapism</li><li>– Hyperkalemia</li><li>– Elevated AST/ALT</li><li>– Osteoporosis</li></ul></li></ul>	<ul><li>Fatal medication errors</li><li>Hypersensitivity</li><li>Hemorrhage<ul><li>– Bleeding disorders</li><li>– Subacute bacterial endocarditis</li><li>– Active ulcerative GI diseases</li><li>– Continuous GI tube drainage</li><li>– Severe HTN</li><li>– History of hemorrhagic stroke</li><li>– Recent invasive procedures including spinal anesthesia</li><li>– Concomitant platelet inhibitors</li><li>– Recent GI bleeding</li><li>– Severe liver disease</li><li>– Age >60 yr</li></ul></li><li>Heparin resistance (>35,000 units/24 hr)</li><li>Thrombocytopenia, HAT, HIT, HITTS</li><li>Hyperkalemia</li><li>Osteoporosis</li><li>Drug interactions including oral anticoagulants and platelet inhibitors</li></ul>	<ul><li>Severe thrombocytopenia</li><li>History (recent) of heparin-induced thrombocytopenia</li><li>Uncontrolled active bleeding except when due to DIC (see Appendix I)</li><li>Suspected intracranial hemorrhage</li><li>Inability to obtain blood coagulation tests at appropriate intervals</li></ul>

Adverse effects—clinical considerations

- Excessive aPTT: result could be a hemidiluted sample, especially if the INR is unexpectedly elevated or Hgb/HCT lower. Consider repeating by peripheral phlebotomy.

- Continued unexpected values: check the bag/add mixture concentration used or vial concentration; verify that patient received it or cross check using an alternative assay such as an ACT, anti-Factor Xa activity, aPTT, or INR. Some individuals for unexplained circumstances may not respond to a particular assay.

Clinical Pearl

- If the correct amount of heparin being administered is unclear, consider replacing with a new bag or syringe that has been verified for accuracy and remeasure labs.

- Bleeding: consider turning off the infusion; reverse with protamine or other blood products as necessary.[31]

- Reversal: see Chapter 7. Heparin rebound can occur after very high doses (cardiothoracic surgery), warranting repeat protamine administration and assessment of continued anticoagulation effects by aPTT or anti-Factor Xa activity measurements.[32]

Heparin-induced thrombocytopenia (HIT) (see Chapter 15)

Table 3-19: ACCP 2008 Recommendations for Platelet Count Monitoring of UFH and LMWH[33]

ACCP 2008 Guidelines for Platelet Count Monitoring			
Heparin	**Risk**	**Platelet Count Monitoring**	**Level**
Yes	>1%	Recommended	1C
Yes	0.1% to 1%	Recommended	2C
UFH	UFH past 100 days	Baseline and within 24 hr	1C

(continued)

Table 3-19: (Continued)

<table>
<tr><th colspan="4">ACCP 2008 Guidelines for Platelet Count Monitoring</th></tr>
<tr><th>Heparin</th><th>Risk</th><th>Platelet Count Monitoring</th><th>Level</th></tr>
<tr><td>Within 30 min of UFH bolus</td><td>Anaphylactoid reaction</td><td>Immediate and compare to prior count</td><td>1C</td></tr>
<tr><td>Therapeutic UFH</td><td></td><td>Every 2–3 days (day 4–14 or until stopping UFH)</td><td>2C</td></tr>
<tr><td>Prophylactic UFH</td><td>Postoperative (HIT risk >1%)</td><td>Every other day (day 4–14 or stopping heparin)</td><td>2C</td></tr>
<tr><td>Prophylaxis</td><td>Medical/OB (HIT risk 0.1% to 1%)</td><td>Every 2–3 days (day 4–14 or stopping heparin)</td><td>2C</td></tr>
<tr><td></td><td>Medical/OB or UFH catheter flush (HIT risk 0.1% to 1%)</td><td>Not recommended</td><td>2C</td></tr>
</table>

SPECIAL POPULATION CONSIDERATIONS

- Low weight/elderly: low weight or elderly patients can potentially be more sensitive or responsive to UFH. "Preset" or fixed, none weight-based dosing, thus has the potential for higher than expected levels of anticoagulation.

- Obesity: see Table 3-9.

- Pregnancy: see Chapter 16.

- Pediatrics: see Chapter 17.

REFERENCES

*Key articles

* 1. Hirsh J, Bauer KA, Donati MB, et al. Parenteral anticoagulants: American College of Chest Physicians Evidence-Based Clinical Practice Guidelines (8th Edition). *Chest.* 2008;133:141S–159S.

2. Kandrotas RJ. Heparin pharmacokinetics and pharmacodynamics. *Clin Pharmacokinet.* 1992;22:359–374.

3. Lexi-Comp Inc. Heparin. Accessed October 21, 2010.

4. Dager W, Roberts J. Heparin, low-molecular-weight heparin and fondaparinux. In: Murphy J, ed. *Clinical Pharmacokinetics.* 5th ed. Bethesda, MD: American Society of Health-System Pharmacists; in press.

5. Bara L, Billaud E, Gramond G, et al. Comparative pharmacokinetics of a low molecular weight heparin (PK 10 169) and unfractionated heparin after intravenous and subcutaneous administration. *Thromb Res.* 1985;39:631–636.

6. Smythe MA, Nutescu EA, Wittkowsky AK. Changes in the USP heparin monograph and implications for clinicians. *Pharmacotherapy.* 2010;30:428–431.

7. Yusuf S, Mehta SR, Chrolavicius S, et al.; Fifth Organization to Assess Strategies in Acute Ischemic Syndromes Investigators. Comparison of fondaparinux and enoxaparin in acute coronary syndromes. *N Engl J Med.* 2006;354:1464–1476.

8. Laslett L, White R. Predictors of the effect of heparin during cardiac catheterization. *Cardiology.* 1995;86:380–383.

* 9. **Raschke RA, Reilly BM, Guidry JR, et al. The weight-based heparin dosing nomogram compared with a "standard care" nomogram. A randomized controlled trial. *Ann Intern Med.* 1993;119:874–881.**

10. Walker AM, Jick H. Predictors of bleeding during heparin therapy. *JAMA.* 1980;244:1209–1212.

11. Anand SS, Yusuf S, Pogue J, et al.; Organization to Assess Strategies for Ischemic Syndromes Investigators. Relationship of activated partial thromboplastin time to coronary events and bleeding in patients with acute coronary syndromes who receive heparin. *Circulation.* 2003;107:2884–2888.

12. Cipolle RJ, Rodvold KA. Heparin. In: Evans WE, Schentag JJ, Jusko WJ, eds. *Applied Pharmacokinetics: Principles of Therapeutic Drug Monitoring. 2nd ed.* Spokane, WA: Applied Therapeutics; 1986:908–943.

13. Morabia A. Heparin doses and major bleedings. *Lancet.* 1986;1:1278–1279.

14. ACC/AHA 2007 Guidelines for the Management of Patients with Unstable Angina/Non–ST-Elevation Myocardial Infarction: executive summary. *Circulation.* 2007; 116:803–877.

15. Harrington RA, Becker RC, Cannon CP, et al. American College of Chest Physicians Evidence-Based Clinical Practice Guidelines (8th ed.): antithrombotic therapy for non–ST-segment elevation acute coronary syndromes. *Chest.* 2008;133: 670S–707S.

16. Goodman SG, Menon V, Cannon CP, et al. American College of Chest Physicians Evidence-Based Clinical Practice Guidelines (8th ed.): acute ST-segment elevation myocardial infarction. *Chest.* 2008;133(6 Suppl):708S–775S.

* 17. **Kearon C, Kahn SR, Agnelli G, et al. American College of Chest Physicians Evidence-Based Clinical Practice Guidelines (8th ed.); antithrombotic therapy for venous thromboembolic disease. *Chest.* 2008;133:454S–545S.**

18. Tanaka KA, Thourani VH, Williams WH, et al. Heparin anticoagulation in patients undergoing off-pump and on-pump coronary bypass surgery. *J Anesth.* 2007;21: 297–303.

19. Yee Yee WP, Norton LL. Optimal weight base for a weight-based heparin dosing protocol. *Am J Health-Syst Pharm.* 1998;55:159–162.

20. Rosborough TK, Shepherd MF. Achieving target anti-Factor Xa activity with a heparin protocol based on sex, age, height, and weight. *Pharmacotherapy.* 2004;24: 713–719.

21. Myzienski AE, Lutz MF, Smythe MA. Unfractionated heparin dosing for venous thromboembolism in morbidly obese patients: case report and review of the literature. *Pharmacotherapy.* 2010;30:105e–112e.

22. Riney JN, Hollands JM, Smith JR, et al. Identifying optimal initial infusion rates for unfractionated heparin in morbidly obese patients. *Ann Pharmacother.* 2010;44: 1141–1151.

* **23.** **Olson JD, Arkin CF, Brandt JT, et al.; College of American Pathologists Conference XXXI on Laboratory Monitoring of Anticoagulation Therapy. Laboratory monitoring of unfractionated heparin therapy. *Arch Pathol Lab Med.* 1998;122:782–788.**

24. Hull RD, Raskob GE, Brant RF, et al. Relation between the time to achieve the lower limit of the APTT therapeutic range and recurrent venous thromboembolism during heparin treatment for deep vein thrombosis. *Arch Intern Med.* 1997;157: 2562–2568.

25. Anand SS, Bates S, Ginsberg JS, et al. Recurrent venous thrombosis and heparin therapy: an evaluation of the importance of early activated partial thromboplastin time results. *Arch Intern Med.* 1999;159:2029–2032.

26. Anand S, Ginsberg JS, Kearon C, et al. The relation between the activated partial thromboplastin time response and recurrence in patients with venous thrombosis treated with continuous intravenous heparin. *Arch Intern Med.* 1996;156: 1677–1681.

27. Raschke R, Hirsh J, Guidry JR. Suboptimal monitoring and dosing of unfractionated heparin in comparative studies with low-molecular-weight heparin. *Ann Intern Med.* 2003;138:720–723.

28. Smith ML, Wheeler KE. Weight-based heparin protocol using anti-Factor Xa monitoring. *Am J Health-Syst Pharm.* 2010;67:371–374.

29. Decousus HA, Croze M, Levi FA, et al. Circadian changes in anticoagulant effect of heparin infused at a constant rate. *Br Med J.* 1985;290:341–344.

30. Fischer KG. Essentials of anticoagulation in hemodialysis. *Hemodial Int.* 2007;11: 178–189.

31. Schulman S, Beyth RJ, Kearon C, et al.; American College of Chest Physicians. Hemorrhagic complications of anticoagulant and thrombolytic treatment. *Chest.* 2008;133(6 Suppl):257S–298S.

32. Teoh KH, Young E, Blackall MH, et al. Can extra protamine eliminate heparin rebound following cardiopulmonary bypass surgery? *J Thorac Cardiovasc Surg.* 2004;128(2): 211–219.

* **33. Warkentin TE, Greinacher A, Koster A, et al.; American College of Chest Physicians. Treatment and prevention of heparin-induced thrombocytopenia. *Chest.* 2008; 133(6 Suppl):340S–380S.**

Low Molecular Weight Heparin and Fondaparinux

4

Edith A. Nutescu

INTRODUCTION

The introduction of the low molecular weight heparins (LMWHs) and the synthetic pentasaccharides had a significant impact on how we administer anticoagulant therapy, particularly in the acute phase. Due to their convenience of use, these agents have been replacing the use of unfractionated heparin (UFH) in many clinical situations.

PHARMACOLOGY AND PHARMACOKINETICS[1-8]

- Three LMWH products are commercially available in the US: dalteparin (Fragmin), enoxaparin (Lovenox), and tinzaparin (Innohep).

- Fondaparinux (Arixtra) is the only commercially available synthetic pentasaccharide.

- All of these agents have an "indirect" anticoagulant effect, requiring antithrombin (AT) to potentiate their activity.

Table 4-1: Mechanism of Action for LMWH and Fondaparinux

LMWHs	Fondaparinux
• Anticoagulant effect is mediated through a specific pentasaccharide sequence that binds to AT and potentiates its activity	• Anticoagulant effect is mediated through a specific pentasaccharide sequence that binds to AT and potentiates its activity
• Inhibit both Factor Xa activity and factor IIa activity, but they are more specific to inhibiting Factor Xa activity than for inhibiting the activity of thrombin (factor IIa)	• Selectively inhibits Factor Xa activity

Table 4-2: Pharmacologic and Clinical Properties of LMWH and Fondaparinux

Property Source	LMWH (chemical or enzymatic depolymerization of UFH)	Fondaparinux (chemical synthesis)
Molecular weight (daltons)	Mean 4,500–5,000	1,728
SC bioavailability	~90%	100%
Activated clotting factors reduced	Factors Xa >IIa	Factor Xa
Binding to proteins other than target	Limited	Limited
Anti-Xa: anti-IIa	2:1 to 4:1	100% anti-Xa
Primary route of elimination	Renal primarily	Renal
Half-life (SC route)	3–5 hr	17–21 hr
Effects of protamine	Partial neutralization	No effect

Clinical Pearl

- Because fondaparinux is a synthetic product, it may be an option in individuals with allergies to animal products or have religious preferences to avoid selected animal derived products.

INDICATIONS, DOSING, AND ADMINISTRATION[1-9]

- Due to their quick onset of action, LMWHs and fondaparinux can be initiated and administered via the SC route, obviating the need for an initial IV bolus dose in cases of acute venous thrombosis (although IV bolus doses have been used in acute arterial thrombosis or in the setting of hemodialysis to protect against thrombosis of the dialysis circuit).

Clinical Pearls

In dosing LMWHs and fondaparinux:

- The actual body weight should be used for dosing of LMWHs and fondaparinux when used for treatment of VTE.[11]

- For LMWHs, restricting the doses to a certain maximum limit or "dose capping" is not recommended when treating VTE. The practice of "dose capping" can lead to under dosing in heavy weight patients and a potential increase in recurrent VTE.

- Dosing of fondaparinux for the treatment of VTE is based on various weight categories (see Table 4-3 below).

Table 4-3: Therapeutic Uses and Recommended Doses for LMWHs and Fondaparinux

Therapeutic Use	Enoxaparin	Dalteparin	Tinzaparin	Fondaparinux
VTE prophylaxis after hip replacement surgery	30 mg SC q 12 hr initiated 12–24 hr after surgery *or* 40 mg SC q 24 hr initiated 10–12 hr prior to surgery	2,500 units SC given 6–8 hr after surgery, then 5,000 units SC q 24 hr *or* 5,000 units SC q 24 hr initiated the evening prior to surgery	75 units/kg SC q 24 hr initiated the evening prior to surgery or 12–24 hr after surgery[a] *or* 4,500 units SC q 24 hr initiated 12 hr prior to surgery[a]	2.5 mg SC q 24 hr initiated 6–8 hr after surgery
VTE prophylaxis after hip fracture surgery	30 mg SC q 12 hr initiated 12–24 hr after surgery[a]	2,500 units SC given 6–8 hr after surgery, then 5,000 units SC q 24 hr[a]	NA	2.5 mg SC q 24 hr initiated 6–8 hr after surgery

(*continued*)

Table 4-3: (Continued)

Therapeutic Use	Enoxaparin	Dalteparin	Tinzaparin	Fondaparinux
VTE prophylaxis after knee replacement surgery	30 mg SC q 12 hr initiated 12–24 hr after surgery	2,500 units SC given 6–8 hr after surgery, then 5,000 units SC q 24 hr[a]	75 units/kg SC q 24 hr initiated the evening prior to surgery or 12–24 hr after surgery	2.5 mg SC q 24 hr initiated 6–8 hr after surgery
VTE prophylaxis after abdominal surgery	40 mg SC q 24 hr initiated 1–2 hr prior to surgery	2,500 units SC 1–2 hr prior to surgery then 2,500 units 12 hr after surgery followed by 5,000 units SC q 24 hr	3,500 units SC q 24 hr initiated 1–2 hr prior to surgery[a]	2.5 mg SC q 24 hr initiated 6–8 hr after surgery
VTE prophylaxis in acute medical illness	40 mg SC q 24 hr	5,000 units SC q 24 hr	NA	2.5 mg SC q 24 hr[a]
Treatment of VTE (DVT +/– PE)	1 mg/kg SC q 12 hr *or* 1.5 mg/kg SC q 24 hr	100 units/kg SC q 12 hr[a] *or* 200 units/kg SC q 24 hr for 1st month, then 150 units/kg SC q 24 hr for months 2 to 6[b]	175 units/kg SC q 24 hr	5 mg SC q 24 hr if weight <50 kg 7.5 mg SC q 24 hr if weight 50–100 kg 10 mg SC q 24 hr if weight >100 kg
Unstable angina or non-Q-wave MI	1 mg/kg SC q 12 hr[c]	120 units/kg SC q 12 hr (maximum dose 10,000 units)	NA	2.5 mg SC q 24 hr[a] Note: UFH was added to prevent thrombus formation on the guidewire (see Table 3-4)

(*continued*)

Table 4-3: (Continued)

Therapeutic Use	Enoxaparin	Dalteparin	Tinzaparin	Fondaparinux
Acute STEMI	**If <75 years of age:** 30-mg single IV bolus plus a 1-mg/kg SC dose followed by 1 mg/kg SC q 12 hr (first two SC doses capped at 100 mg) **If >75 years of age:** 0.75 mg/kg SC q 12 hr (no bolus, first two SC doses capped at 75 mg) All patients should receive aspirin as soon as they are identified as having STEMI and maintained with 75–325 mg once daily unless contraindicated	NA	NA	NA

[a]Non-FDA approved for indication.

[b]Dosing regimen approved for VTE treatment in patients with malignancy.

[c]An additional 30-mg IV bolus with the first SC dose has been studied in clinical trials.

Clinical Pearls

LMWH dose rounding:

Because LMWHs are available in prefilled syringes, approaches of rounding to a convenient syringe size may occur. Considerations in decisions on rounding, or specifying a dose can include the following:

- LMWHs have a wide enough therapeutic window that routine monitoring is not necessary with most uses.

- The weight used can vary between what is reported, different scales, fluid shifts, etc.

- Renal function may influence dosing (especially with enoxaparin) to consider rounding downwards.

- The therapeutic use (i.e., atrial fibrillation) may not have a clear proven benefit or data supporting a specific dosing approach.

- Medication errors and delays in initiating therapy can occur when preparing an individualized unit dose syringe.

- Loss of safety features in the premanufactured syringes.

- Variability occurs between lots.

- Rounding in low weight individuals (i.e., <50 kg) can result in a large percent change in the dose.

- Not all prefilled syringes are graduated.

- Squirting out of the "air bubble" can lead to more bruising at the injection site. Priming the needle in premanufactured LWMHs is not recommended prior to injection.

Timing administration of injections: timing of injections should consider prompt initiation of therapy in acute thrombosis, limiting potential delays or missing a dose secondary to the patient being off the floor or scheduling an anti-Factor Xa activity measurement. For prophylaxis, evening dosing of a once a day regimen may limit missed doses.

MONITORING[1-11]

- LMWHs have a predictable anticoagulant dose response; thus, routine dosage adjustments and monitoring of anticoagulation activity are not required in the majority of patients.

- The PT/INR, aPTT, and ACT are inappropriate laboratory markers to monitor the anticoagulant effect, as they are only minimally affected by LMWHs and fondaparinux.

- LMWHs have minimal effect on Factor IIa; thus, limited prolongation of aPTT may be seen in cases of LMWH overdoses.

Table 4-4: Monitoring Parameters for LMWHs and Fondaparinux

Baseline Monitoring Parameters	Ongoing Monitoring Parameters[a]
Obtain and document baseline labs before initiating therapy	Monitor at least every 3–4 days while on therapy
CBC with platelet count	CBC with platelet count
SCr	SCr
CrCl	CrCl

[a]The frequency of laboratory testing during use in the outpatient care setting has not been established.

Clinical Pearls

Role of anti-Factor Xa activity monitoring:

- Although controversial, measurement of the chromogenic anti-Factor Xa activity has been the most widely used method in clinical practice to measure a patient's response to LMWH or fondaparinux (see Chapter 18).

- While not routinely recommended due to lack of outcomes data, measuring a patient's response to LMWH may be considered in certain high-risk situations such as patients with morbid obesity (weigh more than 150 kg or body mass index more than 50 kg/m^2), very low body weight (weigh less than 50 kg), significant renal impairment (CrCl less than 30 mL/min), neonates and pediatric patients, pregnant women, and in patients who receive extended therapy (>1 month).

- When measuring anti-Factor Xa activity, the sample should be obtained after steady-state concentrations of the LMWH are attained, after the 2nd to 3rd dose.

- Peak concentrations typically occur approximately 4 hours after a subcutaneous dose; thus, timing of the lab draw in relation to dose is critical.

- Trough concentrations can be more useful to rule out drug accumulation, such as in patients with renal failure, and are typically measured just prior to the next dose of the LMWH.

- While there is some variation in the target concentrations reported in the literature, peak anti-Factor Xa activity concentrations of 0.1–0.4 units/mL with twice daily dosing are recommended for prevention of VTE, but a more conservative range is 0.2–0.4 units/mL. For the treatment of VTE, peak anti-Factor Xa activity concentrations of 0.4–1.1 units/mL with twice daily dosing have been suggested, but a more conservative therapeutic range is 0.5–1.0 units/mL. With once daily dosing, as higher doses of a drug are given per dose, peak anti-Factor Xa activity concentrations of 1–2 units/mL have been suggested, but supporting data is even more limited. (For acute coronary syndromes, see Chapter 13.)

- Specific algorithms for dosing adjustments based on anti-Factor Xa activity have not been widely evaluated and are limited at the present time. It is important to check that the time of the anti-Factor Xa activity concentration in relation to the dose is correct ($\sim$4–6 hours after the SC injection for peak or as a predose level for trough in selected settings). One dosing approach has been suggested in pediatric patients that can also be potentially applied in adult populations.

Table 4-5: Sample LMWH Dosing Nomogram Based on Anti-Factor Xa Activity for VTE Treatment

Anti-Factor Xa Activity	Hold Next Dose	Dosage Change	Next Anti-Factor Xa Activity Level
<0.35 units/mL	No	↑ 25%	4 hr after next dose
0.35–0.49	No	↑ 10%	4 hr after next dose

(*continued*)

Table 4-5: (Continued)

Anti-Factor Xa Activity	Hold Next Dose	Dosage Change	Next Anti-Factor Xa Activity Level
0.5–1.0	No	No	Next day, then in 1 week, then monthly
1.1–1.5	No	↓ 20%	Before next dose
1.6–2.0	3 hr	↓ 30%	Before next dose and 4 hr after next dose
>2 International Units/mL	Until anti-Factor Xa activity <0.5 units/mL	↓ 40%	Before next dose and q 12 hr until anti-Factor Xa activity is <0.5 units/mL

Source: adapted from reference 12.

COMMON SIDE EFFECTS, PRECAUTIONS, AND CONTRAINDICATIONS

Table 4-6: Common Side Effects, Precautions, and Contraindications to LMWH and Fondaparinux[13-16]

LMWHs	Fondaparinux
Bleeding	Bleeding
Spinal and epidural hematomas	Spinal and epidural hematomas
Thrombocytopenia	Thrombocytopenia (? HIT)
HIT	
Osteopenia	
Hives/anaphylaxis	

Reversal: see Chapter 7 on the reversal of LMWH or fondaparinux.

LMWHs	Fondaparinux
Protamine can be used as a "partial" reversal agent for the effects of LMWH	No specific antidote exists
Protamine neutralizes approximately 60% of the anti-Factor Xa activity	

(*continued*)

Table 4-6: (Continued)

LMWHs	Fondaparinux
If an LMWH was given in the previous 8 hr, then 1 mg of protamine should be administered for every 100 International Units (or 1 mg) of the LMWH	
If the LMWH dose was given in the previous 8–12 hr, a 0.5-mg dose of protamine should be given for every 100 anti-Factor Xa activity units	
The use of protamine sulfate is not recommended if the LMWH was administered more than 12 hr earlier	

RECOMMENDATIONS FOR TIMING OF LMWH AND FONDAPARINUX IN PATIENTS UNDERGOING NEURAXIAL PROCEDURES[4,14] (ALSO SEE TABLE 8.5)

Table 4-7: Recommendations for the Timing of LMWH or Fondaparinux Administration When Neuraxial Procedures Are Used

Anticoagulant Agent	Minimum Time Between Anticoagulant Dose and Insertion of Spinal Needle or Placement of Epidural Catheter	Minimum Time Between Insertion of Spinal Needle or Placement of Epidural Catheter and Anticoagulant Dose	Minimum Time Between Anticoagulant Dose and Removal of the Epidural Catheter	Minimum Time Between Removal of the Epidural Catheter and Anticoagulant Dose (provided hemostasis has been achieved)
Fondaparinux therapeutic or prophylactic doses	36–48 hr[a]	Avoid while catheter is in place	Ideally avoid while catheter is in place. Just before the next dose and when anticoagulant effect is at minimum	2 hr

(continued)

Table 4-7: (Continued)

Anticoagulant Agent	Minimum Time Between Anticoagulant Dose and Insertion of Spinal Needle or Placement of Epidural Catheter	Minimum Time Between Insertion of Spinal Needle or Placement of Epidural Catheter and Anticoagulant Dose	Minimum Time Between Anticoagulant Dose and Removal of the Epidural Catheter	Minimum Time Between Removal of the Epidural Catheter and Anticoagulant Dose (provided hemostasis has been achieved)
Therapeutic dose LMWH (enoxaparin 1 mg/kg SC q 12 hr or enoxaparin 1.5 mg/kg SC q 24 hr or dalteparin 100 units/kg SC q 12 hr or dalteparin 200 units/kg SC q 24 hr or tinzaparin 175 units/kg SC q 24 hr)	24 hr[a]	Avoid while catheter is in place	Ideally avoid while catheter is in place Just before the next dose and when anticoagulant effect is at minimum	2 hr
Prophylactic dose LMWH (enoxaparin 30 mg SC q 12 hr or enoxaparin 40 mg SC q 24 hr or dalteparin 5,000 units SC q 24 hr)	10–12 hr[a]	Avoid while catheter is in place	Ideally avoid while catheter is in place Just before the next dose and when anticoagulant effect is at minimum	2 hr

[a]Longer elimination times will be required in patients with impaired renal function.

SPECIAL POPULATION CONSIDERATIONS[4,11,16]

Pregnancy and pediatrics

Dosing and monitoring of LMWH in pregnancy (see Chapter 16) and pediatric patients (see Chapter 17) will be covered in those respective chapters.

Morbid obesity dosing considerations for VTE

Total body weight appears to be a good predictor for dosing of LMWHs in obese patients.

Table 4-8: Dosing Consideration for LMWH in Obese Patients[11]

LMWHs
Setting a maximum dose (or "dose capping") when treating patients with VTE is not recommended, and in fact it may result in under dosing of these patients with a potential increase in thrombotic complications
For VTE prophylaxis indications, available data suggest that fixed LMWH doses may not be sufficient in morbidly obese patients and a 25 to 30% dose increase or weight-based dosing of 50 units/kg/day may be considered
Although the Dalteparin Product Information recommends capping the maximum daily dose at 18,000 units for VTE treatment, this raises concerns in clinical practice in patients weighing >100 kg due to the potential of under dosing and heightened risk of thromboembolic complications
Divided daily dosing for enoxaparin (1 mg/kg q 12 hr) has been associated with a lower incidence of recurrent thrombosis compared to 1.5 mg/kg once daily in obesity and cancer
The use of a three times daily regimen to meet various available syringes sizes has not been evaluated.
Limited data with dalteparin or tinzaparin does not address the use of twice daily dosing compared to once daily dosing; decisions may need to consider the patient's weight and available syringe sizes
For enoxaparin: administering SC injections into the thigh in obese patients leads to lower measured anti-Factor-Xa activity compared to administration into the abdomen.

Clinical Pearl

- For morbid obese patients with VTE and good renal function, fondaparinux 10 mg is an alternative therapeutic approach.

Dosing considerations in underweight

Low weight patients (i.e., <50 kg) may be at risk for drug accumulation and bleeding complications when fixed prophylactic doses of LMWH or fondaparinux are administered. Due to a concern of increased bleeding complications, when used for VTE prophylaxis in surgical patients, fondaparinux is contraindicated in patients who weigh less than 50 kg. When used for VTE treatment, the dose of fondaparinux is lowered to 5 mg daily in patients who weigh less than 50 kg.

Dosing considerations in renal dysfunction

As LMWHs are renally eliminated, reduced elimination can result in increased drug concentrations and an increased bleeding risk. The actual degree of accumulation is different for the various LMWHs and fondaparinux as there are differences in their pharmacologic profiles.

Table 4-9: Dosing and Monitoring Considerations for LMWH and Fondaparinux in Patients with Renal Impairment[4,11,16,a]

Anticoagulant	Pharmacokinetic Considerations	Dosing and Monitoring Recommendations	Package Insert Recommendations
Dalteparin	CrCl <30[b] mL/min: no accumulation noted up to 1 week of therapy CrCl 30–50 mL/min: no accumulation noted	CrCl <30[b] mL/min: no dose adjustment needed up to 1 week with prophylaxis doses; for treatment doses consider monitoring anti-Factor Xa activity For use >1 week: consider monitoring of anti-Factor Xa activity and adjust dose if accumulation is noted CrCl 30–50 mL/min: no dose adjustment needed	CrCl <30[b] mL/min: use with caution
Enoxaparin	CrCl <30[b] mL/min: 40% to 50% accumulation noted CrCl 30–50 mL/min: 15% to 20% accumulation noted	CrCl <30[b] mL/min: consider a 40% to 50% dose decrease and subsequent monitoring of anti-Factor Xa activity CrCl 30–50 mL/min: consider a 15% to 20% dose decrease with prolonged use (>10–14 days) and subsequent monitoring of anti-Factor Xa activity	CrCl <30[b] mL/min: prophylaxis—30 mg SC daily treatment—1 mg/kg SC daily
Tinzaparin	CrCl <30[b] mL/min: 20% accumulation noted CrCl 30–50 mL/min: no accumulation noted	CrCl <30[b] mL/min: consider a dose decrease of 20% and subsequent monitoring of anti-Factor Xa activity CrCl 30–50 mL/min: no dose adjustment needed	CrCl <30[b] mL/min: use with caution

(continued)

Table 4-9: (Continued)

Anticoagulant	Pharmacokinetic Considerations	Dosing and Monitoring Recommendations	Package Insert Recommendations
Fondaparinux	CrCl <30[b] mL/min: 55% accumulation noted CrCl 30–50 mL/min: 40% accumulation noted	CrCl <30 mL/min: contraindicated in this population CrCl 30–50 mL/min: if prolonged use (>10 days) drug accumulation may occur and dosing adjustment maybe necessary Could consider measurement of anti-Factor Xa activity to guide with dose adjustment (note: the anti-Factor Xa activity assay in this case has to be specifically calibrated for fondaparinux and many laboratories do not offer this option)	CrCl <30 mL/min: contraindicated CrCl 30–50 mL/min: use with caution[c]

[a]The use of an anti-Factor Xa activity measurement to adjust dosing in the setting of renal insufficiency has not been validated and it is at best a controversial practice. Trough anti-Factor-Xa activity measurements have been considered to assess potential accumulation in patients at increased risk for bleeding.

[b]Data is very limited in patients with a CrCl <20 mL/min. In patients on hemodialysis, limited data is only available for thrombosis prevention in the dialysis circuit but not for the prevention and/or treatment of venous or arterial thrombosis. Thus, until further data is available, UFH is the agent of choice in patients on hemodialysis or with a CrCl <20 mL/min. CrCl measurements in the clinical trials may have used total body weight and thus estimate a value higher than estimated when using the ideal body weight.

[c]Care should be used when fondaparinux is used for an extended time (>7–10 days) in patients with moderate renal impairment (CrCl 30–50 mL/min, as accumulation of the drug has also been reported in these patients at a rate of approximately 40%).

Cancer

- LMWHs are preferred over warfarin for long-term anticoagulation in the setting of cancer and acute thrombosis. Benefits are primarily seen in nonmetastatic disease.

- A higher dose of LMWH (enoxaparin 1 mg/kg twice daily or dalteparin 200 units/kg once daily) during the first 4 weeks has been suggested to provide a more aggressive level on anticoagulation when the risk of recurrent thrombosis is the greatest.

- For enoxaparin, 1 mg/kg twice daily dosing may be preferred over once daily dosing during the initial treatment phase.

- Dalteparin is the only LMWH with an indication for treatment of venous thrombosis in the setting of cancer.

- Benefits of therapy or safety of LMWH use beyond 6 months have not been established at this time.

Elderly

- Renal function can decline with advanced age, requiring in selected situations a reduction in the dose of enoxaparin for treatment uses (this may not be the case with other agents of the class where the degree of accumulation may be lower).

- Consider that some elderly patients can have low body weight where doses of 30–40 mg are closer to a full therapeutic dose.

- Before sending an elderly patient home on an LMWH or fondaparinux, consider the ability to self-inject if arthritis is present.

Critically ill

- Bioavailability for LMWH can be lost in edematous patients or when vasopressors are in use.

- In selected situations, critically ill patients may have low levels of antithrombin (i.e., large trauma, renal failure) thus reducing the level of anticoagulation. Anti-Factor Xa activity measurements using an assay that incorporates AT may not identify this (see Chapter 18).

- No clear data exists on guiding subsequent dosing adjustments for these situations.

REFERENCES

1. Hirsh J, Bauer KA, Donati MB, et al. Parenteral anticoagulants: American College of Chest Physicians Evidence-Based Clinical Practice Guidelines (8th ed.). *Chest.* 2008;133:141S–159S.

2. Wittkowsky AK, Nutescu EA. Thrombosis. In: Koda-Kimble MA, Young LY, Alldredge BK, et al., eds. *Applied Therapeutics: The Clinical Use of Drugs.* 9th ed. Baltimore, MD: Lippincott Williams & Wilkins; 2008:15.1–15.36.

3. Haines ST, Witt D, Nutescu EA. Venous thromboembolism. In: DiPiro J, Talbert R, Yee G, et al. eds. *Pharmacotherapy: A Pathophysiologic Approach.* 7th ed. New York, NY: McGraw-Hill; 2008:331–372.

4. Nutescu EA, Dager W. Heparin, low molecular weight heparin, and fondaparinux. In: Gulseth M, ed. *Managing Anticoagulation Patients in the Hospital.* 1st ed. Bethesda, MD: American Society of Health-System Pharmacists; 2007:177–202.

5. Haines ST, Nutescu EA. Venous thromboembolism. In: Chisholm M, Schwinghammer T, Wells B, et al., eds. *Pharmacotherapy Principles and Practice.* 1st ed. New York, NY: McGraw-Hill; 2007:133–160.

6. Hirsh J, O'Donnell M, Eikelboom JW. Beyond unfractionated heparin and warfarin: current and future advances. *Circulation.* 2007;116(5):552–560.

7. Keam SJ, Goa KL. Fondaparinux sodium. *Drugs.* 2002;62:1673–1685.

8. Nutescu EA, Shapiro NL, Chevalier A, et al. A pharmacologic overview of current and emerging anticoagulants. *Cleve Clin J Med.* 2005;72(suppl 1):S2–S6.

9. Nutescu EA, Wittkowsky AK, Dobesh PP, et al. Choosing the appropriate antithrombotic agent for the prevention and treatment of VTE: a case-based approach. *Ann Pharmacother.* 2006;40:1558–1571.

10. Laposata M, Green D, Van Cott EM, et al. College of American Pathologists Conference XXXI on Laboratory Monitoring of Anticoagulant Therapy: the clinical use and laboratory monitoring of low-molecular-weight heparin, danaparoid, hirudin and related compounds, and argatroban. *Arch Pathol Lab Med.* 1998;122:799–807.

11. Nutescu EA, Spinler SA, Wittkowsky AK, et al. Low molecular weight heparins in renal impairment and obesity: available evidence and clinical practice recommendations across medical and surgical settings. *Ann Pharmacother.* 2009;43:1064–1083.

12. Monagle P Michelson AD, Bovill E, et al. Antithrombotic therapy in children. *Chest.* 2001;119 (suppl 1):344S–370S.

13. Gouin-Thibault I, Pautas E, Siguret V. Safety profile of different low-molecular eight heparins used at therapeutic dose. *Drug Saf.* 2005;28:333–349.

14. Horlocker TT, Wedel DJ, Rowlingson JC, et al. Regional anesthesia in the patient receiving antithrombotic or thrombolytic therapy. *Reg Anesth Pain Med.* 2010;35:64–101.

15. Crowther MA, Warkentin TE. Bleeding risk and the management of bleeding complications in patients undergoing anticoagulant therapy: focus on new anticoagulant agents. *Blood.* 2008;111:4871–4879.

16. Lim W, Dentali F, Eikelboom JW, et al. Meta-analysis: low-molecular-weight heparin and bleeding in patients with severe renal insufficiency. *Ann Intern Med.* 2006;144:673–684.

FIVE

Chapter

5

Parenteral Direct Thrombin Inhibitors

William E. Dager

INTRODUCTION

The parenteral direct thrombin inhibitors (DTIs) act independent of antithrombin and are typically used in situations where unfractionated heparin (UFH) is not recommended such as heparin-induced thrombocytopenia, antithrombin deficiency, or in the setting of acute coronary syndromes. This class of agents works differently then other anticoagulants, despite similar laboratory assessments. Further, due to more limited experience with their use, it is important to approach their management and laboratory assay target ranges as independent of observations with other anticoagulants.

PHARMACOLOGY[1,2]

- The activity of thrombin can be inhibited by currently available DTIs that bind directly to either the catalytic (active) site or substrate recognition site (exocite 1). Thrombin also contains a heparin-binding site (exocite 2).

- All commercially available DTIs directly bind to the catalytic (active) site on thrombin responsible for enzymatic activity.

- Binding to the catalytic (active) site on thrombin inhibits several of the actions of thrombin including cleavage of fibrinogen and platelet activation, both of which are involved in thrombus formation.

- Bivalent DTIs (bivalirudin, desirudin, and lepirudin) also bind to the substrate recognition (exocite 1) on thrombin where fibrinogen can bind.

- DTIs do not bind to exocite 2, and thus are capable of inhibiting the effects of thrombin bound to fibrin (clot bound thrombin).

- DTIs can also block thrombin's ability to activate platelets, stimulate granule release, surface receptor expression and aggregation in addition to a plethora of other factors that mediate vascular integrity.

- Hirudin analogues' (lepirudin and desirudin) ability to tightly bind to thrombin can lead to prolonged inhibition.

- Bivalirudin is enzymatically cleaved by thrombin. This results in loss of activity that is independent of renal or hepatic function. Its effects may not last in stagnant blood. Increased elimination can occur with hemofiltration.

- The onset of bivalirudin on ACT values occurs within 5–10 minutes after a bolus.

- Dabigatran etexilate is an oral DTI (see Chapter 9 for further details).

PHARMACOKINETICS/PHARMACODYNAMICS

Table 5-1: Pharmacokinetics of Available Antithrombin Agents[3–5]

Agent	Argatroban	Bivalirudin	Lepirudin	Desirudin
Source	Synthetic	Analog of hirudin	Leech (hirudo medicinalis)	Recombinant from yeast
Binding to thrombin	3.9×10^{-8} mol/L	1.9 nM	2×10^{-14} M	2.6×10^{-13} M
Route of administration	IV	IV	IV/SC	SC
Plasma half-life (healthy subjects)	31–51 min	25 min	1.3 hr	2 hr
Primary elimination route	Hepatic	Enzymatic	Renal	Renal
Fraction excreted unchanged in the urine (Fe)	16%	20%	35%	40% to 50%
Effect on INR (depends on the amount of DTI present; this may correlate to a elevation in the aPTT or ACT level in the sample)	Moderate	Mild	Small	Small

INDICATIONS/DOSING/ADMINISTRATION

- Postmarketing experiences have suggested lower doing approaches, especially in acutely ill.

The initial dosing regimen for a DTI will depend on the indication for anticoagulation, clinical presentation of the patient, and the desired intensity of parenteral anticoagulation, similar to how heparin is utilized. Specific factors that may influence the dosing include the following:

- Presence of thrombosis
- Impaired organ function
- Presence of active bleeding or risk factors for bleeding

Note that ACT readings with a DTI may vary between low and high response assay methods.

Occasionally, the situation may arise where use of subcutaneous lepirudin or desirudin may be desirable. In such cases, the following dosing can be considered:

- Thrombosis prophylaxis: 15 mg SC q 12 hr (lepirudin or desirudin)
- Treatment doses of 25–50 mg SC q 12 hr have been studied (lepirudin).

aPTT monitoring and dosing titration have been explored. For aPTT values greater than 2 times control, the dose should be held and resumed at a lower amount when the aPTT drops below 2 times control. For line flushing recommendations, see Chapter 15.

Clinical Pearls

Argatroban Dosing in HIT

- Mean dose in Asians (1 mcg/kg/min); lower than doses observed in Hispanic or African Americans[6]
- Critically ill: 0.6 mcg/kg/min vs. noncritical 1.4 mcg/kg/min[7]
- Weight based[7]:
  - Standard: 1.6 mcg/kg/min; adjust in increments of 0.5 mcg/kg/min TBW
  - Hepatic/critical: 0.5 mcg/kg/min; adjust in increments of 0.1 mcg/kg/min; TBW (avoid including excess fluid weight)
  - Wt >50% IBW: initiate at 1 mcg/kg/min

Table 5-2: Dosing and Administration of DTIs for Selected Indications[3,5,7-11]

Indications	Argatroban	Bivalirudin	Lepirudin	Desirudin
HIT: typical IV dosing	No bolus 2 mcg/kg/min Avg: dose in trials 1.6 mcg/kg/min Max: 10 mcg/kg/min Rarely used at rates >3 mcg/kg/min Starting doses of 0.5–1.2 mcg/kg/min have been used in acutely/critically ill patients Reduce dose in hepatic failure aPTT target 1.5–3 times baseline	No indication in HIT; current reports suggest approximately 0.08–0.17 mg/kg/hr depending on treatment goals and the acuity of the patient No bolus aPTT target 1.5–2.5 times control	Mean doses in trials 0.09–0.1 mg/kg/hr Bolus only when acute, life threatening thrombosis is present Option 1 (rarely used): Bolus: 0.4 mg/kg (up to 110 kg to 44 mg) over 15–20 sec Maintenance infusion: 0.15 mg/kg/hr Option 2: Bolus: none unless acute HITTS Maintenance infusion: 0.1–0.15 mg/kg/hr (maximum infusion at 110 kg or 16.5 mg/hr); maintenance infusions <0.1 mg/kg/hr are considered in acutely/critically ill patients; adjust for renal function aPTT target 1.5–2.5 times baseline	NA due to limited data[a]
ACS/PCI/PTCA	Bolus: 350 mcg/kg Infusion: 25 mcg/kg/min IV dosing ACT target: 300–450 sec	Bolus: 0.75 mg/kg Infusion: 1.75 mg/kg/hr IV dosing if needed post-PCI; continue infusion at 0.25 mg/kg/hr (option bolus of 0.1 mg/kg) if the infusion is off more than 2 hr for sheath	Bolus: 0.4 mg/kg Infusion: 0.15 mg/kg/hr ACS infusion over several days; target aPTT 60–100 sec reported	NA due to limited data[a]

(continued)

Table 5-2: (Continued)

Indications	Argatroban	Bivalirudin	Lepirudin	Desirudin
	With GPIIb/IIIa inhibitors: 250 mcg/kg followed by an infusion of 25 mcg/kg/min targeting ACT of 275–450 sec; for ACT <275 sec, a 150-mcg/kg bolus is given	removal, with a aPTT target of approximately 65–70 sec ACT target: none CrCl <30: 1 mg/kg/hr Dialysis: 0.25 mg/kg/hr		
Unstable angina	N/A	Infusion: 0.2 mg/kg/hr IV	N/A	
Deep vein thrombosis prophylaxis following hip replacement surgery	N/A	N/A	N/A	Subcutaneous injection: 15 mg q 12 hr started 5–15 min prior to surgery after regional anesthesia[a]

[a]Desirudin recently became commercially available in the US and has more limited data than other agents.

Table 5-3: Renal, Hepatic, and Hepatorenal Failure Anticoagulation Dosing Under HIT Conditions[3,12,13]

	Argatroban[a]	Bivalirudin	Lepirudin	Desirudin
Hepatic Dose Adjustments	Child Pugh score >6 (See Appendix B) or total bilirubin >1.5 mg/dL Reduce dose to less than or equal to 0.5 mcg/kg/min	Eliminated enzymatically may not need adjustment for hepatic function	No clear data; lower doses in critically ill and hepatic failure may be considered	No clear data; lower doses in critically ill and hepatic failure may be considered
Renal Dose Adjustments **(Hemodialysis See Table 5–4)**	Renal dysfunction dose adjustment unclear No apparent effect of HD on elimination A dosing decrease of 0.1–0.6 mcg/kg/min for every 30-mL/min drop in CrCl in HIT has been reported	Eliminated enzymatically may not need large adjustment for renal dysfunction alone CrCl >60 mL/min: 0.12–0.15 mg/kg/hr; CrCl 30–60 mL/min: 0.06–0.1 mg/kg/hr; CrCl <30 mL/min: 0.03–0.05 mg/kg/hr (Critically ill may require doses on lower end of the range)	CrCl (mL/min): Rate (mg/kg/hr): > 60 0.15 45–60 0.075 30–44 0.045 15–29 0.0225 <15 May depend on dialysis approach; see Table 5-4	CrCl (mL/min): ≥31–60: initiate therapy at 5 mg q 12 hr by subcutaneous injection Monitor aPTT and serum creatinine at least daily; if aPTT exceeds 2 times control: 1. Interrupt therapy until the value returns to less than 2 times control 2. Resume therapy at a reduced dose guided by the initial degree of aPTT abnormality; <31: initiate therapy at 1.7 mg q 12 hr by subcutaneous injection

(continued)

Table 5-3: (Continued)

	Argatroban[a]	Bivalirudin	Lepirudin	Desirudin
		Substantially removed during HD		Monitor aPTT and serum creatinine at least daily; if aPTT exceeds 2 times control: 1. Interrupt therapy until the value returns to less than 2 times control 2. Consider further dose reductions
Hepatorenal Dose Adjustments	Prolonged effects Start with low dose then titrate up Assume initial aPTT is not steady state	Eliminated enzymatically may not need adjustment for hepatic function	Prolonged effects Start with low dose then titrate up Assume initial aPTT is not steady state	Unknown, but a lower dose likely
Monitoring Goal aPTT	1.5–3.0 x control	1.5–2.5 x control	1.5–2.5 x control	Less than 2 x control (DVT prophylaxis)

Abbreviation: x = times. Use patient's baseline aPTT value as the control.

[a]Argatroban is generally preferred over lepirudin in severe renal failure. Bivalirudin may have pharmacokinetic advantages in concurrent hepatic and renal failure.

Table 5-4: Considerations for Dosing DTIs in Hemodialysis[11,13–16]

Agent	Consideration in Hemodialysis (see Table 15-3)
Argatroban	Unclear if dose adjustment are necessary as reports are not consistent
	For anticoagulation to maintain the circuit during intermittent HD only, three regimens have been studied and found equivalent:
	1) 250-mcg/kg bolus with an additional 250-mcg/kg bolus allowed 2 hr later if ACT <140% of baseline 2) 250-mcg/kg bolus followed by 2 mcg/kg/min 3) 2 mcg/kg/min started 4 hr prior to HD with target ACT 140–180 sec
Bivalirudin	When using bivalirudin for therapeutic use (not just to maintain the circuit) it is important to consider that some is dialyzed off, likely necessitating an increase in the rate; The optimal management strategy may depend on the duration of hemodialysis and aPTT value being maintained along with the risk of thrombosis formation during HD; consider aPTT 2 hr into HD to assess a need to temporarily increase the infusion rate during prolonged procedures (>8 hours)
	Initial dose
	For treatment of HIT or antithrombin deficiency in
	1) Intermittent hemodialysis patients: 0.07 mg/kg/hr 2) Extended duration hemodialysis 0.09 mg/kg/hr 3) Continuous renal replacement therapy: 0.07 mg/kg/hr Note: based on total body weight and for infusing during and off dialysis[a]
Lepirudin	When using lepirudin for therapeutic use (not just to maintain the circuit), it is important to consider that hemodialysis or hemofiltration may remove lepirudin; doses as low as 0.005 mg/kg/hr have been used in renal failure requiring HD; the aPTT response may depend on degree of residual renal function present
	For anticoagulation during HD to maintain the circuit only: 0.10 mg/kg IV predialysis

[a]Target aPTT may depend on the dialysis circuit and frequency of thrombosis-related complications. An aPTT of 1.5–2 times baseline aPTT can be considered in place of heparin if anticoagulation is only needed for circuit protection.

DTI Dosing and Management

- Bivalirudin dosing in ACS: the target ACT in the Replace II ACS trial was a bolus to maintain the ACT over 225 seconds. In subsequent ACS trials, ACT monitoring of the bivalirudin was not required.[17]

- Effects of bivalirudin on the ACT can be seen within minutes of a bolus.

- Lepirudin dosing in HIT: no recent trials; bolus only if acute thrombosis is present.[5] Tight binding to thrombin may yield continued antithrombotic effects after aPTT returns to baseline.

- Any DTI: targeting aPTT ratio of 1.5 to 2 x baseline may be considered in absence of acute thromboembolism to minimize bleeding concerns.

MONITORING

Table 5-5: Target aPTT Range in the Setting of HIT

aPTT Range	Clinical Setting
Lower: 1.5–2.0 x baseline	Isolated HIT, AT deficiency or treatment of thromboembolic complications when increased bleeding concerns are present
Higher: 2.0–2.5 x baseline	Argatroban: 2–3 x baseline
	HITTS and limited risk for bleeding

Key points in monitoring DTI regimens

- Differences in sensitivities for aPTT reagents between heparin or DTI may occur and thus the target aPTT range for a DTI will not be the same as heparin nor the same between different DTIs. Furthermore, due to differences in aPTT assays, the target range for a DTI will likely vary between institutions.

- Acutely ill patients such as those with renal, hepatic, or cardiac dysfunction may reach target aPTT values at a dose notably lower than observed in the clinical trials.

- Since most published dosing experiences are based on aPTT monitoring, not serum DTI concentrations, the actual dosing observed may be different due to differences in aPTT assays.

- Other approaches to monitoring DTI infusions include the direct measurement of the DTI serum concentration, use of ecarin clotting times, or use of modified thrombin times.

  - Although more consistent results have been observed with these assays compared to the aPTT, reductions in the incidence of bleeding or thrombosis with their use has not been established.

- Alterations in dosing requirements may be necessary as the dynamic clinical presentation of the patient changes. Measured aPTT values should take this under consideration, and the infusion rate should be adjusted to prevent under or overshooting target goals.[18]

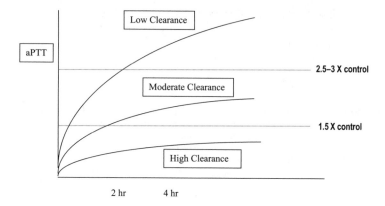

Figure 5-1: Considerations for Measuring aPTT Values at the Initiation of a DTI Infusion

The initial aPTT may depend on plasma clearance. An early aPTT in the upper end of the target range might signal a reduced ability to eliminate the DTI.

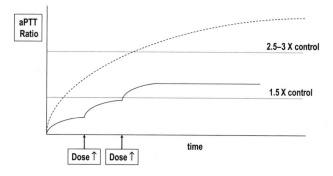

Figure 5-2: Optional Approach to Titrating DTI Infusion into the Target Range in the Presence of Notable Bleeding Concerns

The dotted line represents potential aPTT values above the target in the setting of reduced DTI elimination that is not recognized early in the course of therapy. The solid line describes a strategy of starting a lower infusion rate and titrating upwards to minimize risk of overshooting the target when notable bleeding concerns are present. (Source: adapted from reference 18.)

Table 5-6: Sample Adjustment Scale for a DTI[a]

Agent _____				
Start infusion at _____ (____/hr) Draw aPTT ____hr after starting infusion Draw aPTT/INR/CBC every morning while on infusion			Baseline aPTT _____ Baseline INR _____ Call physician if the rate exceeds _____	
aPTT	Rate adjustment by percentage	Rate adjustment	Repeat aPTT	Comment
Less than ____ sec	Increase infusion rate by 40%	Increase rate _____	4–6 hr	
____ to ____ sec	Increase infusion rate by 20%	Increase infusion _____	4–6 hr	
Goal aPTT ____	No change	No change		Draw aPTT/INR every morning
____ to ____ sec	Decrease infusion rate by 20%	Decrease infusion rate ____	4–6 hr	
Greater than ____ sec	Decrease infusion rate by 40% Hold for 1–2 hr[b]	Decrease infusion rate ____ Hold for 1–2 hr[b]	4–6 hr	[b]For low infusion rates *(defined based on agent)* and aPTT >100 sec *(could vary based on hospital reagent)*, hold 2 hr; if at a higher rate *(defined based on agent)*, hold 1 hr

Clinical thrombosis: target 2.0–2.5 times baseline for lepirudin/bivalirudin (2–3 times baseline argatroban)

No apparent clinical thrombosis: target aPTT 1.5–2/2.5 times baseline

Rate adjustment units (mg/hr, mcg/kg/min, mg/kg/hr) can vary between institutions and the agent used

For argatroban: when using argatroban, adjust initial dose in the following fashion[b]:

– Asian: 1 mcg/kg/min
– Hepatic impairment (Child Pugh >6): 0.5 mcg/kg/min (see Appendix B)
– Critically ill: 0.6–1.0 mcg/kg/min
– Critically ill with multisystem organ impairment: 0.2–0.5 mcg/kg/min
– See Tables 15-2 and 15-3

[a]aPTT target determined by agent, baseline value, and presence of thrombosis.

[b]Use dry weight for calculations in anasarca.

Table 5-7: Monitoring Considerations When Initiating and Adjusting a DTI Regimen

Initiating DTI

- Draw baseline aPTT and INR if not previously done; if a true baseline aPTT is not possible, use laboratory normals to help set targets

- Evaluate renal, liver, and cardiac function for potential reasons to reduce the dose

- Initiate DTI depending on target goals and indication for use

Monitoring DTI (see Figures 15-1 and 15-2)

- Draw aPTT at a predetermined time within 2–6 hr to reduce the risk of overtargeting or undertargeting the selected aPTT goal; note that the initial value reported may not be at steady-state in acutely ill patients

- Adjust dose upwards any aPTT value notably below a ratio of 1.5 x baseline

- Consider adjusting the dose downward if the upper end of the target range is noted shortly after initiating the infusion, or above prior to achieving steady state

- Follow thrombosis progression, platelet count (HIT), patient and HCT (or hemoglobin) for any evidence of bleeding

- If an INR was drawn before starting warfarin while on the DTI, consider an aPTT with it to determine amount of DTI effect on the INR

- A flattening of the aPTT dose response curve has been observed at higher degrees of anticoagulation intensity with minimal change in the aPTT as the DTI concentration increases (see Chapter 18)

- The activated clotting time (ACT) has been used in situations where a higher degree of anticoagulation may be required, such as invasive cardiac or selected surgical procedures (i.e., coronary intervention, coronary bypass, or ECMO)

- The DTI can independently elevate the INR value by interfering with the assay in the laboratory; absent of warfarin, this should not be interpreted as an elevated degree of anticoagulation; the degree of effect on the INR often correlates with the concentration of the DTI present, which is also represented by the intensity of rise in the aPTT; at higher doses, a more pronounced elevation in the INR for any DTI can occur; argatroban generally leads to the largest INR elevations followed by bivalirudin and then lepirudin, which has the least effect on INR

Clinical Pearl

- **Due to the flattening of the aPTT at high concentrations of DTI, following the INR in conjunction with the aPTT can be considered** when very high doses of DTI are being given. If the aPTT is not elevating as the dose is continued to be increased to reach a target aPTT level, but the INR is continuing to rise, you may have experienced the flattening of the aPTT dose response curve. In this situation, since the serum level of the DTI is likely still rising, the INR may now be a guide for assessing dosing titrations.

Transitioning from a DTI to warfarin[3,6,11–23]

Note: aPTT and INR responses to a DTI and warfarin separately vary between assays.

- Draw a baseline INR with a aPTT on DTI therapy alone.

- Initiate warfarin and identify a desired 1.5–2.0 point increase in the INR or pick a preselected INR, which considers the DTI-induced INR prolongation (with minimal change in the aPTT).

- Once the desired number of overlap days and desired platelet recovery has occurred and the INR target is reached, hold the DTI for 4–8 hours and recheck the INR and aPTT.

- After withholding the DTI and the subsequent INR is over 2 with an aPTT close to baseline (indicating the DTI has largely cleared), then the DTI can be discontinued. It may take longer for the effects of a DTI to diminish if a very low infusion rate with aPTT values in the target range, as this suggests slower drug elimination (Figure 15-1). If the INR is less than 2 or in lower portion of the INR range with a continued notable elevation in the aPTT, restarting the DTI infusion may be necessary.

- Another option may be the use of chromogenic factor Xa or factor II to assess if an adequate anticoagulation response with warfarin has occurred.[20–22]

  - Factor X <11% = INR >3.5

  - Factor X of 11% to 42% ~INR 2.0–3.5

  - Factor X >42% = INR <2

  - Factor II targets of 20% to 35% ~INR 2–3

Note: slight differences in the percent range can occur between assay methods.

Table 5-8: Influence of Direct Thrombin Inhibitors on Selected Assays[21]

Agent	Effect
Lepirudin	Increased protein C and protein S
	False positive lupus anticoagulant ratios
	Decrease fibrinogen, factor II, and factor IX
Argatroban	Increased protein C and protein S
	Increased Russell viper venom test (dRVVT)
	Decrease fibrinogen, factor II, and factor IX
Bivalirudin	Increased protein C and protein S
	False positive lupus anticoagulant ratios
	Decreased factor IX

No effect: D-dimer; Von Willebrand's factor; chromogenic plasminogen, protein C, antithrombin (slight elevation observed).

SPECIAL POPULATIONS

Coronary artery bypass grafting (CABG)

- HIT is rare with the exception of recent exposure to heparin.
- Heparin is the anticoagulant of choice in CABG with a pump unless patient has reasons not to use.
- Management options if patient requires CABG
  - Perform procedure without a pump.
  - Delay procedure until heparin antibody cannot be detected (several months).
  - Use alternative anticoagulant.
- Suggested alternative anticoagulant dosing during CABG under HIT conditions

Clinical Pearl

- Since bivalirudin can be cleaved and inactivated by thrombin in stagnant blood, blood clotting in small pockets outside the circulation within the surgical field, unlike with heparin, does not suggest insufficient anticoagulation.

Table 5-9: DTI Dosing Considerations for Open Heart
Surgical Procedures[11,24,25]

Agent	Pump Priming	Bolus	Infusion Rate During CABG	Suggested Target	Adjustment (if needed)
Lepirudin	Add 0.2 mg/kg to priming solution	0.25 mg/kg	0.5 mg/kg	3.0–4.5 mcg/mL	
Bivalirudin with pump[a]	50 mg to priming solution	0.25–1.50 mg/kg/hr	0.53–3.00 mg/kg/hr	Maintain ACT: 2.5 x baseline	
Bivalirudin without pump[a]	–	0.75 mg/kg/hr	1.75 mg/kg/hr	ACT >300 sec	Rate: +/− 0.25 mg/kg/hr or Intermittent bolus: 0.1–0.5 mg/kg; stop 20 min before end of grafting
Argatroban with pump[b]	0.05 mg/kg	0.1 mg/kg bolus	5–10 mcg/kg/min	ACT: 300–400 sec	
Argatroban without pump[b]	5 mg		2–5 mcg/kg/min	ACT: >200 sec	

[a]Hemofiltration can be used to decrease bivalirudin concentrations at end of procedure. In the CHOOSE-ON trial, 50 mg was added to the priming solution with a 1-mg/kg bolus followed by 2.5 mg/kg/hr until 15 minutes before planned going of cardiopulmonary bypass.[24] ACT values targeted 2.5 x baseline or more. Additional bolus doses of 0.1–0.5 mg/kg could be used for subtherapeutic ACT. With the initiation of recirculation, reconnect arterial and venous lines, clamp arterial filter, infuse residual blood, refill cardiopulmonary bypass with saline, recirculate and add a 50-mg bolus followed by continuous infusion of 50 mg/hr into the circuit until determined that CPB was not necessary to reestablish.

[b]Limited case reports with argatroban. Anticoagulation with argatroban has shown to be inconsistent in CABG cases.

- Cessation of anticoagulant: commonly done prior to restoration of flow to grafts.
- If using a cell-saver device during procedure for bivalirudin, add citrate to prevent clotting in the reservoir.
- Hypothermia may slow the removal of bivalirudin and lead to some accumulation.
- Hypothermia induced during surgery may also shut down the clotting cascade. Depending on the situation, anticoagulation may need to reduced or turned off.

Table 5-10: Dosing Considerations for DTIs in Pediatric Patients

Agent	Dose
Argatroban	In normal hepatic function, doses similar to observations in adults may apply; younger patients <6 mo may have lower clearance and require a lower dose; higher doses may be used in selected situations
Lepirudin	A weight-based protocol similar to adults has been successfully used
	0.1 mg/kg/hr (no bolus) if renal function is normal

Use in pediatric patients

- Consider alternative anticoagulant dosing in pediatric patients under HIT conditions.

  - Body weight may be correlated with clearance.

  - Dosing in infants or neonates is unclear.

  - Higher doses may be required during ECMO or invasive procedures including cardiac surgery. Since renal function can decline during ECMO, dosing for lepirudin may need to be lower.

Use in pregnant and lactating patients

Table 5-11: Direct Thrombin Inhibitors in Pregnancy and Lactation

Drug	Category	Pregnancy Info	Lactation Info
Lepirudin	B	Lepirudin crosses the placenta in pregnant rats; however, it is not known if lepirudin crosses the placenta in humans	Enters breast milk; consult prescriber
Bivalirudin	B	Although animal studies have not shown harm to the fetus, safety and efficacy for use in pregnant women have not been established; bivalirudin is used in conjunction with aspirin, which may lead to maternal or fetal adverse effects, especially during the third trimester; use during pregnancy only if clearly needed	Excretion in breast milk unknown; use caution

(continued)

Table 5-11: (Continued)

Drug	Category	Pregnancy Info	Lactation Info
Argatroban	B	Adverse events were not observed in animal studies; there are no adequate and well-controlled studies in pregnant women	Excretion in breast milk unknown/not recommended
		Argatroban should be used in pregnant women only if clearly needed	
Desirudin	C	Found to be teratogenic in rats and rabbits; it has not been evaluated in pregnant women; only use if the benefit clearly outweighs the risk of teratogenicity	Excretion in breast milk unknown/not recommended

Use in ECMO/ECLS patients

Table 5-12: Considerations with Transitioning for UFH to DTI in ECMO (ECLS)

DTI Dose	The dosing depends on the goals of therapy and characteristics of the patient; a bolus has been used in some settings
Switching Over	Stop heparin when DTI infusion is ready to be infused
	Draw aPTT every hour initially; target aPTT may be between 1.5–2.5 or 3 times control
	Watch direction of aPTT change and if it will maintain the target range
	If the change is fairly stable and in target range, consider extending the period between aPTT or ACT draws

The target aPTT or ACT may depend on the ECMO circuit and bedside assessment of the risk for bleeding and thrombosis of the circuit; low flow circuits may warrant a higher target

Newer circuits may be less thrombogenic; however, data on use of lower target ranges is not available

In selected situations, hemofiltration through the ECMO circuit can occur, expediting removal of bivalirudin

For pediatric patients, consider a smaller volume PEDI-TUBE™ to reduce blood loss

Flushing during embolectomy vascular surgery

- Lepirudin: 250 mL of a 0.1-mg/mL solution

SIDE EFFECTS, PRECAUTIONS, CONTRAINDICATIONS

Table 5-13: Side Effects, Precautions, and Contraindications

	Argatroban	Bivalirudin	Lepirudin	Desirudin
Side Effects	>10% *Cardiovascular*—chest pain, hypotension	>10% *Cardiovascular*—hypotension	>10% *Hematologic*—anemia, bleeding from puncture sites, hematoma	>10% *Hematologic*—bleeding, hematoma
	Gastrointestinal— gastrointestinal bleed	*Central nervous system*—pain, headache		2% to 10% Injection site mass
	Genitourinary—genitourinary bleed and hematuria	*Gastrointestinal*—nausea	1% to 10% *Cardiovascular*—CHF, pericardial effusion, ventricular fibrillation	Wound secretion
	1% to 10% *Cardiovascular*—vasodilation, cardiac arrest, ventricular tachycardia, bradycardia, myocardial infarction, atrial fibrillation, angina, CABG-related bleeding, myocardial ischemia, cerebrovascular disorder, thrombosis	*Neuromuscular and skeletal*—back pain	*Central nervous system*—fever	Anemia
		1% to 10% *Cardiovascular*—hypertension, bradycardia, angina	*Dermatologic*—eczema, maculopapular rash	Deep thrombophlebitis
		Central nervous system—insomnia, anxiety, fever, nervousness	*GI*—GI bleeding/rectal bleeding	Nausea
	Central nervous system—fever, headache, pain, intracranial bleeding	*Gastrointestinal*—vomiting, dyspepsia, abdominal pain	*Genitourinary*—vaginal bleeding	0.02% to >2% *Cardiovascular*—hypotension
	Dermatologic—skin reactions	*Genitourinary*—urinary retention	*Hepatic*—transaminases increased	*Central nervous system*—fever, dizziness, cerebrovascular disorder
	Gastrointestinal—nausea, diarrhea, vomiting, abdominal pain		*Renal*—hematuria	*GI*—vomiting, hematemesis

(continued)

Table 5-13: (Continued)

	Argatroban	Bivalirudin	Lepirudin	Desirudin
	Genitourinary—urinary tract infection	*Hematologic*—major hemorrhage; transfusion required, thrombocytopenia	*Respiratory*—epistaxis	*Renal*—hematuria
	Hematologic—hemoglobin decreased, hematocrit decreased	*Local*—injection site pain		*Respiratory*—epistaxis
	Local—bleeding at injection or access site	*Neuromuscular and skeletal*—pelvic pain		*Other*—decreased Hgb, impaired healing, leg pain
	Neuromuscular and skeletal—back pain			*Rare*—anaphylactoid/ anaphylaxis
	Renal—abnormal renal function			
	Respiratory—dyspnea, cough, hemoptysis, pneumonia			
	Miscellaneous—sepsis, infection			
Precautions	Patients with increased risk of hemorrhage: • severe hypertension • lumbar puncture • spinal anesthesia • major surgery • bleeding disorders • GI ulcers hepatic impairment	Thrombus formation Preexisting disease states associated with increased risk of bleeding Elderly patients; increased risk of bleeding events	Severe HTN History recent major surgery History recent major bleeding History of recent CVA	Antibodies from previous exposure severe HTN Hepatic insufficiency/ liver injury Concurrent use with other anticoagulants

(continued)

Table 5-13: (Continued)

	Argatroban	Bivalirudin	Lepirudin	Desirudin
		Avoid IM use due to increased risk of bleeding	Liver dysfunction GI ulceration Bacterial endocarditis Anomaly of vessels or organs Antibody formation—pts with repeat doses may require more monitoring	Antibody formation—pts with repeat doses may require more monitoring
Contraindications	Overt major bleeding Hypersensitivity to argatroban	Active major bleeding Hypersensitivity to bivalirudin or its components	Hypersensitivity to hirudin products Active major bleeding	Hypersensitivity to hirudin products Active major bleeding

Lepirudin-related hypersensitivity reactions[26,27]

- Omission of the bolus dose for lepirudin in the setting of HIT may reduce the risk for a hypersensitivity reaction.
- Rate of anaphylaxis:
  - First exposure: ~0.015%
  - Reexposure to a bolus: ~0.15%
  - Antihirudin antibodies: 40% (3% have dose effects requiring a lower dose)

REFERENCES

*Key articles

1. Kaplan KL. Direct thrombin inhibitors. *Expert Opin Pharmacother.* 2003;4:653–666.

2. Mann MJ, Tseng E, Ratcliffe M, et al. Use of bivalirudin, a direct thrombin inhibitor, and its reversal with modified ultrafiltration during heart transplantation in a patient with heparin-induced thrombocytopenia. *J Heart Lung Transplant.* 2005;24:222–225.

3. **Dager WE, Dougherty JA, Nguyen PH, et al. Heparin-induced thrombocytopenia: a review of treatment options and special considerations. *Pharmacotherapy.* 2007;27:564–587.**

4. Gosselin RC, Dager WE, King JH, et al. Effect of direct thrombin-inhibitors: bivalirudin, lepirudin and argatroban, on prothrombin time and INR measurements. *Am J Clin Path.* 2004;121:593–599.

5. **Warkentin TE, Greinacher A, Koster A, et al. Treatment and prevention of heparin-induced thrombocytopenia. American College of Chest Physicians Evidence-Based Clinical Practice Guidelines (8th ed.). *Chest.* 2008;133:340S–380S.**

6. Hursting MJ, Verme-Gibboney CN. Risk factors for major bleeding in patients with heparin-induced thrombocytopenia treated with argatroban: a retrospective study. *J Cardiovasc Pharmacol.* 2008;52:561–566.

7. Keegan SP, Rolik EM, Ernst NE, et al. Effects of critical illness and organ failure on therapeutic argatroban dosage requirements in patients with suspected or confirmed heparin-induced thrombocytopenia. *Ann Pharmacother.* 2009;43:19–27.

8. Ansara AJ, Arif S, Warhurst RD. A weight-based argatroban dosing nomogram for the treatment of heparin induced thrombocytopenia. *Ann Pharmacother.* 2009;43:9–18.

9. Lubenow N, Eichler P, Leitz T, et al. Lepirudin for prophylaxis of thrombosis in patients with acute isolated heparin-induced thrombocytopenia: an analysis of 3 prospective studies. *Blood.* 2004;104:3072–3077.

10. Huhle G, Hoffmann U, Hoffmann I, et al. A new therapeutic option by subcutaneous recombinant hirudin in patients with heparin-induced thrombocytopenia type II: a pilot study. *Thromb Res.* 2000;99:325–334.

* **11. Hassell K. The management of patients with heparin-induced thrombocytopenia who require anticoagulant therapy. *Chest.* 2005;127:1S–8S.**

12. Hursting MJ, Murray PT. Argatroban anticoagulation in renal dysfunction: a literature analysis. *Nephron Clin Pract.* 2008;109:c80–c94.

13. Fischer KG. Hirudin in renal insufficiency. *Semin Thromb Hemost.* 2002;28:467–482.

14. Kiser TH, Burch JC, Klem PM, et al. Safety, efficacy, and dosing requirement of bivalirudin in patients with heparin-induced thrombocytopenia. *Pharmacotherapy.* 2008;28:1115–1124.

15. Kiser TH, Fish D. Evaluation of bivalirudin treatment for heparin-induced thrombocytopenia in critically ill patients with hepatic and/or renal dysfunction. *Pharmacotherapy.* 2006;26:452–460.

16. Vanholder R, Camez A, Veys N, et al. Pharmacokinetics of recombinant hirudin in hemodialyzed end-stage renal failure patients. *Thromb Haemost.* 1997;77: 650–655.

17. Lincoff AM, Bittl JA, Harrington RA, et al. REPLACE-2 Investigators. Bivalirudin and provisional glycoprotein IIb/IIIa blockade compared with heparin and planned glycoprotein IIb/IIIa blockade during percutaneous coronary intervention: REPLACE-2 randomized trial. *JAMA.* 2003;289:853–863.

18. Dager WE. Considerations for drug dosing post coronary artery bypass graft surgery. *Ann Pharmacother.* 2008;42:421–424.

19. Arpino PA, Hallisey RK. Effect of renal function on the pharmacodynamics of argatroban. *Ann Pharmacother.* 2004;38:25–29.

20. Brown PM, Hursting MJ. Lack of pharmacokinetic interactions between argatroban and warfarin. *Am J Health Syst Pharm.* 2002;59:2078–2083.

21. Gosselin RC, King JH, Janatpour KA, et al. Comparing direct thrombin inhibitors using aPTT, ecarin clotting times, and thrombin inhibitor management testing. *Ann Pharmacother.* 2004;38:1383–1388.

22. Arpino PA, Demirjian Z, Van Cott EM. Use of the chromogenic factor X assay to predict the international normalized ratio in patients transitioning from argatroban to warfarin. *Pharmacotherapy.* 2005;25:157–164.

23. Trask A, Gosselin RC, Diaz J, et al. Warfarin initiation and monitoring with clotting factors II, VII and X levels. *Ann Pharmacother.* 2004;38:251–256.

24. Koster A, Dyke CM, Aldea G, et al. Bivalirudin during cardiopulmonary bypass in patients with previous or acute heparin-induced thrombocytopenia and heparin antibodies: results of the CHOOSE-ON trial. *Ann Thorac Surg.* 2007;83:572–577.

25. Greinacher A. The use of direct thrombin inhibitors in cardiovascular surgery in patients with heparin-induced thrombocytopenia. *Semin Thromb Hemost.* 2004;30: 315–327.

26. Eicher P, Friesen HJ, Lubenow N, et al. Antihirudin antibodies in patients with heparin-induced thrombocytopenia treated with lepirudin: incidence, effects on aPTT, and clinical relevance. *Blood.* 2000;96:2373–2378.

27. Greinacher A, Lubenow N, Eicher P. Anaphylactic and anaphylactoid reactions associated with lepirudin in patients with heparin-induced thrombocytopenia. *Circulation.* 2003;108:2062–2065.

Thrombolytic Considerations When Used with Anticoagulants

Toby C. Trujillo

INTRODUCTION

Today thrombolytic agents such as rt-PA, reteplase, and TNK are crucial agents in the treatment of AMI, stroke, and VTE as well as peripheral arterial thrombosis. Their ability to dissolve a clot, as opposed to preventing clot expansion, is a key distinguishing characteristic from other anticoagulant agents, which makes them valuable options when immediate nonsurgical reperfusion of an occluded artery is warranted. Despite their clinical utility thrombolytic agents carry a high risk of bleeding, especially intracranial hemorrhage, and patient selection must be carefully considered in order to optimize the risk-benefit ratio with these agents.

PHARMACOLOGY AND PHARMACOKINETICS[1-9]

Five thrombolytic agents are commercially available in the US: urokinase, streptokinase, rt-PA (alteplase), reteplase (Retivase), and TNK (TNKase).

Mechanism of action

- All of the available agents exert their effect on the endogenous fibrinolytic system by converting plasminogen to plasmin through hydrolysis of the arginine-valine bond in plasminogen. Plasmin cleaves fibrin and fibrinogen leading to clot dissolution, as well as degrading the procoagulant factors V and VIII.

- Urokinase and streptokinase produce plasminogen activation on a systemic level, leading to global activation of plasminogen to plasmin. With doses used clinically systemic plasmin may be depleted, and fibrin/fibrinogen degradation products may produce a systemic anticoagulant effect.

- Recombinant t-PA, reteplase, and TNK are all fibrin specific thrombolytic agents. As such minimal amounts of plasminogen are converted to plasmin in the absence of fibrin leading to a more localized thrombolytic effect.

- Of note, in patients with plasminogen levels significantly below normal at therapy initiation, it should be anticipated that the therapeutic response from an exogenously administered thrombolytic agent may be blunted or less than expected.

Pharmacologic and clinical properties of thrombolytics

Table 6-1: Characteristics of Available Thrombolytic Agents

Property	Urokinase	Streptokinase	Alteplase (rt-PA)	Reteplase	Tenecteplase (TNK)
Molecular weight, kD	35	47	70	39	70
Half-life, min	13–20	23	4–8	14–18	23–37
Fibrin specificity	Minimal	Minimal	Moderate	Moderate	High
Potential antigenicity	No	Yes	No	No	No
Plasminogen binding	Direct	Indirect	Direct	Direct	Direct
FDA-approved indications	PE	MI, PE, DVT	MI, PE, stroke, catheter occlusion	MI	MI
Patency with TIMI grade 3 flow[a]—90 min	N/A	40% to 50%	46% to 75%	60% to 63%	63%

[a]TIMI grade 3 flow: complete perfusion defined by normal flow, which fills the distal coronary bed completely. TIMI grade 0 flow is no perfusion, with grades 1 and 2 representing partial perfusion of the myocardium.

INDICATIONS, DOSING, AND ADMINISTRATION[10-32]

Depending on the half-life of the compound being used, administration is either by single or multiple IV boluses, or through a continuous IV infusion given for a specified time frame.

Clinical Pearls in Dosing Thrombolytics

- The use of adjunctive antithrombotic therapy (antiplatelet and antithrombin agents) is often needed to maintain patency of the affected artery or vein. However, specific recommendations exist for how and when adjunctive therapies should be initiated in different indications. It is crucial to ensure adjunctive therapies are timed appropriately in relation to thrombolytic administration in order to optimize safety and efficacy.

- Many thrombolytic agents are dosed on body weight (actual body weight), and obtaining an accurate weight prior to the initiation of therapy is crucial to optimize therapy.

MONITORING[10-22]

Monitoring parameters in STEMI

- General
    - Baseline aPTT, PT/INR, hematocrit, platelet count, fibrinogen (streptokinase therapy)
    - Coagulation parameters during therapy: aPTT, PT/INR, fibrinogen level (streptokinase)
    - Vital signs (BP, HR) at baseline and during therapy
    - Bleeding, especially during planned invasive procedures, while lytic state is in effect

Table 6-2: Recommended Doses for Thrombolytic Agents by Patient Population

Patient Group	Urokinase	Streptokinase	Alteplase (rt-PA)	Reteplase	Tenecteplase (TNK)
STEMI	N/A	IV: 1.5 million International Units given IV over 60 min Intracoronary: 20,000 International Units bolus, then 2,000–4,000 International Units/min for 30–90 min	Accelerated infusion regimen: Patients <67 kg: give 15 mg IV over 1–2 min, then 0.75 mg/kg IV over 30 min, then 0.5 mg/kg IV over 1 hr Patients >67 kg: 100 mg IV over 1.5 hr; give 15 mg over 1–2 min, 50 mg over 30 min, then 35 mg over 1 hr 3-hr infusion regimen: Patients <65 kg: 1.25 mg/kg over 3 hr; give 60% of total dose in first hr with 6% to 10% as an IV bolus, then 20%/hr for the next 2 hr Patients >65 kg: 100 mg IV over 3 hr; give 60 mg 1 hr with 6–10 mg as an IV bolus, then 20 mg/hr for the next 2 hr 100 mg IV over 2 hr	10 units IV over 2 min; give second 10-unit dose IV 30 min later unless serious bleeding or anaphylaxis is present	Dose based on weight and given as IV bolus over 5 sec; total dose should not exceed 50 mg <60 kg: 30 mg 60–69 kg: 35 mg 70–79 kg: 40 mg 80–89 kg: 45 mg ≥90 kg: 50 mg

Table 6-2: (Continued)

Patient Group	Urokinase	Streptokinase	Alteplase (rt-PA)	Reteplase	Tenecteplase (TNK)
PE	Load: 4,400 International Units/kg IV over 10 min Maintenance: 4,400 International Units/kg/hr IV for 12 hr	Load: 250,000 International Units/kg IV over 30 min Maintenance: 100,000 International Units/kg/hr IV for 24 hr	Catheter-directed therapy after failed systemic lysis: one single report found success with a range of 10–30 mg total dose administered, in 5–10 mg increments	10 units IV over 2 min; give second 10-unit dose IV 30 min later unless serious bleeding or anaphylaxis present	Catheter-directed therapy after failed systemic lysis: one single report found success with a range of 5–20 mg total dose administered, in 2.5 mg increments
DVT	Load: 4,400 International Units/kg IV over 10 min Maintenance: 4,400 International Units/kg/hr IV for 12 hr	Load: 250,000 International Units/kg IV over 30 min Maintenance: 100,000 International Units/kg/hr IV for 72 hr	Catheter-directed therapy: no single dosing regimen has proven superior to others; dosing options from small reports include • 0.01 mg/kg/hr (max 20 mg in 24 hr) for up to 96 hr • 5-mg bolus, followed by 0.01-mg/kg/hr infusion • 10-mg bolus, followed by 1–2 mg/hr infusion	N/A	N/A

(continued)

Table 6-2: (Continued)

Patient Group	Urokinase	Streptokinase	Alteplase (rt-PA)	Reteplase	Tenecteplase (TNK)
Ischemic stroke	N/A	N/A	Within 3–4.5 hr of symptom onset, recommended *maximum* dose 0.9 mg/kg or 90 mg Patients >100 kg: give 9 mg IV bolus over 1 min, then 81 mg as IV infusion over 1 hr Patients <100 kg: give 0.9 mg/kg IV bolus over 1 min, then 0.81 mg/kg as IV infusion over 1 hr	N/A	N/A
Catheter occlusion	5,000 International Units/2 mL in each IV catheter lumen over 1–2 min; dwell time 1–4 hr then remove; flush catheter with 0.9% NaCl prior to reconnecting tubing; may repeat with 10,000 units if catheter does not clear	N/A	2 mg instilled into the catheter and retained for 30 min to 2 hr; may repeat in 2 hr if catheter still occluded	N/A	N/A

(continued)

Table 6-2: (Continued)

Patient Group	Urokinase	Streptokinase	Alteplase (rt-PA)	Reteplase	Tenecteplase (TNK)
Peripheral arterial occlusion (intra-arterial administration)[a]	240,000 International Units/hr for 2 hr, then 120,000 International Units/hr for 2 hr, then 60,000 International Units/hr for 20 hr or 120,000 International Units IV for 2 hr, then 60,000 International Units/hr until clot is dissolved or 120,000 International Units IV for up to 48 hr	N/A	0.02–0.1 mg/kg/hr for up to 36 hr or Nonweight-based infusion ranging from 1–10 mg/hr, with 2.5 and 5 mg/hr most common doses used; duration variable from 2–24 hr or until clot resolution	One small case series of 15 patients used a dosing regimen of 0.5–1.0 units/hr for 12–32 hr[29] A larger case series of 26 patients used a dose of 0.5–2.0 units/hr (mean 0.9 units/hr) up to a total dose of 20 units (means 20.1 units ± 5.5)[30] A third case series in 81 patients used a 0.5 units/hr infusion for an average of 19.5 hr and a total dose of 10.3 units[31]	N/A

(continued)

Table 6-2: (Continued)

Patient Group	Urokinase	Streptokinase	Alteplase (rt-PA)	Reteplase	Tenecteplase (TNK)
Pleural effusion/empyema		250,000 International Units/100 mL NS instilled intrapleurally for 2–4 hr	N/A	N/A	N/A
Prosthetic valve thrombosis	4,400 International Units/kg IV bolus over 30 min, then 4,400 units/hr or 1.5 million International Units given IV over 3 hr	150,000 International Units to 250,000 International Units loading dose IV over 30 min, then 100,000 units/hr IV or 1.5 million International Units given IV over 3 hr	10 mg IV bolus, then 90 mg IV over 3–5 hr	N/A	N/A

[a]Few randomized trials exist investigating the use of intra-arterial thrombolysis in the setting of peripheral arterial disease. As such, dosing strategies in this population are highly variable as evidenced by the various dosing strategies provided for each agent. Clinicians may encounter dosing regimens that are not accounted for here.

Monitoring parameters in STEMI—Continued

- Therapeutic
    - Resolution of ECG changes
    - Resolution of chest pain
    - Appearance of reperfusion arrhythmias
    - Early cardiac enzyme peak (primarily creatine phosphokinase or CPK)
    - Infarct artery patency—TIMI flow
- Toxic
    - Clinical evidence of bleeding (vascular access site, hematuria, GI bleeding, positive stool guaiac)
    - Intracranial bleeding—impaired cognitive, motor, or sensory function on neurologic exam

Monitoring parameters in PE/DVT

- General
    - Baseline aPTT, PT/INR, hematocrit, platelet count, fibrinogen (streptokinase therapy)
    - Coagulation parameters during therapy: aPTT, PT/INR, fibrinogen level (streptokinase)
    - Vital signs (BP, HR) at baseline and during therapy
    - Oxygen saturation and hemodynamic parameters
- Therapeutic
    - Resolution of symptoms—SOB, chest pain, leg pain, improved hemodynamics
    - Resolution of ECG changes
    - Improved right ventricular function on echocardiogram
- Toxic
    - Clinical evidence of bleeding (vascular access site, hematuria, GI bleeding, positive stool guaiac)
    - Intracranial bleeding—impaired cognitive, motor, or sensory function on neurologic exam

Monitoring parameters in stroke

- General
    - Baseline aPTT, PT/INR, hematocrit, platelet count
    - Coagulation parameters during therapy: aPTT, PT/INR
    - Vital signs (BP, HR) at baseline and during therapy
- Therapeutic
    - Resolution of symptoms—neurologic deficits at presentation
- Toxic
    - Clinical evidence of bleeding (vascular access site, hematuria, GI bleeding, positive stool guaiac)
    - Intracranial bleeding—impaired cognitive, motor or sensory function on neurologic exam

Monitoring parameters in catheter occlusion

- Therapeutic
    - Aspiration of blood or catheter contents
- Toxic
    - Clinical evidence of bleeding (vascular access site, hematuria, GI bleeding, positive stool guaiac)

Monitoring parameters in peripheral arterial occlusion

- General
    - Baseline aPTT, PT/INR, hematocrit, platelet count, fibrinogen (streptokinase therapy)
    - Coagulation parameters during therapy: aPTT, PT/INR, fibrinogen level (streptokinase)
    - Vital signs (BP, HR) at baseline and during therapy
- Therapeutic
    - Resolution of symptoms—leg pain, lower extremity ischemia, restored perfusion
    - Angiographic evidence of improvement

- Toxic
  - Clinical evidence of bleeding (vascular access site, hematuria, GI bleeding, positive stool guaiac)
  - Intracranial bleeding—impaired cognitive, motor or sensory function on neurologic exam

SIDE EFFECTS, PRECAUTIONS, CONTRAINDICATIONS[10-17]

Table 6-3: Contraindications to Thrombolytic Therapy

Absolute Contraindications

- Any prior ICH
- Known structural cerebral vascular lesion (e.g., arteriovenous malformation)
- Known malignant intracranial neoplasm (primary or metastatic)
- Ischemic stroke within 3 months *except* acute ischemic stroke within 4.5 hours
- Suspected aortic dissection
- Active bleeding or bleeding diathesis (excluding menses)
- Significant closed-head or facial trauma within 3 months
- Severe uncontrolled hypertension

Relative Contraindications

- History of chronic, severe, poorly controlled hypertension
- Severe uncontrolled hypertension on presentation (SBP greater than 180 mm Hg or DBP greater than 110 mm Hg)
- History of prior ischemic stroke greater than 3 months, dementia, or known intracranial pathology not covered in contraindications
- Traumatic or prolonged (greater than 10 minutes) CPR or major surgery (within less than 3 weeks)
- Recent (within 2–4 weeks) internal bleeding
- Noncompressible vascular punctures
- For streptokinase: prior exposure (more than 5 days ago) or prior allergic reaction to these agents
- Pregnancy
- Active peptic ulcer
- Current use of anticoagulants: the higher the INR, the higher the risk of bleeding

RISK OF BLEEDING[9-17,33,34]

Patient characteristics that increase the risk of bleeding with thrombolytic agents

- In patients experiencing stroke and myocardial infarction, the most important bleeding complication is intracranial hemorrhage (ICH) (see Table 6-4).

- Due to the low number of patients that have been enrolled in randomized clinical trials for PE (<800 total patients), the actual incidence of intracranial hemorrhage as well as risk factors for bleeding are less well-defined as for other indications.

- Risk factors for bleeding are heavily dependent on the indication for thrombolysis, with patients being treated for stroke having a much higher rate of ICH than patients experiencing STEMI.

- Characteristics predicting increased bleeding in patients with stroke
  - Larger neurologic deficit has been associated with a higher rate of ICH
  - Older age has—in some, but not all analyses—been associated with a higher rate of ICH
  - Diabetes
  - Higher doses of thrombolytic agents

- Characteristics predicting increased bleeding in patients with STEMI
  - Older age
  - Lower body weight
  - Prior stroke
  - Increased systolic or diastolic pressure
  - Female gender

Risk of intracranial hemorrhage between agents

Table 6-4: Rates of Intracranial Hemorrhage Observed in Various Patient Populations

Urokinase	Streptokinase	Alteplase (rt-PA)	Reteplase	Tenecteplase (TNK)
STEMI: N/A— contemporary information not available	STEMI: 0.6% in GUSTO I trial	STEMI: 0.7% for rt-PA vs. 0.6% for streptokinase in GUSTO I trial	STEMI: 0.8% for reteplase vs. 0.4% for streptokinase in INJECT trial	STEMI: 0.9% for TNK vs. 0.9% for rt-PA in ASSENT II study
PE: N/A— contemporary information not available	PE: N/A— contemporary information not available	PE: 3% for rt-PA vs. 0.3% for IV UFH	0.6% for reteplase vs. 0.4% for rt-PA in GUSTO III trial	PE: N/A
DVT: N/A	DVT: N/A	DVT: N/A	PE: N/A	DVT: N/A
Stroke: N/A	Stroke: N/A	Stroke: 6.4% for rt-PA vs. 0.6% for placebo symptomatic ICH within 36 hr in NINDS t-PA study	DVT: N/A	Stroke: N/A
			Stroke: N/A	

DOSING AND MONITORING STRATEGIES FOR ANTICOAGULANT/ ANTIPLATELET AGENTS TO MINIMIZE RISK OF BLEEDING AND OPTIMIZE OUTCOME[9-17,25-28]

Table 6-5: Dosing of Antithrombotic Agents with Thrombolytic Therapy

Patient Group	ASA or ASA + Clopidogrel	UFH	LMWH	Fondaparinux	Bivalirudin
STEMI	ASA: 162–325 mg initial dose using chewable formulation; maintenance dose 81–325 mg daily Clopidogrel: loading dose of 300–600 mg may be considered in patients <75 yr of age; loading dose should be omitted in patients ≥75 yr; maintenance dose of 75 mg daily Recommended for all patients for up to 14 days if no subsequent PCI is performed	Bolus: 60 units/kg, maximum dose 4,000 units Continuous IV infusion: 12 units/kg/hr, maximum initial rate of 1,000 units/hr UFH should be given in conjunction with thrombolytic agents for a minimum of 48 hr; patients receiving fibrin specific agents such as rt-PA, reteplase, and TNK should receive UFH; patients receiving streptokinase should receive UFH only if at high risk of systemic emboli (afib, LV, thrombus)	Enoxaparin is the preferred agent and should be given in conjunction with fibrinolytic agent for a minimum of 48 hr and ideally up to 8 days Patients <75 yr: 30-mg IV bolus followed by 1 mg/kg SC q 12 hr *(maximum of 100 mg for first two doses)* Patients >75 yr: no IV bolus, therapy should be 0.75 mg/kg SC q 12 hr *(maximum of 75 mg for first two doses)* Any patient with CrCl <30 mL/min, regardless of age: maintenance dose should be 1 mg/kg SC q 24 hr	2.5 mg SC once daily started in conjunction with thrombolytic agent; therapy should be continued for minimum of 48 hr and ideally up to 8 days; contraindicated in patients with a CrCl <30 mL/min	N/A

(continued)

Table 6-5: (Continued)

Patient Group	ASA or ASA + Clopidogrel	UFH	LMWH	Fondaparinux	Bivalirudin
PE	N/A	<u>Bolus:</u> 80 units/kg, no recommended maximum dose <u>Continuous IV infusion:</u> 18 units/kg/hr, no recommended maximum dose Therapy may be started with or continued when thrombolytic therapy is initiated; alternatively it is reasonable to initiate therapy after thrombolysis has been administered; in patients who had UFH interrupted for thrombolytic administration, consider the following approach to restarting UFH: • Check the aPTT at the end of lytic infusion • If aPTT is <2 times control, restart UFH at previous infusion rate with no bolus • If aPTT >2 times control, recheck in 4 hr and if acceptable, restart UFH <u>Catheter-directed or local thrombolysis:</u> see DVT	Standard treatment doses of LMWH agents apply Enoxaparin 1 mg/kg SC q 12 hr or daily for patients with a CrCl <30 mL/min *(maximum of 75 mg for first two doses)* Dalteparin 200 International Units/kg SC once daily or 100 International Units/kg SC q 12 hr; caution in patients with CrCl <20 mL/min Tinzaparin 175 units/kg SC once daily; caution in patients with CrCl <20 mL/min Therapy may be started with or continued when thrombolytic therapy is initiated; alternatively it is reasonable to initiate therapy after thrombolysis has been administered	Minimal data are available regarding using fondaparinux with systemic thrombolysis in PE; however, if used, standard treatment doses for VTE could be considered: ≤50 kg: 5.0 mg SC once daily 51–100 kg: 7.5 mg SC once daily ≥100 kg: 10 mg SC once daily	No data available regarding concomitant administration; however, in a patient with active HIT and PE, consider a dose of 0.15–0.25 mg/kg/hr, titrated to an aPTT of 1.5–2.5 times control and continued until warfarin therapy is therapeutic; these recommended doses come from ACS and HIT data

(continued)

Table 6-5: (Continued)

Patient Group	ASA or ASA + Clopidogrel	UFH	LMWH	Fondaparinux	Bivalirudin
DVT	N/A	Systemic thrombolysis: follow recommendations for PE Catheter-directed or local thrombolysis: UFH dosing in this setting is not standardized; often lower intensities of anticoagulation were reported in studies as compared to standard DVT/PE dosing (often less than 1,000 units/hr); in addition, goal aPTT used in the literature include 1.2–1.7 times baseline, 1.5–2.5 times baseline, up to 80–100 sec	Systemic thrombolysis: follow recommendations for PE Catheter-directed or local thrombolysis: minimal information available, recommend utilizing dosing strategies found under PE	Systemic thrombolysis: follow recommendations for PE Catheter-directed or local thrombolysis: minimal information available, recommend utilizing dosing strategies found under PE	No data available regarding concomitant administration; however, in a patient with active HIT and PE, would recommend a dose of 0.15–0.25 mg/kg/hr, titrated to an aPTT of 1.5–2.5 times control and continued until warfarin therapy is therapeutic; these recommended doses come from ACS and HIT data

(continued)

Table 6-5: (Continued)

Patient Group	ASA or ASA + Clopidogrel	UFH	LMWH	Fondaparinux	Bivalirudin
Ischemic stroke	ASA: therapy initiation should be withheld for a minimum of 24 hr after the administration of thrombolysis; thereafter, ASA 325 mg as an initial dose is recommended Clopidogrel: a dose of 75 mg daily is only recommended if ASA cannot be used with the same timing constraints as discussed above	Therapeutic anticoagulation with UFH is not recommended in the previous 48 hr, or 24 hr after thrombolysis for ischemic stroke; UFH for VTE prophylaxis may be initiated 24 hr after thrombolysis	Therapeutic anticoagulation with LMWH is not recommended in the previous 48 hr, or 24 hr after thrombolysis for ischemic stroke; LMWH for VTE prophylaxis may be initiated 24 hr after thrombolysis	N/A	N/A
Catheter occlusion	N/A	N/A	N/A	N/A	N/A

(continued)

Table 6-5: (Continued)

Patient Group	ASA or ASA + Clopidogrel	UFH	LMWH	Fondaparinux	Bivalirudin
Peripheral arterial occlusion (intra-arterial) administration)	N/A	UFH generally administered concomitantly with intra-arterial thrombolytic; dosing in trials generally consisted to a 3,000–5,000 unit bolus, followed by a 600–1,000 units/hr continuous infusion titrated to a defined goal aPTT	N/A	N/A	N/A
Pleural effusion/empyema	N/A	N/A	N/A	N/A	N/A
Prosthetic valve thrombosis	N/A	N/A	N/A	N/A	N/A

REFERENCES

*Key articles

1. Verstraete M. Third-generation thrombolytic drugs. *Am J Med.* 2000;109:52–58.

2. Tsikouris JP, Tsilouris AP. A review of available fibrin-specific thrombolytic agents used in acute myocardial infarction. *Pharmacotherapy.* 2001;21(2):207–217.

3. Stringer KA. Biochemical and pharmacologic comparison of thrombolytic agents. *Pharmacotherapy.* 1996;16(5, part 2):119–126.

4. Simpson D, Siddiqui AA, Scott LJ, et al. Reteplase. A review of its use in the management of thrombotic occlusive disorders. *Am J Cardiovasc Drugs.* 2006;6(4):265–285.

5. Modi N, Eppler S, Breed J, et al. Pharmacokinetics of a slower clearing tissue plasminogen activator variant, TNK-tPA, in patients with acute myocardial infarction. *Thromb Haemost.* 1998;79:134–139.

6. Morse MA, Todd JW, Stouffer GA. Optimizing the use of thrombolytics in ST-segment elevation myocardial infarction. *Drugs.* 2009;69(14):1945–1966.

7. Tanswell P, Modi N, Combs D, et al. Pharmacokinetics and pharmacodynamics of tenecteplase in fibrinolytic therapy of acute myocardial infarction. *Clin Pharmacokinet.* 2002;41(15):1229–1245.

8. Todd JL, Tapson VF. Thrombolytic Therapy for Acute Pulmonary Embolism. *Chest.* 2009;135:1321–1329.

9. Wittkowsky AK, Nutescu EA. Thrombosis. In: Koda-Kimble MA, Young LY, Alldredge BK, et al., eds. *Applied Therapeutics: The Clinical Use of Drugs.* 9th ed. Baltimore, MD: Lippincott Williams & Wilkins; 2008:15.1–15.36.

10. Antman EM, Anbe DT, Armstrong PW, et al. ACC/AHA guidelines for the management of patients with ST-elevation myocardial infarction: a report of the American College of Cardiology/American Heart Association Task Force on Practice Guidelines (Committee to Revise the 1999 Guidelines for the Management of Patients With Acute Myocardial Infarction). 2004. Available at www.acc.org/ clinical/guidelines/stemi/index.pdf.

11. Antman EM, Hand M, Armstrong PW, et al. 2007 focused update of the ACC/AHA 2004 Guidelines for the Management of Patients with ST-Elevation Myocardial Infarction: a report of the American College of Cardiology/American Heart Association Task Force on Practice Guidelines. *J Am Coll Cardiol.* 2008;51:(2):210–247.

12. Kushner FG, Hand M, Smith SC Jr, et al. 2009 focused updates: ACC/AHA guidelines for the management of patients with ST-elevation myocardial infarction (updating the 2004 guideline and 2007 focused update) and ACC/AHA/SCAI guidelines on percutaneous coronary intervention (updating the 2005 guideline and 2007 focused update): a report of the American College of Cardiology Foundation/American Heart Association Task Force on Practice Guidelines. *Circulation.* 2009;120: 2271–2306.

* 13. **Kearon C, Kahn SR, Agnelli G, et al. Antithrombotic therapy for venous thromboembolic disease: American College of Chest Physicians Evidence-Based Clinical Practice Guidelines (8th ed.).** *Chest.* **2008;133:454S–545S.**

14. Haines ST, Witt D, Nutescu EA. Venous thromboembolism. In: DiPiro J, et al., eds. *Pharmacotherapy.* 7th ed. New York, NY: McGraw-Hill; 2008:331–372.

* 15. **Adams HP Jr, del Zoppo G, Alberts MJ, et al. Guidelines for the early management of adults with ischemic stroke: a guideline from the American Heart Association/ American Stroke Association Stroke Council, Clinical Cardiology Council, Cardiovascular Radiology and Intervention Council, and the Atherosclerotic Peripheral Vascular Disease and Quality of Care Outcomes in Research Interdisciplinary Working Groups.** *Stroke.* **2007;38:1655–1711.**

* 16. **del Zoppo GJ, Saver JL, Jauch EC, et al. Expansion of the time window for treatment of acute ischemic stroke with intravenous tissue plasminogen activator.** *Stroke.* **2009;40:2945–2948.**

17. Albers G, Amarenco P, Easton D, et al. Antithrombotic and thrombolytic therapy for ischemic stroke: American College of Chest Physicians Evidence-Based Clinical Practice Guidelines (8th ed.). *Chest.* 2008;133:630S–669S.

18. Semba CP, Bakal CW, Calis KA, et al. Alteplase as an alternative to urokinase. Advisory panel on catheter-directed thrombolytic therapy. *J Vasc Interv Radiol.* 2000;11(3):279–287.

19. Ouriel K, Veith FJ, Sasahara AA. A comparison of recombinant urokinase with vascular surgery as initial treatment for acute arterial occlusion of the legs. *N Engl J Med.* 1998;338(16):1105–1111.

20. Ponec D, Irwin D, Haire WD, et al. Recombinant tissue plasminogen activator (alteplase) for restoration of flow in occluded central venous access devices: a double blind placebo-controlled trial—the cardiovascular thrombolytic to open occluded lines (COOL) efficacy trial. *J Vasc Interv Radiol.* 2001;12(8):951–955.

21. Semba CP, Murphy TP, Bakal CW, et al. Thrombolytic therapy with the use of alteplase (rtPA) in peripheral arterial occlusive disease: review of the clinical literature. *J Vasc Interv Radiol.* 2000;11(2 Pt 1):149–161.

22. Sugimoto K, Hofmann LV, Razavi MK, et al. The safety, efficacy, and pharmacoeconomics of low-dose alteplase compared with urokinase for catheter-directed thrombolysis of arterial and venous occlusions. *J Vasc Surg.* 2003;37(3):512–517.

23. Chin NK, Lim TW. Controlled trial of intrapleural streptokinase in the treatment of pleural empyema and complicated parapneumonic effusions. *Chest.* 1997;111:275–279.

24. Bonow RO, Carabello BA, Chatterjee K, et al. ACC/AHA 2006 guidelines for the management of patients with valvular heart disease: a report of the American College of Cardiology/American Heart Association Task Force on Practice Guidelines. *Circulation.* 2006;114:e84–e231.

25. Baekgaard N, Broholm R, Just S, et al. Long-term results using catheter-directed thrombolysis in 103 lower limbs with acute iliofemoral venous thrombosis. *Eur J Vasc Endovasc Surg.* 2010;39(1):112–117.

26. Vik A, Holme PA, Singh K, et al. Catheter-directed thrombolysis for treatment of deep venous thrombosis in the upper extremities. *Cardiovasc Intervent Radiol.* 2009;32(5):980–987.

27. Enden T, Kløw NE, Sandvik L, et al.; CaVenT study group. Catheter-directed thrombolysis vs. anticoagulant therapy alone in deep vein thrombosis: results of an open randomized, controlled trial reporting on short-term patency. *J Thromb Haemost.* 2009;7(8):1268–1275.

28. Kuo WT, van den Bosch MA, Hofmann LV, et al. Catheter-directed embolectomy, fragmentation, and thrombolysis for the treatment of massive pulmonary embolism after failure of systemic thrombolysis. *Chest.* 2008;134(2):250–254.

29. Davidian MM, Powell A, Benenati J, et al. Initial results of reteplase in the treatment of acute lower extremity arterial occlusions. *J Vasc Interv Radiol.* 2000;11:289–294.

30. Ouriel K, Katzen B, Mewissen M, et al. Reteplase in the treatment of peripheral arterial and venous occlusions: a pilot study. *J Vasc Interv Radiol.* 2000;11:849–854.

31. Hanover TM, Kalbaugh CA, Gray BH. Safety and efficacy for the treatment of acute arterial occlusion: complexity of the underlying lesion predicts outcome. *Ann Vasc Surg.* 2005;19:817–822.

32. Robertson I, Kessel DO, Berridge DC. Fibrinolytic agents for peripheral arterial occlusion. *Cochrane Database Syst Rev.* 2010;3:CD001099.

33. **Meijer KM, Schulman S. Determinants of bleeding risk in patients on antithrombotic and antifibrinolytic agents.** *Semin Thromb Hemost.* **2008;34(8):762–771. Epub 2009 Feb 12.**

34. **Schulman S, Beyth RJ, Kearon C, et al. Hemorrhagic complications of anticoagulant and thrombolytic treatment: American College of Chest Physicians Evidence-Based Clinical Practice Guidelines (8th ed.).** *Chest.* **2008;133:257S–298S.**

Note: the following key articles are not cited in the text.

Mehta RH, Alexander JH, Van de Werf F, et al. Relationship of incorrect dosing of fibrinolytic therapy and clinical outcomes. *JAMA.* **2005;293:1746–1750.**

Sobel M, Verhaeghe R; American College of Chest Physicians; American College of Chest Physicians. Antithrombotic therapy for peripheral artery occlusive disease: American College of Chest Physicians Evidence-Based Clinical Practice Guidelines (8th ed.). *Chest.* **2008;133(6 Suppl):815S–843S.**

Anticoagulation Reversal

7

John A. Dougherty, Lance J. Oyen, William E. Dager

INTRODUCTION

Bleeding, or concerns for bleeding during anticoagulation therapy, may at times create a need to lower or completely reverse the existing intensity of anticoagulation. Besides holding the anticoagulant or managing the bleeding directly, additional agents may be considered to counter the effects of the anticoagulant. Such agents may directly reverse the anticoagulants pharmacological effects or independently drive normal coagulation (hemostasis). Multiple factors are involved in finding the optimal approach to minimize bleeding consequences while limiting the risk for a thrombotic event. This chapter will provide insights into developing a strategy for reversing anticoagulation.

REVERSAL CONSIDERATIONS

Questions that need to be answered when deciding the best approach to reverse the effects of an anticoagulant:

- Is the goal to stop active bleeding?
- Or is the goal to prevent bleeding?

Once these questions are answered, the clinician should consider the following:

- Pharmacodynamic and pharmacokinetic properties of potential reversal agents
- Current degree of anticoagulation
- Target level of anticoagulation
- Desired timing of the onset of anticoagulation reversal
- Desired duration of anticoagulation reversal

- Desired outcome of the therapy plan versus the risks (i.e., Is the risk of the active bleeding or prevention of bleeding high enough to risk the use of agents that could cause embolic complications?)
- If multiple agents need to be used in combination to meet reversal goals
- Options to reestablish anticoagulation with prolonged reversal effects for a given strategy
  - Example: patients with a high risk for thrombosis (cancer with multiple thromboembolic events) and end-stage renal disease may have fewer options to reinitiate anticoagulation (i.e., potential bridging agents that are renally excreted may not be optimal), and excessive reversal (10 mg vitamin K for three doses in a warfarin patient) may create challenges in reestablishing anticoagulation.

Patient-specific considerations when developing a reversal plan

General considerations for developing a reversal strategy

- Is the patient anemic, thrombocytopenic, or bleeding?
- Does the patient have risk factors for bleeding?
- What is the clinical impact of blood loss?
  - Is the baseline Hgb/HCT sufficient to minimize consequences of blood loss?
  - Is the baseline Hgb/HCT low or is there a situation present limiting the ability to transfuse?
  - Do preexisting disease states create additional clinical risks from blood loss?
- Is the patient receiving antithrombotic and/or antiplatelet therapy?
  - How long will it take for the effects to dissipate?
  - Is there a plan to continue or reinitiate therapy?
- Has a reversal agent already been given?

RISK FACTORS FOR BLEEDING

Table 7-1: Risk Factors for Increased Anticoagulant Bleeding[1]

Category	Characteristics
Anticoagulation	Quality (out of range versus in goal)
	Presence of multiple anticoagulants or antiplatelet agents
	Organ dysfunction (e.g., hepatic failure, renal failure, etc.) creating reduced capacity for hemostasis to occur
Patient	Anemia
	Genetic coagulopathy disorders
	Prior bleeding
	Cancer
	Chronic renal insufficiency
	Uncontrolled hypertension
	Malignancy
	Alcohol abuse
	Previous stroke
	Age >70 yr old
	Organ failure reducing anticoagulant clearance
	Reduced platelet count or function
Procedures	Invasive procedure disrupting vascular integrity
	Recent procedure (bleeding risk is higher closer to surgery)
	Drains at site
	Anticoagulation required for the procedure (e.g., bypass, vascular catheterization)
	Vascular irregularities (e.g., aneurysm)

Considerations for reversing anticoagulation during invasive procedures:

- Closed-cavity (pericardial, spinal, CNS, ocular, etc.) regions where small amounts of blood can pool and create notable risk for complications
- Feasibility to transfuse
- Presence of drains or ability to intervene to manage bleeding

REVERSAL OPTIONS

Steps for developing a plan to reverse anticoagulation effects:

1. Assess laboratory validity (Do the results accurately describe the situation?) (see Chapter 18)

   - Is the value believable? (see Chapter 18)
     - Dilution of sample
     - Sample sent or drawn incorrectly (e.g., sample degradation, alteration)
   - Occurrence of an unexpected value (single value not supported by a trend or clinical explanation)
   - Does the observed value match the clinical presentation?
     - Recheck or validate if time permits
   - Is an interacting factor influencing a result? (see Chapter 18)
   - False INR elevation (see Table 18-7)
     - Lupus anticoagulant
     - Direct thrombin inhibitor
     - Heparin in absence of a neutralization step
     - Hepatic failure
   - False aPTT elevation (see Table 18-7)
     - Sampling technique
   - False anti-Factor Xa activity level elevation
     - Was the test calibrated to the agent that is being measured?
     - Does clinical urgency allow time to recheck the questioned value prior to implementing a reversal plan?
   - Can an alternative test confirm the observation (anti-Factor Xa activity or aPTT to confirm a unexpected low ACT)

2. Consider clinical reason for reversal and timeline assessment for new goal levels

   - Determine the appropriate approach for the current issue (see Table 7-2)
   - If the patient is bleeding, what is the acute bleeding issue?
   - Assessment of thrombosis risk with loss of anticoagulation versus bleeding concerns (see Table 7-3)
   - How fast must the anticoagulant effects be reversed? (see Table 7-3)

- If the bleeding event or risk with the procedure is life-threatening (i.e., intracranial hemorrhage) or capable of causing permanent disabling consequences (ocular bleeding), immediate/urgent reversal may be necessary.

- If major bleeding, but not life-threatening (i.e., drop in hemoglobin, see Appendix J) is occurring, immediate reversal may or may not be needed depending on the clinical situation and options available to support the patient's needs.

- What degree of reversal is necessary (complete, partial, or bringing excessive effects back into a safe value)? (See Tables 7-4, 7-5, and 7-6.)

- Complete reversal may be desired if major bleeding is occurring or is anticipated to occur (during high-risk planned procedure).

- Partial reversal may be considered (i.e., INR <2 or <1.5) when bleeding concerns are present, but not high enough when balanced with thrombosis concerns to warrant full reversal (common when using reversal to facilitate procedures).

- Bring excessive values down (here, the goal may be to drop the INR, aPTT, or ACT back into the target range faster than would occur simply by holding the agent).

Table 7-2: Approaches to Reversing Anticoagulation Effects (approach may include complete or partial reduction of anticoagulation)

Approach	Consideration
Holding the anticoagulant	Goal is hours to days naturally reducing pharmacologic effects
	Depends on urgency to reverse effect and patient's ability to eliminate the effects of the agent within the desired time period
Antidote	Administration of an agent that directly inhibits the pharmacologic affects of an anticoagulant
	Goal is minutes to hours reducing pharmacologic effects, usually when a patient is at high risk of harm or that harm is already occurring
Establishing hemostasis	Administration of an agent (i.e., a procoagulant) that promotes normal coagulation

(*continued*)

Table 7-2: (Continued)

Approach	Consideration
Revision of the anticoagulation approach	Goal is to reduce therapy target usually related to changes in risk acceptance Usually does not involve an antidote

Table 7-3: Assessment of the Bleeding vs. Thrombosis Risk

	Syndrome or Indication	Timeline	Hemostatic Goal	Rebound Risk
Urgent	Life-threatening or bleeding that may lead to damage a vital organ; active bleeding or presumed bleeding with hypotension, tachycardia, hematoma, swollen joints, other signs or symptoms that suggest immediate consequences; may include selected emergent invasive procedures where immediate reversal is necessary	Minutes to hours	Onset within minutes to hours for emergent symptoms (e.g., ICH); normal indices achieved rapidly and maintained for 24–72 hr (e.g., INR = 1, aPTT back to baseline)	High; minimize with repeat doses of rapid acting reversal agent and consider combining with agents with prolonged action (e.g., vitamin K)
Semiurgent	Plan for emergent invasive medical procedure causative of bleeding	Hours to days	Therapeutic anticoagulation level or lower usually in 24–72 hr; reserve for patients with risk factors for bleeding or the procedure is high risk for bleeding	Moderate; reversal should cover duration of risk window such as procedure duration and removal of invasive devices

3. Develop a reversion plan (see next section)

REVERSAL PLAN

Table 7-4: Considerations for **Urgent** Reversal of Anticoagulation Effects

Goal: minimal active anticoagulation for major or life-threatening hemorrhage but without protracted antagonism beyond immediate 24–72 hr unless longer period of reversal necessary (repeat invasive procedure planned or under consideration)

Large doses of vitamin K can delay reinitiating anticoagulation with warfarin for days to weeks, potentially requiring bridge therapy; as the severity of the bleeding increases, the importance of prolonged reversal diminishes as an extended duration of low INRs may be desirable

- If an immediate surgical procedure associated with a high risk of bleeding complications or life threatening bleed, which cannot delay therapy, choice of reversal and/or hemostasis therapy with effects in minutes is ideal; this may include both therapy for emergent reversal, and prevention of rebound of anticoagulant effect

Goal: minimal to no active anticoagulant effect with a return of anticoagulation indices (aPTT or INR) to baseline; dose of reversal therapy may be adapted to the current intensity of anticoagulation level if there is a desire to avoid prolonged effects when continued concerns for thrombosis are present; replacement of impaired coagulant factors if necessary for incomplete reversal with antidotes; for instance, use of rFVIIa, fresh frozen plasma (FFP), or PPC for emergent hemostasis (not drug antidote) plus 10 mg IV vitamin K to prevent rebound effects in warfarin induced life-threatening hemorrhage

- Generally goal of reversal is at least 24–72 hr, but as long as a life threatening bleeding issues are present, long-term anticoagulation may not be an immediate concern; for instance, with warfarin vitamin K IV 10 mg may be repeated if necessary; for SC LMWH or SC UFH, prolonged infusion of protamine may be necessary

Table 7-5: Considerations for **Semiurgent** Reversal of Anticoagulation Effects

Goal: lower end of target range for minimally invasive procedure to subtherapeutic goal for highly invasive, bleeding-inducing procedures; for patients with high bleeding risks (see below), intensity of new goal may be adjusted to a lower target during the period of increased bleeding concern; for instance, INR reversal from 6 may be reduced to 2.5–3.5 for patient goal without other risks, but to perhaps 2.0–2.5 for the procedure if patient has additional risk factors for bleeding

- Low-risk procedure or high risk for bleeding; goal: low goal range but not complete reversal of anticoagulant effect; relatively lower dose of reversal therapy and selection of therapy where rebound effects acceptable

(*continued*)

Table 7-5: (Continued)

- Administering rapid onset agents too far in advance may minimize reversal effect secondary to subsequent decline in effects and rebound in level of anticoagulation; for instance, a common mistake in the use of FFP for a procedure like a pacemaker lead placement is to infuse until the desired INR is obtained but then have a significant delay from that time until the procedure occurs, allowing for the INR to rebound (increase); this can be avoided by initiating FFP within 4–6 hr of the procedure and continuing it up to the time of the procedure

Table 7-6: Considerations in **Nonurgent** Reversal of Anticoagulant Effects

- Generally therapeutic level is goal with minimal intervention (e.g., holding the anticoagulant; oral vitamin K reversal plus holding the anticoagulant for a day)

- Generally holding therapy for 3–4 half-lives, accounting for any organ clearance compromise; for warfarin therapy, holding for 1–2 days and restarting at a lower dose is often sufficient

- Monitor pertinent labs or clinical features of bleeding; reassess further need for reversal

- Decline in anticoagulant effects may be relative to the anticoagulant dose, with patients receiving higher anticoagulant doses for the same goal level able to clear out the anticoagulant faster than those on lower chronic doses at the same measured effect

Onset and offset of agents to reverse warfarin (Figure 7-1)

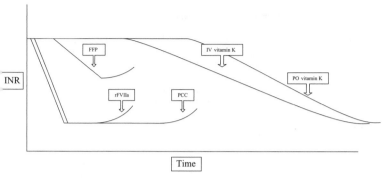

Figure 7-1: Description of the Duration of Effect for Various Agents in Reversing Vitamin K Antagonists

This figure illustrates the potential rebound in INR when administering various reversal strategies that have a shorter duration of effect compared to warfarin. The effects of rFVIIa and PCC are rapid; however, the shorter half-life of factor VII leads to an earlier rebound compared to PCC. For FFP, there is a delay in the partial effects secondary to the time to administer and amount given. Rebound from FFP begins shortly after the end of infusion. For vitamin K, the IV form has an earlier onset; however, the impact of the oral form begins to catch up at 24 hours. The degree and timing of rebound may depend on the dose administered and how high the INR is.

Monitor for bleeding or recalcitrant bleeding

Table 7-7: Considerations for Monitoring the Impact of the Reversal Approach

Factor	Monitoring Considerations
Bleeding	• Vital signs, hematocrit or hemoglobin, platelets • Signs of bleeding: physical assessment, wound sites, urine and stool for occult blood
Intensity of anticoagulation	• aPTT, anti-Factor Xa activity, INR, ACT, platelet count, and fibrinogen (patients with serious bleeding); other testes may be available depending on the setting; see Chapter 18

(continued)

Table 7-7: (Continued)

Factor	Monitoring Considerations
	• Assess potential impact should rebound in anticoagulant effect if using a reversal strategy that has a shorter duration of effect than the anticoagulant being reversed
Impaired drug elimination	Organ functions studies consistent with prolonged anticoagulation effects after holding because of a reduction in elimination (LFTs, renal function, cardiac output)

Table 7-8: Factors Impacting Extent and Speed of Reversal

Consideration of risk for thrombosis	• Thrombotic event (TE) history, number, location, and severity of the event(s) • Recent TE event • Hereditary risk factors/hypercoagulable state • Risk score (example: CHADS2) for stroke-related risk in AF (see Chapter 12)[2]
Requirement of bridge therapy prior to a procedure when thrombosis concerns are notable	Ability to provide a bridging agent should be assessed (see Chapter 8) • Ability to afford product and desired duration • Safety of the therapy or related risks • Ability to provide followup management • Patient ability to administer • Dose adjusted for organ function • Bleeding risk of a continued effect at time of the procedure
Patient risk factors for continued or worsening bleeding (not reversal) Angina/ACS, altered mental status, pulmonary insufficiency, dialysis efficacy	• Additional invasive procedures Additional complications may be a concern should continued bleeding or drop in Hgb/Hct occur

(continued)

Table 7-8: (Continued)

Magnitude/Intensity of current anticoagulation effect	Current intensity of anticoagulant effects Degree of reversal • Return to target goals • Below target or return to baseline
Dose of anticoagulation agent	Higher doses of the anticoagulant required to maintain typical therapy targets may reverse faster (possible increase in clearance); e.g., the INR may drop faster in patients requiring higher weekly warfarin dosing than those on lower low weekly doses
Estimation of patient's ability to eliminate the anticoagulant	Pharmacokinetics of the anticoagulant Presence of organ dysfunction
Predictability of reversal agent effects	• Route of administration • Bioavailability • Dose-response relationship

Clinical Pearl

• Assay errors during collection or measuring can occur. Single "critical" values could be misleading compared to values observed with a supporting tend from previous measurements. If clinical symptoms do not support the laboratory measurement, consider rechecking the value prior to implementing a different management plan. Adding an alternate test may be considered in selected situations.

AGENT SPECIFIC CONSIDERATIONS

Unfractionated heparin[3]

- Short half-life (90 minutes) with effects typically lost 3–4 hours after stopping the infusion but potentially longer with large doses (e.g., after boluses, cardiac procedures or SC administration)

    - Rebound from tissues can occur after large doses used during cardiopulmonary bypass.

- Monitoring with activated partial thromboplastin time (aPTT) or anti-Factor Xa activity with normal therapeutic dosing or activated clotting time (ACT) when very high intensity dosing (e.g., catheterization lab, operating room)

    - Note: return to baseline on high range ACT may still yield a VTE treatment target aPTT value.

    - aPTT or anti-Factor Xa activity level may be necessary to determine full reversal.

    - Pharmacologic effects rapidly reversed with protamine (see Table 7-11).

PARENTERAL ANTI-FACTOR XA ACTIVITY ANTAGONISTS (LOW MOLECULAR WEIGHT HEPARINS AND FONDAPARINUX)

Low molecular weight heparins (LMWHs)

- Value of anti-Factor Xa activity monitoring in face of reversal has not been established.

    - Note: 1 mg enoxaparin ~100 anti-Factor Xa activity units

- Protamine ~60% effective; side effects similar[4]

    - Dosing (see Table 7-10)

        - If used, other strategies to consider include blood products (i.e., FFP, cryoprecipitate) to normalize and replace clotting factors.

- Recalcitrant to protamine or imminent life threatening bleeding, rFVIIa (dose not established), or PCC (see below) can be considered. Repeat doses of protamine may need to be considered if activity is prolonged from reduced elimination in renal insufficiency.

Fondaparinux

* Long half-life (17–21 hours)
* No definitive antidote data, but some limited short-term effect may exist with rFVIIa and may be a consideration in life-threatening situations.[5-7] Activated PCC hypothetically may have an effect (see PCC section below).
* Protamine may not effectively reverse fondaparinux given the lack of sites on the molecule to elicit an effect, and similar hypersensitivity precautions would still be a concern if used.

DIRECT THROMBIN INHIBITORS

Agents

* Lepirudin, argatroban, bivalirudin, desirudin, dabigatran
* Warfarin with parenteral DTI may elevate the INR value of the warfarin anticoagulation.
    * Elevated INR values secondary to DTI in the absence of warfarin may not reflect excessive loss of systemic vitamin K dependent clotting factors; thus, vitamin K should not be used for reversal if no warfarin has been given.
    * The INR, aPTT, ecarin clotting time, or thrombin time may also be elevated with oral DTIs. The INR's ability to reflect a level of anticoagulant effect is unclear.
* Prolonged effect due to reduced elimination in impaired cardiac, hepatic, or renal function require prolonged monitoring for recurrent bleeding or ongoing bleeding risk.
* In patients with normal organ function patients, the parenteral DTI half-life is short and effects will minimize within 3–4 hours of stopping.
    * In the presence of organ failure, effects of the DTI may last longer after holding secondary to slower elimination.
        * Dabigatran etexilate is approximately 80% renally cleared.
        * Hemodialysis can remove approximately $2/3$ of dabigatran.[8]
    * DTIs administered by the SC or oral route may have longer durations of actions.
    * Drug interactions with the oral agents may prolong their effects.
* Bivalirudin: no reliable data on reversal agents; however, low dose rFVIIa has been used along with ultrafiltration with some effect.[9] More data is needed to verify this concept.

Warfarin

No bleeding present, but elevated INR

- If no invasive procedure is planned, reversal with vitamin K may not alter outcomes (see Table 7-14).

Procedure/surgery planned-INR reversal within hours

- IV phytonadione provides a faster decrease in the INR over oral with some effects observed as early as 4 hours after IV administration.[10] In this situation, it may be used more to reduce degree of anticoagulation after the procedure, but it will not facilitate the procedure. A more rapid acting agent will be needed.

Greater than 24 hours

- Oral phytonadione provides a decrease in the INR starting within 24 hours.

Table 7-9: Dose for Method of Reversal[a]

	Dose for Method of Reversal			
	Often used in combination		Addition of either rFVIIa or PCC can be considered, not both	
Clinical Scenario	**FFP**	**Vitamin K**	**rFVIIa**	**PCC**
• Life threatening bleeding	10–20 mL/kg IV	10 mg IV[b] administer slow over 30 min	10–40 mcg/kg	25–50 International Units/kg
• Acute situations requiring invasive procedure within 6–24 hr	10–15 mL/kg IV (NR for fluid overloaded heart failure patients)	Dose dependent on INR, 0.5–3 mg IV for goal INR <3; this depends on the degree of reversal planned, the initial INR, the goal INR from reversal, and the dose of warfarin involved	NR	25–50 International Units/kg
• Minor bleeding	NR	1–5 mg PO; dose based on INR	NR	NR

(continued)

Table 7-9: (Continued)

Clinical Scenario	Dose for Method of Reversal			
	Often used in combination		Addition of either rFVIIa or PCC can be considered, not both	
	FFP	Vitamin K	rFVIIa	PCC
• Elective procedure in greater than 24 hr	0–15 mL/kg IV	1–5 mg PO; dose based on INR (NR for patients with higher risk of thrombosis [i.e., valves patients])	NR	NR

Abbreviation: NR = not recommended.

[a]The table provides modalities to reverse the effects of vitamin K antagonists. The modalities are not always complete in their reversal but provide strategies to decrease the drug's effects.[11-16]

[b]The vitamin K dose of 10 mg IV assumes a goal for full reversal and limited concerns to reinitiate a vitamin K antagonist for a period of time (>1 week). Consider the timing of the procedure and potential rebound with rFVIIa, FFP, or PCC. Doses for these agents just prior to the procedure may provide a higher period of hemostasis over administration earlier. Vitamin K may be warranted to maintain reversal postprocedure.

Clinical Pearls

- The dose of vitamin K to reverse warfarin will depend on how high the INR is and the targeted value after reversal. Only a small change in the percent of activated clotting factors is required to drop critical values into the target range (and thus a small amount of vitamin K required) compared to dropping the INR value below the therapeutic range or back to baseline where a larger dose of vitamin K may be considered.

- One strategy when a patient is not bleeding is to consider low dose vitamin K dose with a followup INR later (e.g., 12 hours). If the INR has dropped sufficiently, then no additional dose may be needed. If not a sufficient drop, the dose can be repeated. FFP can also be administered shortly prior to the procedure.

Thrombolytics

- No clear antidote exists; however, blood products and aminocaproic acid have been used.[17]

- Blood product replacement and replacement of factors (e.g., FFP, cryoprecipitate (if low fibrinogen), and/or PRBC) especially in hemorrhage.

AGENTS TO REVERSE ANTICOAGULATION

Table 7-10: Mechanism/Pharmacology/Pharmacokinetics of Agents for Anticoagulation Reversal[13]

Reversal Agent	Mechanism	Kinetics	Dose	Rebound of Anticoagulant
Protamine	Combines chemically with heparin molecules to form inactive salt	Onset within 5 min Duration is irreversible and dose dependent Rebound of anticoagulation may occur with subcutaneous heparin or LWMH doses	See Table 7-11	Likely with subcutaneous dosing associated with later delivery, but not related to loss of effect
Fresh frozen plasma (FFP)	Contains all coagulant factors, including II, VII, IX, and X but in diluted form compared to other options Requires activation of factors in vivo	Onset in 1–4 hr depending on dose and magnitude of anticoagulation Duration of effect 6 hr or less	10–20 mL/kg IV	~4–6 hr

(*continued*)

Table 7-10: (Continued)

Reversal Agent	Mechanism	Kinetics	Dose	Rebound of Anticoagulant
Prothrombin complex concentrates (PCC)	Contains coagulant factors, including II, IX, and X and some with VII, in concentrations 25 times that of FFP Requires activation of factors in vivo A few products (i.e., FEIBA) contain activated factors (see PCC section)	Onset within 10–15 min Duration of effect 12–24 hr Used with vitamin K for longer reversal of warfarin	25–50 International Units/kg IV; this may vary between products (best to review your formulary specific choice to determine dosing used in studies)	~12 hr
Recombinant activated factor seven (rFVIIa)	Selective replacement of rFVIIa, which activates extrinsic clotting pathway resulting in thrombin formation	Onset within 10 min Duration of effect 4–6 hr Used with FFP to limit INR (with warfarin) rebound and vitamin K extends to >24 hr	10–90 mcg/kg IV No dose ranging trials are available in this setting; low doses of 1 mg have normalized the INR within 15 min	6–12 hr
Vitamin K	Cofactor for hepatic production of Factors II, VII, IX, and X	Onset PO 12–24 hr or IV 4–12 hr SC and IM not recommended Duration dependent on warfarin intensity INR rebound occurring in days	Up to 10 mg IV/PO	Dose dependent

CONSIDERATIONS FOR DRUG ADMINISTRATION

• Protamine: typically reserved for life-threatening bleeds during UFH or LMWH therapy or to prevent risks of bleeding after very large UFH doses.

Table 7-11: Protamine for Reversal of Heparins[3,13]

	Dose	Comment
Unfractionated heparin	• <u>For IV heparin:</u> 1 mg/100 units of heparin, maximum of 50 mg at rate not to exceed 5 mg/min; If >60 min after holding the UFH infusion, 0.5 mg/100 units; If >2 hr, 0.25 mg/100 units; may give additional protamine if warranted after at least 10 min • <u>For subcutaneous heparin (treatment dosing):</u> 25–50 mg IV infusion over 8–16 hr (with bleeding/ high risk of bleeding: aPTT at goal, use 25 mg; if elevated aPTT, use 50 mg and recheck aPTT)	Because the half-life of IV heparin is relatively short (~60–90 min) with effects dissipating rapidly after stopping the IV infusion, consider calculating the dose of protamine sulfate from the amount of heparin administered within the preceding few hours (e.g., from a continuous IV infusion of heparin at 1,250 units/hr approximately 30 mg of protamine sulfate would be used) <u>After an IV UFH bolus and bleeding (or high risk):</u> 1 mg/100 units of UFH if aPTT at goal; 1.5 mg/100 units of UFH if the aPTT is elevated Infuse at 5 mg/min After large doses in cardiac bypass graft surgery and initial protamine reversal, redistribution of heparin out of tissues to the plasma may lead to a rebound heparin effect where additional protamine may be considered when bleeding concerns are present[18] Neutralization of SC UFH may require a prolonged infusion of protamine sulfate The APTT (or ACT) can be used to assess the effectiveness of protamine sulfate neutralization
LMWH	• Protamine 1 mg/100 anti-Factor Xa activity units IV at 5 mg/min within 8 hr of dose	Tinzaparin >dalteparin >enoxaparin (in order of effect) for neutralization by protamine; any clinical significance of this between agents is unknown[4]

(continued)

Table 7-11: (Continued)

	Dose	Comment
	• If 8 hr or more after dose, 0.5 mg/100 anti-Factor Xa activity units • Consider repeat dose of 0.5 mg/100 anti-Factor Xa activity units if bleeding continues	Enoxaparin 1 mg ~100 anti-Factor Xa activity units

• Protamine can be administered undiluted in emergency situations, but dilution in D5W or NS is preferred.

Table 7-12: Risks Associated with Protamine Use[3,19]

Cardiac effects (hypotension, shock, bradycardia)

Pulmonary edema

Pulmonary vasoconstriction

Flushing

Urticaria

Angioedema

Leucopenia

Thrombocytopenia

• Caution: hypersensitivity reactions are potentially higher in patients with allergy to fish, prior use of protamine insulin, or prior vasectomy; consider corticosteroids or histamine antagonist to treat reactions

VITAMIN K (PHYTONADIONE)

Factors to consider in determining a vitamin K reversal dose:

• Pregnancy category C

• The liver needs to be capable of producing clotting factors.

• Very small amounts of vitamin K can drop a critical INR value (>6) to the target range.[20]

- It may take more vitamin K to reverse the INR below 2 or 1.5 as a greater number of active clotting factors are needed per INR unit change (see Chapter 18).

- Individuals very sensitive to warfarin may have larger INR declines compared to less sensitive patients for the same vitamin K dose.[21]

- At higher initial INR values, small changes in clotting factors create larger changes in the subsequent INR value.

Clinical Pearls

- At lower INR values, a larger change in the percent of activated clotting factors is necessary to see a rise in the value (INR of 2–3 will be ~25–40% of normal). INR values over 6 will be less than 10% of normal activated clotting factors. At this level, small changes in the number of activated clotting factors will lead to larger changes in the INR.

- For reversal of high INR values, small increases in the number (or percent of normal) of activated clotting factors will lead to a larger drop in the INR compared to the amount of activated clotting factors needed to drop the INR below 2, or back to baseline. Thus, small doses of vitamin K may drop a high INR into the therapeutic range, but a larger dose may be necessary to drop the INR below 2.

- If the patient is very sensitive to warfarin, a larger drop per a set dose of vitamin K may occur compared to a patient requiring higher doses of warfarin and the same INR.

- Of additional note is that for a given INR, the value may drop faster independent of vitamin K in individuals requiring a higher dose of warfarin.

Reversing an elevated INR with vitamin K may depend on presence of bleeding. In a recent analysis assessing bleeding and thrombotic–related outcomes in clinically stable, nonbleeding patients with no plan for an invasive procedure, use of vitamin K solely to drop the INR was not associated with improving outcomes (see Table 7-13).[22]

Table 7-13: Assessment of 1.25 mg Vitamin K Orally vs. Placebo in Reversal If INR Values Between 4.5–10 in Nonbleeding Patients[22]

	Day 7			Day 30			Day 90		
	Vitamin K	Placebo	p	Vitamin K	Placebo	p	Vitamin K	Placebo	p
Any bleeding	7.9%	9.2%	0.52	11.5%	12.7%	0.63	15.8%	16.3%	0.86
Major bleeding	-	-	-	-	-	-	2.5%	1.1%	0.22
Thromboembolism	0.3%	0.3%	1.00	0.6%	0.3%	0.62	1.1%	0.8%	0.72
Death	0	0.3%	1.00	0.3%	1.4%	0.22	2.0%	1.9%	0.94

Vitamin K 2.5 mg PO appears to be an effective reversal strategy in nonbleeding outpatients with INR values over 10.[23]

Table 7-14: Vitamin K Products Commonly Used for Reversal

Dosing Form	Administration Considerations	Comments
Injectable	• Available as 10 mg/mL or 1 mg/0.5 mL concentration • Physically compatible in NS, D5W, or D5WNS • Administer under light sensitive conditions (protect from light) • Recommended to infuse at a rate not exceeding 1 mg/min • Clinical application: infuse IV in 50 mL of compatible fluid over 30–60 min	• Subcutaneous administration not preferred because of erratic absorption and delay in onset of effect compared to IV or PO (see Table 7-15) • Not recommended as intramuscular administration because of potential for hematoma since patient is anticoagulated • IV doses of 0.1–0.5 mg appear to be as effective as higher doses to reduce excessive INR values into the target range, with over reversal less likely with the lower dose[24] • Anaphylactoid, (and rarely anaphylaxis) reactions can occur (see Table 7-18)
Oral	• Available as 5-mg unscored tablet • IV form can be administered orally	– Clinical application: to give doses less than 5 mg, the intravenous formulation that is diluted (cherry syrup is one option) orally to give a more accurate dose

Table 7-15: Reversal of Warfarin with Oral vs. SC Vitamin K[25]

Note: PO appears to work faster, minimizing any reasons for administering by the SC route.

Mean INR	1 mg PO N = 26	1 mg SC N = 25
Initial INR	5.6	6.2
INR day 1	2.9	4.2
INR day 2	2.2	3.1
INR day 3	2.7	2.8

Table 7-16: Reversal of Warfarin with IV vs. PO Vitamin K[26]

Target INR	2.5 mg PO	0.5 mg IV
INR 2–4	6 hr: 0% 12 hr: 35% 24 hr: 87%	6 hr: 46% 12 hr: 67% 24 hr: 67%
% INR at 24 hr <2.0	7%	29%
% INR at 24 hr >4.0	4%	4%

Note: baseline was INR 6–10.

Table 7-17: Assessment of IV Vitamin K Formulation Administered PO for Nonurgent Reversal of Anticoagulation[27]

Initial INR	8-11.9	12-20	> 20
Vitamin K dose	2.5 mg	5 mg	5 mg
Day 1 (~14 hr)–INR -% INR 2.0–4.9 -% INR <2	3.5 77% 8%	3.0 52% 17%	2.9 44% 29%

Note: differences in clotting factors present between an INR of 8 to >20 is very small.

Table 7-18: Adverse Effects Observed with Parenteral Vitamin K

Adverse Event
Hypersensitivity reactions including anaphylaxis (IV route)
Flushing sensations
Profuse sweating
Changes in taste
Dizziness
Hypotension
Dyspnea
Cyanosis
Pain/swelling/tenderness at injection site
• <u>On repeated injections:</u> erythematous, indurated, and pruritic plaques have occurred, rarely progressing to scleroderma-like lesions; most dermatological effects have occurred following intramuscular injections
Hyperbilirubin (newborns)

Vitamin K dispensing:

• Dispense IV doses in a piggyback bag to assure slower infusion rates.

• Use caution with availability of 10-mg vials outside the pharmacy (i.e., available in the automated dispensing cabinets). If the pharmacy is able to turn around a dose (noting that the onset of effect is several hours and that more rapid acting agents can be used if necessary), consider the benefits of pharmacy assessment of the dose and route along with the need for other interventions to minimize the potential for over or under reversal and delay in the use of other adjuncts (FFP, PCC, or rFVIIa). When pharmacy services are not available, consider procedures that address safety and dosing concerns.

FRESH FROZEN PLASMA (FFP)[13,14]

• Fluid portion of 1 unit of blood centrifuged, separated, and frozen at −18°C within 6 hours of collection

• The general dose for FFP is 10–20 mL/kg.

• A unit typically equals about 200 mL of FFP.

- 1 mL of FFP contains about 1 unit of each coagulation factor. The INR of FFP is 1.0.
- The expected response depends on patient's predose level of coagulation factors.
- Thawing (generally 30 minutes), storage, and donor dependence limitation
- Primary use is for temporary reversal. Partial reversal of warfarin therapy (in emergency or high risk for bleeding scenarios where anticoagulation must be resolved by replacing vitamin K dependent factors) includes risk of rebound anticoagulation occurring 4–6 hours after dose. It is most commonly administered with adjunctive therapy such as IV vitamin K and potentially rFVIIa or PCC, especially for subtherapeutic goals and critical bleeding.
- Primary use is for emergency or high risk for bleeding scenarios where anticoagulation must be reversed, but where target is still goal range INR (2.0–3.5) and *not* complete reversal.
- Volume associated with FFP may cause volume-related complications (fluid overload, cardiogenic shock) and limit its utility in a life-threatening bleeding situation (can't be infused quickly enough).
- Risk of transfusion reaction (see Appendix K for transfusion-related reactions) should be monitored.
- Transmission of blood borne pathogens is very low risk.
- Additional benefit in hemorrhagic shock, providing volume in addition to factor replacement often along with platelets and/or red blood cells.

PROTHROMBIN COMPLEX CONCENTRATES (PCC)[14,15]

- Dosed on Factor IX units, but caution that the order does not confuse PCC with Factor IX, which is a single factor only[15]
- Prothrombin complex concentrate, also known as PCC or FIXCC, contains factors II, VII, IX, and X and some also include proteins C and S. Some are low in Factor VII (PCC 3) and others have relatively equal amounts of all four (PCC 4).[28]
    - PCC3: contains therapeutic concentrations of Factors II, IX, and X; may contain other factors such as Protein C, S, and Factor VII to lesser concentrations
    - PCC4: contains therapeutic concentrations of Factors II, VII, IX, and X; may contain other factors such as Protein C or Protein S to lesser concentrations

- Activated PCC (i.e., FEIBA) provides selected clotting factors in the activated form.[13] The proposed advantage of using activated PCC is that it can work below anti-Factor Xa activity and II in the common pathway of the clotting cascade (thus below the sites of activity of the anticoagulants).[29]

- Heparin and antithrombin have been added to some PCC products to minimize accumulation of factor II and X effects, which may last longer and cause thromboembolism.

- Factor components are 25 times more concentrated than that of the plasma concentration.

- No refrigeration or thawing is required, but reconstitution is necessary.

- Fluid effects and transfusion reactions are potential adverse reactions, but the most severe is thrombosis.

- Rapid administration makes administration simple. See related product information for maximum infusion rate.

- Onset of effects is generally complete reversal of warfarin-induced, elevated INR within 10–30 minutes.[30-33]

- Adverse effects:

  - Allergic reactions

  - Transfusion-related reactions (see Appendix K)

  - Thromboembolism (potentially increased when repeat or high doses are used)

    - PCC3 and PCC4 seem similar in rates of thromboembolic events (both more likely at higher doses).

- HIT (in theory for those products containing heparin—know your formulary product).

Dosing

Warfarin

- See Table 7-9 regarding warfarin-induced elevation, combinations of phytonadione, and other products.

- Dosing varies by specific product and studies using the product. In most studies, 25–50 units (Factor IX equivalent) per kg or 500 International Units was used. Be familiar with institution-specific products and be aware of the evidence and dosing for those agents prior to use.

- Dose based on degree of INR; weight adjusted in combination has been more effective than standard dosing (e.g., 500 International Units)[34]

Combined with other reversal agents

- Rebound INR increase can occur in 12–24 hr especially if used without IV phytonadione. The addition of vitamin K should be considered (generally 10 mg IV) in life-threatening, nonsurgically repairable bleeds or with the need for prolonged complete reversal such as intracranial hemorrhage.
- Phytonadione should be continued in life-threatening or emergent bleeding situations when using PCC.[35]
- Intravenous phytonadione is predominately used in emergent situations with PCC and FFP compared to oral phytonadione.
- FFP with PCC, if using a PCC3, has been suggested to augment factor VII levels.[36]
  - This addition of FFP may be a consideration when using PCC products deficient in factor VII.
- Generally administration of PCC in the high INR situation can result in low normal goal range or subtherapeutic anticoagulation (<2.0).
- The risk for thromboembolic complications may be higher when using PCC and rFVIIa, either together or in addition to other agents such as aminocaproic acid.
- Understand your options and products available including dosing and/or available evidence. Each is different.[15]
- Several approaches to individualize the PCC dose have been explored.[37] The approach used should consider the agents available, personal experiences with their use, and available published experiences. Multiple approaches have been explored and examples are provided below. Dose is based on factor level.
  - International Units requested = kg weight X (target factor level–current factor level)[38]
    - Infusion rate 100 International Units/min
- Dose based on the observed INR
  - Dose of PCC (Beriplex) for initial INR[39]
    - 25 International Units/kg for INR of 2.0–3.9
    - 35 International Units/kg for INR 4.0–6.0
    - 60 International Units/kg for INR >6.0

- – Based on weight (kg) and observed INR[34]
  - – Refer to the reference for several dosing tables described.
  - – PCC was Cofact.

LMWH/fondaparinux

- Prothrombin complex concentrates (PCC) may have a role in protamine recalcitrant reversal.[29]
  - – FEIBA: the ability of FEIBA to work downstream of anti-Factor Xa activity in the common pathway in the coagulation cascade has been postulated with limited evidence as a advantage in reversing anticoagulation when in the presence of an anti-Factor Xa activity inhibitor (fondaparinux analyzed). Dose of FEIBA proposed is 25 units/kg.
    - – Note: PCC products contain clotting factors. FEIBA differs from other PCCs in that some of the factors present are already in an activated form. The activated factors may produce immediate thrombin generation in the presence of an anti-Factor Xa activity inhibitor such as fondaparinux.[29]

Clinical Pearl

- Several PCC products are currently available. Be familiar with the products available for use. Differences between products do exist. Some are PCC3, where an additional transfusion of other blood products may be considered. Some products contain additional substances including heparin, which may be of concern for patients with a history of HIT. The duration of effect and potential for inducing thrombosis may be related to the dose given. Generally, rFVIIa should be avoided in individuals receiving a PCC.

RECOMBINANT FACTOR VIIA (ACTIVATED rFVIIA)

- Available in vials that contain 1 mg, 2 mg, and 5 mg of activated rFVIIa
- Common approaches used for hemostasis in presence of an anticoagulant: 10–40 units/kg IV, but doses as high as 90 units/kg have been used.[13,16]
  - – Dose may depend on the risk of bleeding complications and thrombosis.
  - – No dose ranging trials in this setting are available.

- – Lower doses have recently been explored out of concern for thromboembolic concerns with the rFVIIa.
- High cost (approximately $1,000 per mg)
- No refrigeration, easy to store, quick preparation and administration
- Use diluent that is provided in product packaging.
- Administer within 3 hours of preparation.
- Administer as bolus over 2–5 minutes.
- Flush line with NS.
- Hemostatic effects observed within 5–15 minutes (allows potential titration to effects by starting with lower doses if time permits).
- Rebound in the INR for warfarin patients can occur in 12–24 hours when rFVIIa is used alone. Prolonged reduction in the INR can be accomplished by adding vitamin K. FFP and IV vitamin K may be a consideration to provide continued reversal until the full onset of vitamin K effects (see Figure 7-1).
- Observations from a small registry suggest a potential benefit when used with other antidotes to reestablish hemostasis during LMWH and UFH therapy.[40]
- No direct comparisons to PCC are available.

Table 7-19: Adverse Events Associated with the Use of rFVIIa Outside Hemophiliacs

• Thromboembolism	The reported incidence of thromboembolism may be higher than observed in the hemophiliac population due to increased embolic risks for embolism
	Black box warnings with off label use: arterial and venous thrombotic and thromboembolic events following administration of rFVIIa have been reported during postmarketing surveillance; clinical studies have shown an increased risk of arterial thromboembolic adverse events with rFVIIa when administered outside the current approved indications; fatal and nonfatal thrombotic events have been reported; discuss the risks and explain the signs and symptoms of thrombotic and thromboembolic events to patients who will receive rFVIIa; monitor for signs or symptoms of activation of the coagulation system and for thrombosis
• Hypersensitivity	

REFERENCES

*Key articles

1. Smythe MA, Dager WE, Patel NM. Managing complications of anticoagulant therapy. *J Pharm Pract.* 2004;17:327–346.

2. Gage BF, Waterman AD, Shannon W, et al. Validation of clinical classification schemes for predicting stroke: results from the National Registry of Atrial Fibrillation. *JAMA.* 2001;285:2864–2870.

3. Hirsh J, Bauer KA, Donati MB, et al. Parenteral anticoagulants: American College of Chest Physicians Evidence-Based Clinical Practice Guidelines (8th ed.). *Chest.* 2008;133(Suppl):141S–159S.

4. Crowther MA, Berry LR, Monagle PT, et al. Mechanisms responsible for the failure of protamine to inactivate low-molecular-weight heparin. *Br J Haematol.* 2002;116: 178–186.

5. Bijsterveld NR, Moons AH, Boekholdt M, et al. Ability of recombinant factor VIIa to reverse the anticoagulant effect of the pentasaccharide fondaparinux in healthy volunteers. *Circulation.* 2002;106:2550–2554.

6. Lisman T, Bijsterveld NR, Adelmeijer J, et al. Recombinant factor VIIa reverses the in vitro and ex vivo anticoagulant and profibrinolytic effects of fondaparinux. *J Thromb Haemost.* 2003;1:2368–2373.

7. Young G, Yonekawa KE, Nakagawa PA, et al. Recombinant activated factor VII effectively reverses the anticoagulant effects of heparin, enoxaparin, fondaparinux, argatroban, and bivalirudin ex vivo as measured using thromboelastography. *Blood Coagul Fibrinolysis.* 2007;18:547–553.

8. Stangier J, Rathgen K, Stähle H, et al. Influence of renal impairment on the pharmacokinetics and pharmacodynamics of oral dabigatran etexilate: an open-label, parallel-group, single-centre study. *Clin Pharmacokinet.* 2010;49:259–268.

9. Stratmann G, deSilva AM, Tseng EE, et al. Reversal of direct thrombin inhibition after cardiopulmonary bypass in a patient with heparin-induced thrombocytopenia. *Anesth Analg.* 2004;98:1635–1639.

10. Watson HG, Baglin T, Laidlaw SL, et al. A comparison of the efficacy and rate of response to oral and intravenous Vitamin K in reversal of over-anticoagulation with warfarin. *Br J Haematol.* 2001;115:145–149.

* **11. Leissinger CA, Blatt PM, Hoots K, et al. Role of prothrombin complex concentrates in reversing warfarin anticoagulation: a review of the literature. *Am J. Hematol.* 2008;83:137–143.**

12. Garcia D, Crowther MA, Ageno W. Practical management of coagulopathy associated with warfarin. *BMJ.* 2010;340:c1813.

* **13. Schulman S, Bijsterveld NR. Anticoagulants and their reversal. *Transfus Med Rev.* 2007;21:37–48.**

14. Goldstein JN, Rosand J, Schwamm LH. Warfarin reversal in anticoagulated-associated intracerebral hemorrhage. *Neurocrit Care.* 2008;9:277–283.

15. Levy JH, Tanaka KA, Dietrich W. Perioperative hemostatic management of patients treated with vitamin K antagonists. *Anesthesiology.* 2008;109:918–926.

16. Dager WE, Regalia R, Williamson D, et al. Reversal of elevated international normalized ratios and bleeding with low-dose recombinant activated factor VIIa in patients receiving warfarin. *Pharmacotherapy.* 2006;26:1091–1098.

17. Goldstein JN, Marrero M, Masrur S, et al. Management of thrombolysis-associated symptomatic intracerebral hemorrhage. *Arch Neurol.* 2010;67:965–969.

18. Teoh KH, Young E, Blackall MH, et al. Can extra protamine eliminate heparin rebound following cardiopulmonary bypass surgery? *J Thorac Cardiovasc Surg.* 2004;128: 211–219.

19. Hiong YT, Tang YK, Chui WH, et al. A case of catastrophic pulmonary vasoconstriction after protamine administration in cardiac surgery: role of intraoperative transesophageal echocardiography. *J Cardiothorac Vasc Anesth.* 2008;22:727–731.

20. Shetty HGM, Backhouse G, Bentley DP, et al. effective reversal of warfarin-induced excessive anticoagulation with low dose vitamin k1. *Thromb Haemost.* 1992;67: 13–15.

21. White RH, McKittrick T, Hutchinson R, et. al. Temporary discontinuation of warfarin therapy: changes in the international normalized ratio. *Ann Intern Med.* 1995;122: 40–42.

22. Crowther MA, Ageno W, Garcia D, et al. Oral vitamin K versus placebo to correct excessive anticoagulation in patients receiving warfarin: a randomized trial. *Ann Intern Med.* 2009;150:293–300.

23. Crowther MA, Garcia D, Ageno W, et al. Oral vitamin K effectively treats international normalised ratio (INR) values in excess of 10. Results of a prospective cohort study. *Thromb Haemost.* 2010;104:118–121.

24. Whitling AM, Bussey HI, Lyons RM. Comparing different routes and doses of phytonadione for reversing excessive anticoagulation. *Arch Intern Med.* 1998;158: 2136-2140.

25. Crowther MA, Douketis JD, Schnurr T, et al. Oral vitamin K lowers the international normalized ratio more rapidly than subcutaneous vitamin K in the treatment of warfarin-associated coagulopathy. A randomized, controlled trial. *Ann Intern Med.* 2002;137:251–254.

26. Lubetsky A, Yonath H, Olchovsky D, et al. Comparison of oral vs intravenous phytonadione (vitamin K1) in patients with excessive anticoagulation: a prospective randomized controlled study. *Arch Intern Med.* 2003;163:2469–2473.

27. Baker P, Gleghorn A, Tripp T, et al. Reversal of asymptomatic over-anticoagulation by orally administered vitamin K. *Br J Haematol.* 2006;133:331–336.

28. Hellstern P, Beeck H, Fellhauer A, et al. Factor VII and activated-factor-VII content of prothrombin complex concentrates. The PCC Study Group. *Vox Sang.* 1997;73: 155–161.

* **29. Desmurs-Clavel H, Huchon C, Chatard B, et al. Reversal of the inhibitory effect of fondaparinux on thrombin generation by rFVIIa, aPCC and PCC. *Thromb Res.* 2009;123:796–798.**

30. Yasaka M, Oomura M, Ikeno K, et al. Effect of prothrombin complex concentrate on INR and blood coagulation system in emergency patients treated with warfarin overdose. *Ann Hematol.* 2003;82:121–123.

31. Yasaka M, Sakata T, Naritomi H, et al. Optimal dose of prothrombin complex concentrate for acute reversal of anticoagulation. *Thromb Res.* 2005;115:455–459.

32. Yasaka M, Sakata T, Minematsu K, et al. Correction of INR by prothrombin complex concentrate and vitamin K in patients with warfarin related hemorrhagic complication. *Thromb Res.* 2003;108:25–30.

33. Markis M, Greaves M, Phillips WS, et al. Emergency oral anticoagulation reversal: the relative efficacy of infusions of fresh frozen plasma and clotting factor concentrate on correction of the coagulopathy. *Thromb Haemost.* 1997;77:477–480.

* **34. van Aart L, Eijkhout HW, Kamphuis JS, et al. Individualized dosing regimen for prothrombin complex concentrate more effective than standard treatment in the reversal of oral anticoagulant therapy: an open, prospective randomized controlled trial. *Thromb Res.* 2006;118:313–320.**

35. Ansell J, Hirsh J, Hylek E, et al. The pharmacology and management of the vitamin K antagonists: the eighth ACCP conference on antithrombotic and thrombolytic therapy. *CHEST.* 2008;133(Suppl);160S–198S.

* **36. Baker RI, Coughlin PB, Gallus AS, et al. Warfarin reversal consensus guidelines on behalf of the Australasian Society of Thrombosis and Haemostasis. *Med J Aust.* 2004;181:492–497.**

* **37. Bershad EM, Suarez JI. Prothrombin complex concentrates for oral anticoagulant therapy-related intracranial hemorrhage: a review of the literature. *Neurocrit Care.* 2010;12:403–413.**

38. Boulis N, Bobek M, Schmaier A, et al. Use of factor IX complex in warfarin-related intracranial hemorrhage. *Neurosurgery.* 1999;45:1113–1119.

39. Preston FE, Laidlaw ST, Sampson B, et al. Rapid reversal of oral anticoagulation with warfarin by a prothrombin complex concentrate (Beriplex): efficacy and safety in 42 patients. *Br J Haematol.* 2002;116:619–624.

40. Ingerslev J, Vanek T, Culic S. Use of recombinant factor VIIa for emergency reversal of anticoagulation. *J Postgrad Med.* 2007;53:17–22.

Transitions in Care; Periprocedural Bridging and Transitions Between Agents

8

John Fanikos

INTRODUCTION

Patients who receive long-term antiplatelet (AP) therapy or oral anticoagulation with vitamin K antagonists (VKA) commonly transition from the ambulatory setting to the hospital and back again. This clinical scenario often requires antithrombotic therapy changes. Each transition point (hospital admission, procedure, unit transfer, discharge to home, or long-term care) represents an opportunity to assess medication regimens for errors, omissions, and treatment adjustments. Emphasis on abbreviating hospital stay and reducing costs further magnifies the need for seamless conversion between oral and parenteral antithrombotic therapies. As these patients transition, either electively or urgently, the diagnosis and indications for anticoagulant therapy should be evaluated (Figure 8-1). Surgical and invasive procedures add additional levels of complexity where VKA and AP therapy may be continued, interrupted, or replaced with short-term parenteral or "bridge" therapy. Since there is not a standardized definition of "bridging," most regimens have been developed from observational studies. Physician and patient preference will play a role in determining whether therapy is continued, stopped, or replaced with an alternative agent.

PERIPROCEDURAL BRIDGING PRINCIPLES

- Determine thromboembolism risk with interruption of anticoagulant and/ or AP therapy.

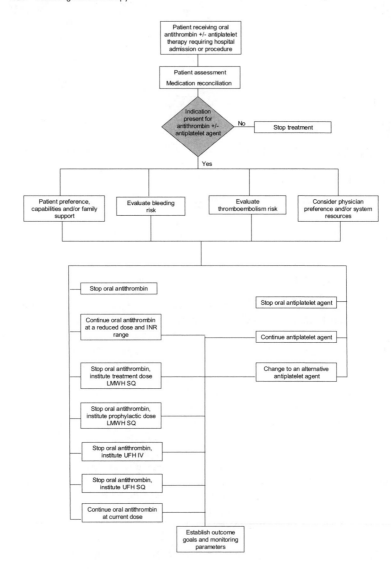

Figure 8-1: Patient Assessment and Outcome Goals

- Assess bleeding risk
  - Associated with parenteral antithrombotic therapy
  - Associated with surgical or invasive procedure
- Weigh risk vs. benefits
  - Consider patient and physician's goals and preferences

PERIPROCEDURAL THROMBOEMBOLIC RISK ASSESSMENT

- Patients should undergo a thorough assessment for thromboembolism using risk stratification.[1]
- Identify level of thromboembolism risk based on underlying disease and comorbidities.

Table 8-1: Risk Assessment and Stratification for Venous and Arterial Thromboembolism During the Periprocedural Period[1]

INDICATION FOR ANTICOAGULATION OR ANTIPLATELET THERAPY

		Arterial Thrombosis		Venous Thrombosis	
TE Risk Category	**Event Rate**	**Mechanical Heart Valves or Stents**	**Atrial Fibrillation**	**Venous Thrombo-embolism**	**Thrombophilia**
High risk	>10% per yr 1% per yr	Mitral valve prosthesis Caged ball or tilting disc aortic valve prosthesis Stroke or TIA within 6 mo Bare metal stent implantation within 1 mo, drug-eluting stent within 12 mo	$CHADS_2$ score ≥5 Stroke or TIA within 3 mo Rheumatic valvular heart disease	DVT or PE within 3 mo	Protein C deficiency Protein S deficiency Antithrombin deficiency Homozygous factor V Leiden gene mutation Homozygous prothrombin gene mutation

(continued)

Table 8-1: (Continued)

INDICATION FOR ANTICOAGULATION OR ANTIPLATELET THERAPY

		Arterial Thrombosis		Venous Thrombosis	
TE Risk Category	Event Rate	Mechanical Heart Valves or Stents	Atrial Fibrillation	Venous Thrombo-embolism	Thrombophilia
Moderate risk	5% to 10% per yr	Bileaflet aortic valve prosthesis plus • atrial fibrillation • prior stroke • prior TIA • hypertension • diabetes • CHF • age ≥75	CHADS$_2$ score 3 or 4	DVT or PE within 3–12 mo Recurrent DVT or PE Active cancer or cancer treatment within 6 mo	Heterozygous factor V Leiden gene mutation Heterozygous prothrombin gene mutation
Low risk	<5% per yr	Bileaflet aortic valve prosthesis and no other risk factors for stroke	CHADS$_2$ score of 0 to 2 (and no prior stroke or TIA)	Single VTE event >12 mo and no other risk factors	Hyperhomocysteinemia Elevated Factors VIII, IX, XI

Abbreviations: DVT = deep vein thrombosis; PE = pulmonary embolism; TIA = transischemic attack; TE = thromboembolism.

CHADS$_2$ scoring: please see Chapter 12. Congestive heart failure = 1 point; hypertension = 1 point; age over 75 = 1 point; diabetes mellitus = 1 point; prior stroke = 2 points.

Determining procedural risk of hemorrhage

- Assess the risk of bleeding from the procedure.[2,3]

- Incidence of hemorrhage will depend on the procedure and occur in as many as 11.9% of patients during routine surgery. Published bleeding rates include the following:
    - Thoracic surgery 33.7%
    - Abdominal surgery 11.4%
    - Other major surgery 14.3%

- Two thirds of bleeding events will occur within 48 hours after the intervention.
- Procedures in closed areas or cavities carry a high risk for hemorrhagic complications:
  - Pericardial region (related to pacemaker/internal cardiac defibrillator (ICD) insertion)
  - Spinal (related to trauma from lumbar puncture or epidural placement)
  - Urologic procedures (involving the retroperitoneum or bladder lumen)

Table 8-2: Procedural Risk of Hemorrhage[2,3]

Category of Bleeding Risk	Invasive or Surgical Procedure
Low or minimal bleeding risk	Arthrocentesis
	Arthroscopy
	Biopsy (prostate, bladder, thyroid, breast, lymph node, pancreas)
	Bronchoscopy +/− biopsy
	Cataract eye surgery
	Central venous catheter removal
	Coronary angiography +/− percutaneous coronary intervention (radial less bleeding risk than femoral)
	Dental hygiene or extraction (single or multiple)
	Electrophysiologic testing
	Joint and soft tissue injections
	Noncoronary angiography
	Gastrointestinal endoscopy or colonoscopy with or without biopsy
Moderate	Intra-abdominal surgery
	• Abdominal hernia repair, abdominal hysterectomy, appendectomy, bowel resection, cholecystectomy, polypectomy

(*continued*)

Table 8-2: (Continued)

Category of Bleeding Risk	Invasive or Surgical Procedure
	Orthopedic surgery
	• Hip replacement surgery, knee replacement, shoulder surgery, foot surgery hand surgery, carpal tunnel repair
	Vascular surgery
	• Endarterectomy, carotid bypass surgery
	Other
	• Axillary node dissection
	• Dental surgery
	• Dilation and curettage
	• ICD or pacemaker insertion
	• Hemorrhoidal surgery or hydrocele repair
	• Noncataract eye surgery
	• Skin cancer excision
	• Sternotomy wire removal
High	Thoracic surgery
	• Abdominal aortic aneurysm repair, heart valve replacement, coronary artery bypass, lung surgery (lobectomy, wedge resection, segmentectomy, pneumonectomy)
	Cancer surgery
	• Urologic, gynecologic, head and neck, colorectal, breast
	Orthopedic
	• Bilateral knee replacement
	Neurosurgical
	• Cancer surgery of brain or spinal column, laminectomy
	Other
	• Transurethral prostate resection
	• Renal or hepatic biopsy

PERIPROCEDURAL BLEEDING RISK ASSESSMENT

- The procedure itself is one of the most important risk factors for bleeding.
- Consider patient risk factors and comorbidities that may impact oral or parenteral anticoagulation and increase procedural and postprocedural bleeding risk.
- Patients should undergo a thorough assessment for bleeding risk.

Table 8-3: Major Patient Risk Factors and Comorbidities Increasing Bleeding Risk with Anticoagulation[4-7]

Risk Factor or Comorbidity	Explanation
Increasing age	Risk increases as age increases over 55 years
History of bleeding	Higher risk with more recent bleeding event (e.g., gastrointestinal, intraocular, hematuria, etc.)
Vascular disease	Prior stroke or peripheral vascular disease
Renal dysfunction	Creatinine clearance[a] <90 mL/min or serum creatinine >1.2 mg/dL associated with higher risk
Hepatic dysfunction	Associated with altered coagulation function and a higher risk of bleeding with worsening liver function
Congestive heart failure	Exacerbations may alter anticoagulant response and pharmacodynamics
Anemia	Hematocrit, <30% or hemoglobin <13 g/dL males, <12 g/dL females is associated with higher risk
Cancer	Bleeding risk correlates with the extent of cancer
Hypotension	Systolic blood pressure <100 mm of Hg
Hypertension	Systolic blood pressure >200 mm of Hg
Female	Predictor of higher risk, exact mechanism is unknown
Diabetes mellitus	Impacts many risk factors that increase bleeding risk

[a]Calculated using Cockcroft-Gault formula.

- Various prognostic and scoring indices for bleeding exist for initiating VKA therapy, in-hospital risk, and postprocedural risk.[4-7]
- Consider using an appropriate bleeding index to identify patient's risk level for bleeding.

TRANSITIONING FROM ORAL ANTICOAGULATION TO PARENTERAL THERAPY

- Based on thromboembolism and bleeding risk, devise a "bridge" strategy.[1]
- Planning and timely intervention can tailor anticoagulant therapy and thereby balance thromboembolism and bleeding risk.
- When warfarin is restarted, often the maintenance dose is utilized. When there is a desire for earlier "measured" INR response, another option is to start with an increased dose for the initial 2–3 days (≈50% increase in the maintenance dose), then follow with the usual maintenance dose.
- Low molecular weight heparin (LMWH) prophylactic doses have never been studied in the arena of preventing arterial thromboembolism. Thus, when bridging for atrial fibrillation and mechanical heart valves, therapeutic dosing is usually preferred.
- Registry data suggest "bridging" may be unnecessary for the vast majority of patients in an anticoagulation management service with warfarin continued uninterrupted or at a lower intensity.[8-12]
- Patients receiving higher weekly warfarin doses are likely to eliminate the drug faster and return to baseline INR earlier than those patients on low weekly warfarin doses.
- Standardized LMWH "bridge" regimens often result in significant residual anticoagulant activity shortly before surgery.[13]
- Patients with impaired renal function are likely to have delayed LMWH clearance.
- Residual LMWH activity, as measured by anti-Factor Xa testing, can last 24 hours after a dose.
- Consider any events during the intraoperative and immediate postoperative period (excessive bleeding or bleeding vessels that required intervention) that may impact reinitiating anticoagulation.

- The decision to restart anticoagulation after a procedure must be made in consultation with the surgeon or proceduralist.
- Duration of LMWH bridging may be significantly longer (12 days) than that seen in reported clinical trials.[14]
- Tailoring a LMWH regimen to patients risk using a reduced dose (70 anti-Factor Xa units/kg twice daily) in high-risk patients or a prophylactic dose regimen in low-to-moderate risk patients provides a low incidence of thromboembolic rates (0.4%) and a low incidence of major bleeding (1.2%).[15]

Table 8-4: Risk Assessment for Thromboembolism[1,a]

TE Risk Category	Bleeding Risk		
	Very Low or Low	**Moderate or Intermediate**	**High or Very High**
Low risk	Continue warfarin therapy through hospitalization and/or procedure: • Adjust dose based on target INR Continue AP therapy through hospitalization and/or procedure	Continue warfarin therapy through hospitalization and/or procedure: • Adjust dose based on target INR; warfarin can be held if needed; parenteral bridging is rarely needed preprocedure and VTE prophylaxis doses with parenteral anticoagulants can be considered postprocedure Continue AP therapy through hospitalization and/or procedure	Stop warfarin therapy 5–7 days before procedure: • Allow INR to return to normal • IF INR is >1.5 1–2 days before surgery, give vitamin K 1 mg orally Stop clopidogrel, prasugrel, or cilostazol 5–10 days before surgery; continue aspirin therapy through hospitalization and/or procedure if at high risk for coronary events Postprocedure: restart warfarin the day of or after the procedure; restart AP therapy approximately 24 hr after the procedure. VTE prophylaxis doses with parenteral anticoagulants can be considered

(continued)

Table 8-4: (Continued)

TE Risk Category	Bleeding Risk		
	Very Low or Low	**Moderate or Intermediate**	**High or Very High**
Moderate risk	Continue warfarin therapy through hospitalization and/or procedure: • Adjust dose based on target INR Continue AP therapy through hospitalization and/or procedure	Stop warfarin 5 days before surgery Allow the INR to return to normal Consider "bridge" therapy 2 days preprocedure: • Prophylactic or therapeutic dose LMWH (therapeutic preferred for valves and atrial fibrillation) Stop LMWH dosing 24 hr before surgery: • If once daily LMWH used, the last dose should be half the total daily dose Continue AP therapy through hospitalization and/or procedure Postprocedure: restart parenteral anticoagulation 24 hr postoperative; consider initial prophylactic LMWH dosing if later escalation to therapeutic dosing is planned; restart warfarin the day of or after the procedure	Stop warfarin 5–7 days before surgery Allow the INR to return to normal Begin "bridge" therapy 2 days preprocedure: • Prophylactic or therapeutic dose LMWH (therapeutic preferred for valves and atrial fibrillation) Stop LMWH dosing 24 hr before surgery: • If once daily LMWH used, the last dose should be half the total daily dose Stop clopidogrel, prasugrel, or cilostazol 5–10 days before surgery Continue aspirin therapy through hospitalization and/or procedure if at high risk for coronary events Postprocedure: restart parenteral anticoagulation 24 hr postoperative; consider initial prophylactic LMWH dosing if later escalation to therapeutic LMWH is planned; restart warfarin the day of or after the procedure; restart AP therapy approximately 24 hr after the procedure

(continued)

Table 8-4: (Continued)

TE Risk Category	Bleeding Risk		
	Very Low or Low	**Moderate or Intermediate**	**High or Very High**
High risk	Continue warfarin therapy through hospitalization and/or procedure: • Adjust dose based on target INR Continue AP therapy through hospitalization and/or procedure	Stop warfarin 5 days before surgery; allow the INR to return to normal Begin "bridge" therapy 2 days preprocedure: • Therapeutic dose LMWH • Therapeutic adjusted IV UFH Stop LMWH dosing 24 hr before surgery: • If once daily LMWH used, the last dose should be half the total daily dose Discontinue IV UFH 4–6 hr before surgery Continue AP therapy through hospitalization and/or procedure Postprocedure: restart parenteral anticoagulation 24 hr postoperative; consider initial prophylactic LMWH dosing if later escalation to therapeutic parenteral anticoagulation is planned; restart warfarin the day of or after the procedure	Stop warfarin 5–7 days before surgery; allow the INR to return to normal; begin "bridge" therapy 2 days preprocedure: • Therapeutic dose LMWH • Therapeutic adjusted IV UFH Stop LMWH dosing 24 hr before surgery: • If once daily LMWH used, the last dose should be half the total daily dose Discontinue IV UFH 4–6 hr before surgery Stop clopidogrel, prasugrel, or cilostazol 5–10 days before surgery Continue aspirin therapy through hospitalization and/or procedure if at high risk for coronary events Postprocedure: restart therapeutic dose UFH/LMWH 48–72 hr postoperative; prophylactic dose UFH/LMWH could be considered earlier provided hemostasis is achieved; restart warfarin the day of or after the procedure; restart AP therapy approximately 24 hr after the procedure

Abbreviation: TE = thromboembolic.

[a]Please note that individual patient situations could cause significant variation from this proposed table. Further, postoperative parenteral anticoagulant and AP therapies should not be started until adequate hemostasis is achieved.

- Low dose vitamin K 1 mg can be given to normalize INR the day before surgery without conferring warfarin resistance postoperative.[16]

- Dual AP therapy should be continued for 1 month with a bare metal stent (BMS) and for up to 12 months or more with drug-eluting stent (DES) insertion.[17]

- The greatest risk for acute stent thrombosis with interruption of dual AP therapy is in the first 14 days after implantation.[18]

- Postoperative stent thrombosis can occur as late as 4 years after DES implantation.[19]

Steps to consider in transitioning anticoagulation therapy for periprocedural bleeding

- Operationalize an individualized plan for the patient (Figure 8-2).

CONSIDERATIONS IN USING ANTICOAGULANT/ ANTIPLATELET THERAPY IN CONJUNCTION WITH NEURAXIAL ANESTHESIA

- Ensure safe transition with anticoagulation through neuraxial (spinal or epidural) procedural anesthesia (Table 8-5).

- Avoid risks of spinal hematoma.
  - Incidence with no anticoagulant; 1:220,000 with epidural anesthesia and 1:2,320,000 with spinal anesthesia
  - Incidence with heparin; 1:70,000 with epidural anesthesia and 1:100,000 with spinal anesthesia

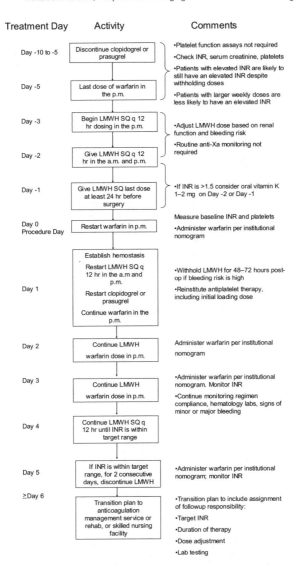

Treatment Day	Activity	Comments
Day -10 to -5	Discontinue clopidogrel or prasugrel	•Platelet function assays not required
		•Check INR, serum creatinine, platelets
Day -5	Last dose of warfarin in the p.m.	•Patients with elevated INR are likely to still have an elevated INR despite withholding doses
		•Patients with larger weekly doses are less likely to have an elevated INR
Day -3	Begin LMWH SQ q 12 hr dosing in the p.m.	•Adjust LMWH dose based on renal function and bleeding risk
Day -2	Give LMWH SQ q 12 hr in the a.m. and p.m.	•Routine anti-Xa monitoring not required
Day -1	Give LMWH SQ last dose at least 24 hr before surgery	•If INR is >1.5 consider oral vitamin K 1–2 mg on Day -2 or Day -1
Day 0 Procedure Day	Restart warfarin in p.m.	Measure baseline INR and platelets
		•Administer warfarin per institutional nomogram
Day 1	Establish hemostasis Restart LMWH SQ q 12 hr in the a.m and p.m. Restart clopidogrel or prasugrel Continue warfarin in the p.m.	•Withhold LMWH for 48–72 hours post-op if bleeding risk is high
		•Reinstitute antiplatelet therapy, including initial loading dose
Day 2	Continue LMWH warfarin dose in p.m.	Administer warfarin per institutional nomogram
Day 3	Continue LMWH warfarin dose in p.m.	•Administer warfarin per institutional nomogram. Monitor INR
		•Continue monitoring regimen compliance, hematology labs, signs of minor or major bleeding
Day 4	Continue LMWH SQ q 12 hr until INR is within target range	
Day 5	If INR is within target range, for 2 consecutive days, discontinue LMWH	•Administer warfarin per institutional nomogram; monitor INR
≥Day 6	Transition plan to anticoagulation management service or rehab, or skilled nursing facility	•Transition plan to include assignment of followup responsibility:
		•Target INR
		•Duration of therapy
		•Dose adjustment
		•Lab testing

Figure 8-2: Periprocedural Patient Activities

Table 8-5: Guidelines for Regional Anesthesia with Anticoagulation or Antiplatelet Use[20]

AGENT OR CLASS

Neuraxial Anesthesia Technique	Fibrinolytic Therapy	UFH Prophylaxis	Intravenous UFH	LMWH Prophylaxis	LMWH Therapeutic	Warfarin	Antiplatelet Therapy
Epidural or spinal anesthesia needle or catheter insertion	Avoid fibrinolytic administration for at least 10 days after puncture If patients are to receive fibrinolytic therapy, neuraxial anesthesia techniques should be avoided	5,000 units SC BID dosing is considered acceptable The safety of 5,000 units SC TID dosing has not been established	Delay heparin administration until 1 hr after needle placement	Presence of blood during needle and catheter placement delays initiation of LMWH 24 hr		Stop warfarin at least 4–5 days prior to procedure INR should be checked prior to insertion if warfarin given more than 24 hr earlier	Stop GP IIb/IIIa inhibitors 8 hr (eptifibatide, tirofiban) to 48 hr (abciximab) prior to needle placement
				Pre-op LMWH prophylaxis dosing: delay needle placement at least 10–12 hr after the LMWH dose Post-op LMWH daily dosing: administer first LMWH dose 6–8 hr post-op; administer second dose no sooner than 24 hr after the first dose Post-op LMWH BID dosing: first LMWH dose no earlier than 24 hr postop; indwelling catheters should be removed prior to BID LMWH initiation	Pre-op LMWH therapeutic doses: delay needle placement by at least 24 hr after LMWH dose; indwelling catheters should be removed prior to LMWH initiation	INR must be normal prior to needle placement Patients receiving warfarin therapy during epidural analgesia should have INR monitored daily	Stop clopidogrel 7 days prior to needle placement Stop ticlopidine 14 days prior to needle placement

Table 8-5: (Continued)

Neuraxial Anesthesia Technique	Fibrinolytic Therapy	UFH Prophylaxis	Intravenous UFH	LMWH Prophylaxis	LMWH Therapeutic	Warfarin	Antiplatelet Therapy
Epidural or spinal anesthesia catheter removal	No recommendation If fibrinolytic therapy is given, monitor fibrinogen level recovery as guidance	No contraindications	Remove indwelling catheter 2–4 hr after the last heparin dose Reheparinize 1 hr after catheter removal	Catheter removal a minimum of 10–12 hr after last LMWH dose Administer first dose 2 hr after catheter[a] removal	Catheter removal a minimum of 24 hr after the last dose of LMWH	Check INR prior to catheter removal Catheters should ideally be removed when INR is below 1.5 but removal can be cautiously considered if INR 1.5–3.0	Catheters must be removed prior to initiating eptifibatide, tirofiban, abciximab, clopidogrel, or ticlopidine

[a]Epidural clinical pearls. Many health systems choose to avoid LMWH prophylaxis in conjunction with indwelling epidural catheters due to the complex requirements needed to do it safely. Many health systems consider delaying warfarin re-initiation until catheter is removed to avoid complications in catheter removal.

CONVERTING FROM INTRAVENOUS ANTICOAGULATION TO SUBCUTANEOUS THERAPY

- During hospitalization patients may require transition between parenteral therapies or as a "bridge" to VKA.

- Consider differences in pharmacokinetic properties of UFH and LMWH (or fondaparinux).

- Avoid concurrent use of parenteral anticoagulant agents to ensure safety.

- When transitioning from IVUFH to an alternative parenteral anticoagulant agent with rapid onset of activity, it may be preferable to wait a selected period of time before initiating the alternative therapy in patients at increased risk of bleeding.

- Because of potential distractions and logistic considerations, consider stopping the UFH at the same time as initiating any new anticoagulant unless an atypical clinical situation is present.

Table 8-6: Practical Considerations for Transitioning Between Various Parenteral Anticoagulants

Conversion from adjusted-dose IV UFH infusion to adjusted-dose SC UFH	• Calculate the 24-hr IV UFH dose requirement needed to maintain therapeutic aPTT • Increase the total 24-hr UFH dose requirement by 10% to 20% (SC dosage requirements are higher than IV) • Divide the dose calculated above by 2 to determine the initial q12 hr SC dosing requirement • Discontinue IV UFH and initiate the first SC UFH dose (as calculated above) within 1 hr • Check aPTT or anti-Factor Xa activity level at 6 hr after first SC dose • Adjust further SC UFH doses based on aPTT or anti-Factor Xa activity level • Ensure a heparin 10,000- or 20,000-unit/mL concentration is available (ensure your dispensing procedures ensure the safe use of these agents due to the well-known neonatal intensive care heparin errors)
Conversion from IV UFH infusion to SC LMWH (or SC fondaparinux)	• Calculate the appropriate LMWH (or fondaparinux) dose based on the specific indication for use and patient weight • Discontinue IV UFH

(*continued*)

Table 8-6: (Continued)

	• Initiate the first SC LMWH (or fondaparinux) dose within 1 hr
	• If aPTT drawn within the last 6 hr is greater than 100 sec or an anti-Factor Xa activity level greater than 1 International Unit/mL, wait 2 hr before administering LMWH (or fondaparinux)
Conversion from SC LMWH (or fondaparinux) to IV UFH infusion	• Calculate the appropriate IV UFH dose based on indication for use and patient weight
	• Discontinue SC LMWH (or fondaparinux)
	• Omit bolus or loading dose
	• Initiate IV UFH 1–2 hr before the next scheduled LMWH or fondaparinux dose administration:
	a. When switching from SC LMWH given q 12 hr, initiate IV UFH at 10–11 hr after last LMWH dose
	b. When switching from SC LMWH given q 24 hr, initiate IV UFH at 22–23 hr after last LMWH dose
	c. When switching from SC fondaparinux given q 24 hr, initiate IV UFH at 22–23 hr after last fondaparinux dose
	d. Evaluate patient's renal status and if impaired, the IV UFH dosing initiation intervals suggested in a–c above need to be extended accordingly
	• Check aPTT or anti-Factor Xa activity level at 6 hr after initiating the IV UFH infusion
	• Adjust further UFH doses based on aPTT or anti-Factor Xa activity level and dosing nomogram
Conversion from SC LMWH (or fondaparinux) to adjusted-dose SC UFH	• Calculate the adjusted-dose SC UFH dosing requirements: the recommended initial dose is 250 units/kg SC given q 12 hr
	• Ensure a heparin 10,000- or 20,000-unit/mL concentration is available (see the above precaution on these dosing forms)
	• Discontinue SC LMWH (or fondaparinux)
	• Initiate SC UFH at the time the next SC LMWH (or fondaparinux) dose is scheduled to be administered:
	a. When switching from SC LMWH given q 12 hr, initiate SC UFH at 12 hr after last LMWH dose
	b. When switching from SC LMWH given q 24 hr, initiate SC UFH at 24 hr after last LMWH dose
	c. When switching from SC fondaparinux given q 24 hr, initiate SC UFH at 24 hr after last fondaparinux dose

(continued)

Table 8-6: (Continued)

	d. Evaluate patient's renal status; if impaired, the SC UFH dosing initiation intervals suggested in a–c above need to be extended accordingly
	• aPTT or anti-Factor Xa activity level should be drawn at 6 hr (mid-interval) after the first SC UFH dose
	• Subsequent SC UFH doses should be adjusted based on aPTT or anti-Factor Xa activity level and dosing nomogram
Conversion between prophylactic fixed dose UFH to LMWH (or fondaparinux) or LMWH (or fondaparinux) to UFH	• For patients receiving prophylactic SC UFH q 8 or 12 hr, discontinue UFH
	• Evaluate patient's renal status and determine appropriate LMWH (or fondaparinux) dose and interval
	• Administer LMWH (or fondaparinux) at the next scheduled dose administration time
	• Continue LMWH dosing per prescribed regimen
	• For patients receiving prophylactic SC LMWH (or fondaparinux) q 12 or 24 hr, discontinue LMWH (or fondaparinux)
	• Administer UFH at the next scheduled dose administration time
	• Continue UFH dosing q 8 or 12 hr per prescribed regimen

TRANSITIONING FROM PARENTERAL ANTICOAGULATION TO ORAL VKA THERAPY

- For patients with active thrombosis, UFH or LMWH is administered concurrently and overlapped with warfarin for at least 5 days and until the INR has reached a therapeutic range for 24 hours.
- INR ranges will vary depending on indication for anticoagulation.
- For warfarin naïve patients, initiation nomograms can avoid excessive anticoagulation and rapidly achieve target INR with a starting dose between 5 and 10 mg.[21–23]
- For previously treated warfarin patients, re-initiate therapy at prior chronic maintenance dose.
- Warfarin loading doses are not warranted and may elevate the patient's risk of bleeding.
- Elderly patients with comorbidities or recent surgery should initiate warfarin with a dose ≤5 mg.
- For younger, heavier patients, consider larger initial doses (5.0–7.5 mg).
- Consider clinically significant disease states and drug–drug interactions.

- INR monitoring starts, at the latest, after the first initial 2–3 VKA doses. Unstable patients in the hospital should have daily monitoring.

- Warfarin maintenance doses are adjusted based on the cumulative weekly dosage with increases or decreases of no more than 10% to 20% of the weekly dose. Any variation in doses from day-to-day should be spread evenly over the week.

NOVEL ANTICOAGULANTS PENDING FOOD AND DRUG ADMINISTRATION APPROVAL

- Orally active agents that target thrombin (factor IIa) and factor Xa are in late stages of drug development for a wide variety of thromboembolic indications including both prevention and treatment.

- Novel agents are administered in fixed doses and do not require coagulation monitoring.

- Dabigatran etexilate and rivaroxaban are approved in the European Union and Canada for VTE prophylaxis in patients undergoing elective hip or knee replacement surgery.

- Other similar factor Xa inhibitors (apixaban, betrixaban, edoxaban, eribaxaban) and antithrombin inhibitors (AZD 0837, MCC-977) agents are in earlier phases of development.

- Agents vary in their site of action, onset, duration, and elimination.

Table 8-7: Comparison of Pharmacodynamic Properties of Novel Anticoagulants[24–26]

Agent	Target Clotting Factor	Reversible Binding to Catalytic Site	Bioavailability	Food Effect	t_{max} (hr)	$t_{1/2}$ (hr)	Renal Excretion	Agents for Reversal
Rivaroxaban	Xa	Yes	60% to 80%	Delayed absorption	1.25–3.0	7.0–7.6	36%	rFVIIa
Apixaban	Xa	Yes	66%	Not reported	1.0–3.0	8.0–15.0	25%	Not reported
Dabigatran	IIa	Yes	6.5%	Delayed absorption	1.25–3.0	12.0–17.2	80%	rFVIIa, APPC

Abbreviations: t_{max} = time to reach maximum plasma concentrations; $t_{1/2}$ = half-life; rVIIa = recombinant activated factor VII; APPC = activated prothrombin complex concentrate.

TRANSITION TO NOVEL ANTICOAGULANTS

- For guidance on dosing and therapy transitions, follow the dosing and treatment schemas from published clinical trials.[27–30]

- In the absence of information, evaluate concomitant therapies based on actual half-lives needed for wash out of the initial agent and the onset of action of the second drug.

- Medications following first order or linear elimination at the end of one $t_{1/2}$, 50% of the medication is eliminated, and at the end of five $t_{1/2}$'s, 97% of the drug is eliminated.

- Data are still emerging with limited information in special populations (elderly, obese, organ dysfunction, etc.).

Table 8-8: Practical Considerations for Transitioning Between Various Novel Anticoagulants[24–31]

Conversion from adjusted-dose IV UFH infusion to oral rivaroxaban, dabigatran, or apixaban	Consider pharmacodynamics: IV UFH ($t_{1/2}$ = 60 min) Consider t_{max} for oral agent Stop IV UFH infusion Rivaroxaban, dabigatran,[30] or apixaban: 1. Administer first oral dose of rivaroxaban, dabigatran, or apixaban at the time of UFH discontinuation 2. Continue novel antithrombotic agent per prescribed regimen
Conversion from SC LMWH (or SC fondaparinux) therapeutic dosing to oral rivaroxaban, dabigatran, or apixaban	Consider pharmacodynamics: LMWH ($t_{1/2}$ = 6–7 hr), fondaparinux ($t_{1/2}$ = 17–21 hr) SC Consider t_{max} for oral agent Rivaroxaban, dabigatran, or apixaban: 1. Give rivaroxaban, dabigatran, or apixaban 0–2 hr before next LMWH (or fondaparinux) dose 2. Stop all following parenteral doses 3. Continue novel antithrombotic agent per prescribed regimen

(*continued*)

Table 8-8: (Continued)

Converting from prophylactic dose SC UFH, LMWH (or fondaparinux) to oral rivaroxaban, dabigatran, or apixaban prophylactic dose	Stop current parenteral prophylaxis agent Rivaroxaban, dabigatran, or apixaban: 1. Administer rivaroxaban, dabigatran, or apixaban orally at the time of the next scheduled parenteral dose 2. Continue dosing per prescribed regimen
Converting from direct thrombin inhibitor (bivalirudin, argatroban, or lepirudin) IV infusion to oral therapeutic dose rivaroxaban, dabigatran, or apixaban	Consider pharmacodynamics: bivalirudin (t$\frac{1}{2}$ = 25 min), argatroban (t$\frac{1}{2}$ = 45 min), lepirudin (t$\frac{1}{2}$ = 60 min) IV[26] Consider t_{max} for oral agent Aim for oral agent t_{max} to correspond to direct thrombin inhibitor elimination Rivaroxaban, dabigatran, or apixaban: 1. Administer first rivaroxaban, dabigatran, or apixaban oral dose 1 hr prior to bivalirudin infusion cessation or immediately at cessation of argatroban or lepirudin infusion 2. Evaluate patient's renal and hepatic status; if impaired, extend initiation interval accordingly
Converting from warfarin to oral rivaroxaban, dabigatran, or apixaban	For all novel agents: 1. Give final warfarin dose 2. Wait 2–3 days 3. When INR <2.0, give first dose of rivaroxaban, dabigatran, or apixaban
Converting from oral therapeutic dose rivaroxaban, dabigatran, or apixaban to adjusted-dose IV UFH infusion	Discontinue novel oral agent Wait 2–5 half-lives estimating 75% to 97% of the drug will washout UFH will peak in 4–6 hr after infusion initiation Rivaroxaban: 1. Wait 1–2 days 2. Calculate the appropriate IV infusion UFH dose based on indication for use and patient weight 3. Omit bolus or loading dose 4. Evaluate patient's renal status; if impaired, the IV UFH dosing initiation interval needs to be extended accordingly

(continued)

Table 8-8: (Continued)

	5. Check aPTT or anti-Factor Xa activity level at 6 hr after initiating the IV UFH infusion
	6. Adjust further UFH doses based on aPTT or anti-Factor Xa activity level and dosing nomogram
	Dabigatran:
	1. Wait 12–24 hr
	2. Calculate the appropriate IV infusion UFH dose based on indication for use and patient weight
	3. Omit bolus or loading dose
	4. Evaluate patient's renal status; if impaired, the IV UFH dosing initiation interval needs to be extended accordingly
	5. Check aPTT or anti-Factor Xa activity level at 6 hr after initiating the IV UFH infusion
	6. Adjust further UFH doses based on aPTT or anti-Factor Xa activity level and dosing nomogram
	Apixaban:
	1. Wait 2–3 days
	2. Calculate the appropriate IV infusion UFH dose based on indication for use and patient weight
	3. Omit bolus or loading dose
	4. Check aPTT or anti-Factor Xa activity level at 6 hr after initiating the IV UFH infusion
	5. Adjust further UFH doses based on aPTT or anti-Factor Xa activity level and dosing nomogram
Converting oral rivaroxaban, dabigatran, or apixaban to LMWH (or fondaparinux)	Discontinue novel oral agent
	Consider peak activity for LMWH (3–5 hr) or fondaparinux (3 hr)
	Calculate the appropriate LMWH (or fondaparinux) dose based on the specific indication for use and patient weight
	Rivaroxaban:
	1. Wait 1–2 days
	2. Calculate the appropriate LMWH/fondaparinux dose based on indication for use and patient weight

(continued)

Table 8-8: (Continued)

	3. Evaluate patient's renal status; if impaired, the LMWH dosing initiation interval needs to be extended accordingly
	Dabigatran:
	1. Wait 12 hr for patients with a creatinine clearance ≥30 mL/min; wait 24 hr for patients with a creatinine clearance <30 mL/min
	2. Calculate the appropriate LMWH/fondaparinux dose based on indication for use and patient weight
	Apixaban:
	1. Wait 2–3 days
	2. Calculate the appropriate LMWH/fondaparinux dose based on indication for use and patient weight
	3. Evaluate patient's renal and hepatic status; if impaired, the LMWH dosing initiation interval needs to be extended accordingly

REFERENCES

1. Douketis JD, Berger PB, Dunn AS, et al. The perioperative management of antithrombotic therapy. American College of Chest Physicians Evidence-Based Clinical Practice Guidelines (8th ed.). *Chest*. 2008;133:299S–339S.

2. Douketis JD, Johnson JA, Turpie AG. Low-molecular-weight heparin as bridging anticoagulation during interruption of warfarin. Assessment of a standardized periprocedural anticoagulation regimen. *Arch Intern Med*. 2004;164:1319–1326.

3. Torn M, Rosendaal FR. Oral anticoagulation in surgical procedures: risks and recommendations. *Br J Surg*. 2003;123:676–682.

4. Ruiz-Giménez N, Suárez C, González R, et al. Predictive variables for major bleeding events in patients presenting with documented acute venous thromboembolism. Findings from the RIETE Registry. *Thromb Haemost*. 2008;100:26–31.

5. Wells PS, Forgie MA, Simms M, et al. The outpatient bleeding risk index. *Arch Intern Med*. 2003;163:917–920.

6. Subherwal S Bach RG, Chen AY, et al. Baseline risk of major bleeding in non–ST-segment–elevation myocardial infarction. The CRUSADE (Can Rapid risk stratification of Unstable angina patients Suppress ADverse outcomes with Early implementation of the ACC/AHA guidelines) bleeding score. *Circulation*. 2009;119:1873–1882.

7. Nikolsky E, Mehran R, Dangas G, et al. Development and validation of a prognostic risk score for major bleeding in patients undergoing percutaneous coronary intervention via the femoral approach. *Eur Heart J.* 2007;28:1936–1945.

8. Garcia DA, Regan S, Henault LE, et al. Risk of thromboembolism with short-term interruption of warfarin therapy. *Arch Intern Med.* 2008;168:63–69.

9. Wanzi OM, Beheiry A, Fahmy T, et al. Atrial fibrillation in patients with therapeutic international normalized ration. Comparison of strategies of anticoagulation management in the periprocedural period. *Circulation.* 2007;116:2531–2534.

10. Beldi G, Beng L, Siegel G, et al. Prevention of perioperative thromboembolism in patients with atrial fibrillation. *Br J Surg.* 2007;94:1351–1355.

11. Bonow RO, Carabello BA, Chatterjee K, et al. ACC/AHA 2006 Guidelines for the management of patients with valvular heart disease: executive summary. A report of the American College of Cardiology/American Heart Association Task Force on Practice Guidelines. *Circulation.* 2006;114:450–452.

12. Larson BJG, Zumberg MS, Kitchen CS. A feasibility study of continuing dose-reduced warfarin for invasive procedures in patients with high thromboembolic risk. *Chest.* 2005;127:922–927.

13. O'Donnell MJ, Kearon C, Johnson J, et al. Brief communication: Preoperative anticoagulant activity after bridging low-molecular-weight heparin for temporary interruption of warfarin. *Ann Intern Med.* 2007;146:184–187.

14. Eerhake JP, Merz JC, Cooper JV. The duration of anticoagulation bridging therapy in clinical practice may significantly exceed that observed in clinical trials. *J Thromb Thrombolysis.* 2007;23:107–113.

15. Pengo V, Cucchini U, Denas G, et al. Standardized low-molecular-weight heparin bridging regimen in outpatients on oral anticoagulants undergoing invasive procedure or surgery. An inception cohort study. *Circulation.* 2009;119:2920–2927.

16. Woods K, Douketis JD, Kathirgamanathan K, et al. Low-dose oral vitamin k to normalize the international normalized ratio prior to surgery in patients who require temporary interruption of warfarin. *J Thromb Thrombolysis.* 2007;24:93–97.

17. Grines CL, Bonow RO, Casey DE, et al. Prevention of premature discontinuation of dual antiplatelet therapy in patients with coronary artery stents. A science advisory from the American Heart Association, American College of Cardiology, Society for Cardiovascular Angiography and Interventions, American College of Surgeons, and American Dental Association, With Representation From the American College of Physicians. *Circulation.* 2007;115:813–818.

18. Collet JP, Montalescot G. Premature withdrawal of and alternative therapies to dual oral Antiplatelet therapy. *Eur Heart J.* 2006;8(Suppl):G46–G52.

19. Spahn DR, Howell SJ, Delabays A, et al. Coronary stents and perioperative antiplatelet regimen: dilemma of bleeding and stent thrombosis. *Br J Anaesth.* 2006;96:657–677.

20. Horlocker TT, Wedel DJ, Rowlingson JC, et al. Regional anesthesia in the patient receiving antithrombotic or thrombolytic therapy (American Society of Regional

Anesthesia and Pain Medicine evidence-based guidelines, third edition). *Reg Anesth Pain Manag.* 2010;35:64–101.

21. Harrison L, Johnston M, Massicotte MP, et al. Comparison of 5 mg and 10 mg loading doses in initiation of warfarin therapy. *Ann Intern Med.* 1997;126:133–136.

22. Crowther MA, Ginsberg JB, Kearon C, et al. A randomized trial comparing 5 mg and 10 mg loading doses. *Arch Intern Med.* 1999;159:46–48.

23. Kovacs MJ, Roger M, Anderson DR, et al. Comparison of 10 mg and 5 mg warfarin initiation nomograms together with low molecular weight heparin for outpatient treatment of acute venous thromboembolism. *Ann Intern Med.* 2003;138:714–719.

24. Eriksson BI, Quinlan DJ, Weitz JI. Comparative pharmacodynamics and pharmacokinetics of oral direct thrombin and factor Xa inhibitors in development. *Clin Pharmacokinetics.* 2009;48:1–22.

25. Turpie AGG. New oral anticoagulants in atrial fibrillation. *Eur Heart J.* 2007;29:155–165.

26. Di Nisio M, Middeldorp S, Büller HR. Direct thrombin Inhibitors. *N Engl J Med.* 2005;353:1028–1040.

27. Mega JL, Braunwald E, Mohanavelu S, et al. Rivaroxaban versus placebo in patients with acute coronary syndromes (ATLAS ACS-TIMI 46): a randomized, double blind, phase II trial. *Lancet.* 2009;374:29–38.

28. Connolly SJ, Ezekowitz, MD, Yusuf S, et al. RE-LY Steering Committee and Investigators. Dabigatran versus warfarin in patients with atrial fibrillation. *N Engl J Med.* 2009;361:1139–1151.

29. Alexander JH, Becker RC, Bhatt DL, et al. APPRAISE Steering Committee and Investigators. Apixaban, an oral, direct, selective factor Xa inhibitor, in combination with antiplatelet therapy after acute coronary syndromes. Results of the Apixaban for Prevention of Acute Ischemic and Safety Events (APPRAISE) trial. *Circulation.* 2009;119:2877–2885.

30. Schulman S, Kearon C, Kakkar AK, et al. The RE-COVER Study Group. Dabigatran versus warfarin in the treatment of acute venous thromboembolism. *N Engl J Med.* 2009;361:2342–2352.

31. Ezekowitz MD, Connolly SJ, Parekh A, et al. Rationale and design of RE-LY: randomized evaluation of long-term anticoagulant therapy, warfarin, compared with dabigatran. *Am Heart J.* 2009;157:805–810.

KEY ARTICLES

Birnie D, Healey JS, Kranh A, et al. Bridge or continue coumadin for device surgery: a randomized controlled trial rationale and design. *Curr Opin Cardiol.* 2008;24: 82–87.

Dunn AS, Spyropoulos AC, Turpie AG. Bridging therapy in patients on long-term oral anticoagulants who require surgery: the Prospective Peri-operative Enoxaparin Cohort Trial (PROSPECT). *J Throm Haemos.* 2007;5:2211–2218.

Jaffer AK, Ahmed M, Brotman DJ, et al. Low-molecular-weight-heparins as periprocedural anticoagulation for patients on long-term warfarin therapy: a standardized bridging therapy protocol. *J Thromb Thrombolysis*. 2005;20:11–16.

O'Riordan JM, Margey RJ, Blake G, et al. Antiplatelet agents in the perioperative period. *Arch Surg*. 2009;144:69–76.

Rivas-Gandara N, Ferreira-Gonzalez I, Tornos P. Enoxaparin as bridging anticoagulant in cardiac surgery. *Heart*. 2008;94:205–210.

Seshadri N, Goldhaber SZ, Elkayam U, et al. The clinical challenge of bridging anticoagulation with low-molecular-weight heparin in patients with mechanical prosthetic heart valves: an evidence-based comparative review focusing on anticoagulation options in pregnant and nonpregnant patients. *Am Heart J*. 2005;150:27–34.

Spyropoulos AC, Douketis JD. Guidelines for antithrombotic therapy: periprocedural management of antithrombotic therapy and use of bridging anticoagulation. *Intnl Angiol*. 2008;27:333–343.

Spyropoulos AC, Frost FJ, Hurley JS, et al. Costs and clinical outcomes associated with low-molecular-weight heparin vs unfractionated heparin for perioperative bridging in patients receiving long-term oral anticoagulant therapy. *Chest*. 2004;125:1642–1650.

Thachil J, Gatt A, Martlew. Management of surgical patients receiving anticoagulation and antiplatelet agents. *Br J Surg*. 2008;95:1437–1448.

Wiegand WKH, LeJeune D, Boguschewski GF, et al. Pocket hematoma after pacemaker or implantable cardioverter defibrillator surgery. Influence of patient morbidity, operation strategy, and perioperative antiplatelet/anticoagulation therapy. *Chest*. 2004;126: 1177–1186.

NINE

Chapter

9

New Oral Anticoagulants

Ann K. Wittkowsky

INTRODUCTION

Considerable effort has been devoted to developing new oral anticoagulants that are as safe and effective as warfarin but that do not require routine anticoagulation monitoring and have practical advantages with respect to drug interactions, dietary considerations, disease state influences, etc. Three agents—dabigatran, rivaroxaban, and apixaban—are nearing approval in the US.

PHARMACOLOGY

The new oral agents are inhibitors of either factor IIa (dabigatran) or factor Xa (rivaroxaban, apixaban). They directly inhibit fIIa or fXa, without going through indirect mechanism like inhibiting vitamin K-dependent clotting factor synthesis (warfarin) or accelerating the action of antithrombin against factor Xa and/or factor IIa (heparin, low molecular weight heparins [LMWHs], fondaparinux). While theoretical arguments have been made regarding the potential superiority of either factor Xa or factor IIa as a target, only head-to-head clinical trials will resolve these questions.

Clinical Pearl

- Compared to traditional anticoagulants (i.e., heparin, warfarin), the new oral anticoagulants have a wider therapeutic window and more predictable dose-response; thus, these agents are not expected to require routine anticoagulation monitoring and frequent dosage adjustments in the majority of the patients.

Table 9-1: Selected New Oral Antithrombotic Agents in Development

	DABIGATRAN	**RIVAROXABAN**	**APIXABAN**
Mechanism of action	Direct factor IIa inhibitor	Direct factor Xa inhibitor	Direct factor Xa inhibitor
Manufacturer	Boehringer-Ingelheim	Bayer with Ortho McNeil	Pfizer with Bristol Myers Squibb
Brand name	Pradaxa (Europe) Pradax (Canada)	Xarelto (Europe and Canada)	Not yet assigned
Approval status	2008—approved in Europe/Canada for VTE prophylaxis in orthopedic surgery 2010—approved in US for stroke prevention in atrial fibrillation	2008—approved in Europe/Canada for VTE prophylaxis in orthopedic surgery 3/09—FDA advisory panel approval for VTE prophylaxis in orthopedic surgery 2011—submitted to FDA for stroke prevention in atrial fibrillation	Not yet approved

UPDATE OF PUBLISHED PHASE 3 CLINICAL TRIALS

The new oral anticoagulants are being investigated for a variety of indications, including prevention and treatment of venous thromboembolism (VTE), stroke prevention in atrial fibrillation, and acute coronary syndromes. Doses of each drug may be different for specific indications.

Table 9-2: Ongoing and Completed Phase III Clinical Trials Involving New Anticoagulants[a]

	Dabigatran		Rivaroxaban		Apixaban	
	Completed	Ongoing	Completed	Ongoing	Completed	Ongoing
Prevention of VTE in total hip replacement	RE-MOBILIZE RE-MODEL	RE-NOVATE-11	RECORD-1 RECORD-2		ADVANCE-3	
Prevention of VTE in total knee replacement	RE-NOVATE		RECORD-3 RECORD-4		ADVANCE-1 ADVANCE-2	
Prevention of VTE in acute medical illness				MAGELLAN		ADOPT
Treatment of VTE	RE-COVER	RE-MEDY RE-COVER-11 RE-SONATE	EINSTEIN-DVT EINSTIN-EXT	EINSTEIN-PE		AMPLIFY AMPLIFY-EXT
Stroke prevention in atrial fibrillation	RE-LY		ROCKET-AF		AVERROES	ARISTOTLE
Acute coronary syndromes		RE-DEEM		ATLAS	APPRAISE	

[a]See www.clinicaltrials.gov for details.

Table 9-3: Prevention of Venous Thromboembolism in Orthopedic Surgery

	DABIGATRAN			RIVAROXABAN				APIXABAN	
	RE-MOBILIZE[1] (n=2615)	RE-MODEL[2] (n=2101)	RE-NOVATE[3] (n=3494)	RECORD 1[4] (n=4541)	RECORD 2[5] (n=2509)	RECORD 3[6] (n=2531)	RECORD 4[7] (n=3148)	ADVANCE-1[8] (n=3195)	ADVANCE-2[9] (n=3057)
Target population	TKR	TKR	THR	THR	THR	TKR	TKR	TKR	TKR
Test therapies	D 150 or 220 mg every day	D 150 or 220 mg every day	D 150 or 220 mg every day	R 10 mg every day	R 10 mg every day	R 10 mg every day	R 10 mg every day	A 2.5 mg BID	A 2.5 mg BID
First dose of test therapy	6–12 hr post-op (½ dose)	1–4 hr post-op (½ dose)	1–4 hr post-op (½ dose)	6–8 hr post-op	6–8 hr post-op	6–8 hr post-op	6–8 hr post-op	12–24 hr post-op	12–24 hr post-op
Reference therapy	Enoxaparin 30 mg BID	Enoxaparin 40 mg every day	Enoxaparin 40 mg every day	Enoxaparin 40 mg every day	Enoxaparin 40 mg every day	Enoxaparin 40 mg every day	Enoxaparin 30 mg BID	Enoxaparin 30 mg BID	Enoxaparin 40 mg every day
First dose of reference therapy	12–24 hr post-op	Evening before surgery	Evening before surgery	12 hr pre-op	12 hr pre-op	12 hr pre-op	12–24 hr post-op	12–24 hr post-op	12 hr pre-op
Treatment duration	12–15 days	6–10 days	28–35 days	35 days	R 35 days E 14 days	14 days	14 days	12 +/– 2 days	12 +/– 2 days

(continued)

Table 9-3: (Continued)

	DABIGATRAN			RIVAROXABAN				APIXABAN	
	RE-MOBILIZE[1] (n=2615)	RE-MODEL[2] (n=2101)	RE-NOVATE[3] (n=3494)	RECORD 1[4] (n=4541)	RECORD 2[5] (n=2509)	RECORD 3[6] (n=2531)	RECORD 4[7] (n=3148)	ADVANCE-1[8] (n=3195)	ADVANCE-2[9] (n=3057)
Primary endpoint	Total VTE + all-cause mortality	Total VTE + all-cause mortality	Total VTE + all-cause mortality	Total VTE + all-cause mortality	Total VTE + all-cause mortality	Total VTE + all-cause mortality	Total VTE + all-cause mortality	Total VTE + all-cause mortality	Total VTE + all-cause mortality
Incidence of primary endpoint	D 150: 33.7% (p=0.02 vs. enoxaparin) D 220: 31.1% (p<0.001 vs. enoxaparin) Enoxaparin 25.7%	D 150: 40.5% D 220: 36.4% Enoxaparin 37.7%	D 150: 8.6% D 220: 6.0% Enoxaparin 6.7%	R 1.1% (p<0.001) Enoxaparin 3.7%	R 2.0% (p<0.001) Enoxaparin 9.3%	R 9.6% (p<0.001) Enoxaparin 18.9%	R 6.9% (p=0.012) Enoxaparin 10.1%	A 9.0% (p=0.06) Enoxaparin 8.8%	A 15.1% (p<0.001) Enoxaparin 24.4%
Analysis	D is inferior to enoxaparin	D is noninferior to enoxaparin	D is noninferior to enoxaparin	R is superior to enoxaparin	Extended R is superior to short-term enoxaparin	R is superior to enoxaparin	R is superior to enoxaparin	A is *not* noninferior to enoxaparin	A is superior to enoxaparin

Source: revised from reference 14.

Table 9-4: Bleeding Complications

	DABIGATRAN			RIVAROXABAN				APIXABAN	
	RE-MOBILIZE[1] (n=2615)	RE-MODEL[2] (n=2101)	RE-NOVATE[3] (n=3494)	RECORD 1[4] (n=4541)	RECORD 2[5] (n=2509)	RECORD 3[6] (n=2531)	RECORD 4[7] (n=3148)	ADVANCE-1[8] (n=3195)	ADVANCE-2[9] (n=3057)
Major bleeding	D 150 mg 0.6% D 220 mg 0.6% Enoxaparin 1.4%	D 150 mg 1.3% D 220 mg 1.5% Enoxaparin 1.3%	D 150 mg 1.3% D 220 mg 2.0% Enoxaparin 1.6%	R 0.3% Enoxaparin 0.1%	R 0.1% Enoxaparin 0.1%	R 0.6% Enoxaparin 0.5%	R 0.7% Enoxaparin 0.3%	A 0.7% (p=0.05) Enoxaparin 1.4%	NR
Definition of major bleeding	Fatal bleeding; bleeding leading to ≥2 g/dL fall in Hbg or transfusion of ≥2 units of blood; retroperitoneal, intracranial, intraocular or intraspinal bleeding; or bleeding leading to treatment cessation or reoperation			Fatal bleeding; bleeding into a critical organ (e.g., retroperitoneal, intracranial, intraspinal, intraocular); bleeding requiring reoperation; clinically overt bleeding *outside the surgical site* leading to ≥2 g/dL fall in Hbg or transfusion of ≥2 units of blood				Fatal bleeding; bleeding leading to ≥2 g/dL fall in Hbg or transfusion of ≥2 units of blood; retroperitoneal, intracranial, intraocular or intraspinal bleeding; or bleeding leading to treatment cessation or reoperation	
Major or clinically relevant bleeding	NR	NR	NR	NR	NR	NR	NR	A 2.9% (p=0.03) Enoxaparin 4.3%	A 3.5% (p=0.09) Enoxaparin 4.8%
Definition of major or clinically relevant bleeding	Not used			Not used				See above and below	

(continued)

Table 9-4: (Continued)

	DABIGATRAN			RIVAROXABAN				APIXABAN	
	RE-MOBILIZE[1] (n=2615)	RE-MODEL[2] (n=2101)	RE-NOVATE[3] (n=3494)	RECORD 1[4] (n=4541)	RECORD 2[5] (n=2509)	RECORD 3[6] (n=2531)	RECORD 4[7] (n=3148)	ADVANCE-1[8] (n=3195)	ADVANCE-2[9] (n=3057)
Clinically relevant nonmajor bleeding	D 150 mg 2.5% D 220 mg 2.7% Enoxaparin 2.4%	D 150 mg 6.8% D 220 mg 5.9% Enoxaparin 5.3%	D 150 mg 4.7% D 220 mg 4.2% Enoxaparin 3.5%	R 2.9% Enoxaparin 2.4%	R 3.3% Enoxaparin 2.7%	R 2.7% Enoxaparin 2.3%	R 2.6% Enoxaparin 2.0%	A 2.2% Enoxaparin 3.0%	NR
Definition of clinically relevant nonmajor bleeding	Skin hematoma ≥25 cm²; wound hematoma ≥100 cm²; epistaxis >5 min; macroscopic hematuria lasting ≥24 hr if associated with an intervention; spontaneous rectal bleeding; gingival bleeding >5 min; any other bleeding judged as clinically significant by investigator			Not defined	"events such as" multiple source bleeding, unexpected hematoma >25 cm²; excessive wound hematoma	Not defined	Multiple source bleeding, unexpected hematoma >25 cm²; excessive wound hematoma; epistaxis 5 min; macroscopic hematuria; gingival bleeding >5 min; rectal bleeding; coughing or vomiting blood; vaginal bleeding:	Clinically overt bleeding that did not meet the criteria for major bleeding, including epistaxis requiring intervention, GI bleeding (endoscopically confirmed, hematemesis or melena), hematuria persisting >24 hr, bruising/ecchymosis; hematoma; hemoptysis	

(continued)

Table 9-4: (Continued)

	DABIGATRAN			RIVAROXABAN				APIXABAN	
	RE-MOBILIZE[1] (n=2615)	RE-MODEL[2] (n=2101)	RE-NOVATE[3] (n=3494)	RECORD 1[4] (n=4541)	RECORD 2[5] (n=2509)	RECORD 3[6] (n=2531)	RECORD 4[7] (n=3148)	ADVANCE-1[8] (n=3195)	ADVANCE-2[9] (n=3057)
Nonmajor bleeding	NR	NR	NR	R 5.8% Enoxaparin 5.8%	R 6.5% Enoxaparin 5.5%	R 4.3% Enoxaparin 4.4%	R 10.2% Enoxaparin 9.2%	NR	NR
Definition of nonmajor bleeding	Not used			Clinically relevant nonmajor bleeding, hemorrhagic wound complications, and other nonmajor bleeding	Any bleeding event not adjudicated as major bleeding	Clinically relevant nonmajor bleeding, hemorrhagic wound complications, and other nonmajor bleeding	Hemorrhagic wound complications and other nonmajor bleeding	blood in semen; intra-articular bleeding with trauma; surgical site bleeding	NR
Minor bleeding	NR	D 150 mg 8.4% D 220 mg 8.8% Enoxaparin 9.9%	D 150 mg 6.2% D 220 mg 6.1% Enoxaparin 6.4%	NR	NR	NR	NR	A 2.4% Enoxaparin 2.5%	NR

(continued)

Table 9-4: (Continued)

	DABIGATRAN			RIVAROXABAN				APIXABAN	
	RE-MOBILIZE[1] (n=2615)	RE-MODEL[2] (n=2101)	RE-NOVATE[3] (n=3494)	RECORD 1[4] (n=4541)	RECORD 2[5] (n=2509)	RECORD 3[6] (n=2531)	RECORD 4[7] (n=3148)	ADVANCE-1[8] (n=3195)	ADVANCE-2[9] (n=3057)
Definition of minor bleeding	Bleeding not meeting the criteria for major bleeding or clinically significant nonmajor bleeding			Not used				Clinically overt bleeding not meeting criteria for major or clinically significant nonmajor bleeding	

Source: reprinted with permission from reference 14.

Clinical Pearl

- Timing of the administration of the first dose of novel oral antico-agulants after orthopedic surgery is a balancing act between the goal of attaining maximal efficacy for VTE prevention and the goal of minimizing the risk of bleeding at the surgical site. Administering the first dose shortly after surgery allows for reduced VTE recurrence but may result in higher bleeding complications. Thus, care should be used in appropriate timing of the first to dose to attain the ideal window between efficacy and safety concerns.

Table 9-5: Stroke Prevention in Atrial Fibrillation[10]

	Dabigatran 110 mg BID (n=6015)	Dabigatran 150 mg BID (n=6076)	Warfarin to INR 2.0–3.0 (n=6022)
Mean duration of followup	2 yr		
Mean CHADS2 score	2.1	2.2	2.1
Time-in-therapeutic range	NA	NA	64%
Stroke or systemic embolism	1.53 %/yr (p<0.001 for noninferiority vs. warfarin)	1.11 %/yr (p<0.001 for noninferiority vs. warfarin)	1.69 %/yr
All cause mortality	3.75 %/yr	3.64 %/yr	4.13 %/yr
Major bleeding	2.71 %/yr (p=0.003 vs. warfarin)	3.11 %/yr (p=0.31 vs. warfarin)	3.36 %/yr
Intracranial hemorrhage	0.23 %/yr (p<0.001 vs. warfarin)	0.30 %/yr (p<0.001 vs. warfarin)	0.74 %/yr
Minor bleeding	13.16 %/yr (p<0.001 vs. warfarin)	14.84 %/yr (p=0.005 vs. warfarin)	16.37 %/yr

Clinical Pearl

- Based on the results of the RELY study, dabigatran shows promise as a more convenient and less complex to use anticoagulant for the long-term treatment of stroke prevention in patients with atrial fibrillation.[10]

Table 9-6: Pharmacokinetics/Pharmacodynamics[11,14]

	DABIGATRAN	RIVAROXABAN	APIXABAN
Molecular weight	628 daltons	436 daltons	460 daltons
Protein binding	35%	92% to 95%	87%
Volume of distribution	60–70 L	50 L	"Low"
Time to maximum serum concentrations	1.25–3.0 hr	2.4 hr	3.0–3.5 hr
Elimination half-life	12–14 hr	5–9 hr	8–15 hr
Activation	Prodrug dabigatran etexilate converted to active drug dabigatran via hydrolysis	None	None
Metabolism	Conjugation	Oxidation (via CYP3A4 [18%] and CYP2J2 [14%]) and CYP-independent hydrolytic cleavage [14%]	Oxidation (via CYP3A4) and conjugation
Renal excretion of unchanged drug	80%	36% via p-glycoprotein and breast cancer resistance protein	25%
Dialyzable	Yes	Not expected	Unlikely

Clinical Pearl

- The degree of renal excretion varies among the novel oral anticoagulants and it is expected that these agents will require specific dosage adjustments and careful monitoring based on the degree of renal impairment present (see Table 9-4.)[1]

CLINICAL USE

Limited data are available regarding the use of these new oral antithrombotic agents in patients with renal impairment or hepatic dysfunction. In general, all published clinical trials have intended to exclude patients with creatinine clearances less than 30 mL/min and patients with Child Pugh Class C hepatic failure. As well, limited information is available regarding the influence of food and concurrent medications on these agents.

Table 9-7: Use in Renal Impairment[11,14]

	DABIGATRAN	RIVAROXABAN	APIXABAN
CrCl 80–100	110 mg every day x 1 then 220 mg every day for VTE prophylaxis 150 mg BID for stroke prevention in AF	10 mg every day for VTE prophylaxis 20 mg every day for stroke prevention in AF	2.5 mg BID
CrCl 50–80	No adjustment recommended 1.5 x increase in AUC	44% increase in AUC No adjustment recommended	Not reported
CrCl 30–50	3.2 x increase in AUC 75 mg every day x 1 then 150 mg every day "use with caution" for VTE prophylaxis No dosing adjustment recommended for stroke prevention in AF	52% increase in AUC No adjustment recommended	Not reported

(*continued*)

Table 9-7: (Continued)

	DABIGATRAN	RIVAROXABAN	APIXABAN
CrCl 15–29	6.3 x increase in AUC 2 x increase in T1/2 Contraindicated in VTE prophylaxis 75 mg BID dose adjustment for stroke prevention in AF	64% increase in AUC "use with caution"	Not reported
CrCl <15	Contraindicated	"Use not recommended"	Not reported

Table 9-8: Use in Hepatic Dysfunction[11,14]

	DABIGATRAN	RIVAROXABAN	APIXABAN
Effect on AST/ALT	Similar to enoxaparin in clinical trials	Similar to enoxaparin in clinical trials	Similar to enoxaparin in clinical trials
Use in moderate hepatic failure **(Child Pugh B)**	No change in AUC	127% increase in AUC "use with caution"	Not reported
Use in severe hepatic failure **(Child Pugh C)**	Excluded from clinical trials	Excluded from clinical trials	Not reported

Table 9-9: Dietary Considerations[11–14]

	DABIGATRAN	RIVAROXABAN	APIXABAN
Effect of food	Delayed Tmax	0.5-hr delay in Tmax 41% increase in Cmax 28% increase in AUC Decreased interpatient variability in AUC and Cmax	Not reported

(*continued*)

Table 9-9: (Continued)

	DABIGATRAN	RIVAROXABAN	APIXABAN
Effect of gastric pH	None	None	Not reported
Effect of antacids	None	None	Not reported
Effect of H2 receptor antagonists	None	None	Not reported
Effect of proton pump inhibitors	22% decrease in Cmax 33% decrease in AUC Not considered clinically relevant	None	Not reported
Recommended administration	Take with or without food	Take with food or within 2 hr of eating	Not reported

Clinical Pearl

- Although the list of drug interactions associated with the new oral anticoagulants appears to be more limited compared to warfarin, care should still be used and patients screened for potential interacting medications via the specified pathways in Table 9-10.

Table 9-10: Drug Interactions[11,14]

	DABIGATRAN	RIVAROXABAN	APIXABAN
Anticoagulant agents	Increased risk of bleeding	Increased risk of bleeding	Increased risk of bleeding
Antiplatelet agents	Increased risk of bleeding	Increased risk of bleeding	Increased risk of bleeding

(continued)

Table 9-10: (Continued)

	DABIGATRAN	RIVAROXABAN	APIXABAN
CYP3A4 inhibitors reported	Not applicable	Ketoconazole (100% inc AUC/Cmax) Ritonavir (100% inc AUC/Cmax) Clarithromycin (50% inc AUC/Cmax) Erythromycin (30% inc AUC/Cmax)	Not yet reported
CYP3A4 inducers reported	Not applicable	Rifampin (50% dec AUC)	Not yet reported
p-GP inhibitors reported	Amiodarone (50% ↑AUC) Ketoconazole (150% ↑AUC) Verapamil 1 hr before dabigatran (250% ↑AUC) Verapamil/dabigatran concurrent (170% ↑ AUC) Verapamil 2 hr after dabigatran (no change) Clarithromycin (use with caution) Quinidine (contraindicated)	Ketoconazole (100% inc AUC/Cmax) Ritonavir (100% inc AUC/Cmax) Clarithromycin (50% inc AUC/Cmax) Erythromycin (30% inc AUC/Cmax)	Not yet reported
p-GP inducers reported	Rifampin (60% ↓ AUC)	Not yet reported	Not yet reported

Table 9-11: Dabigatran Considerations for Use

US/FDA-Approved Indication	Stroke Prevention in Atrial Fibrillation
Dosage availability	75-mg and 150-mg oral capsules
	Do not chew, break, or open capsules (this can substantially increase the bioavailability)
	Once opened, capsules in each bottle expire in 30 days
Dosage form	Capsules contain multiple drug pellets containing a tartaric acid core (coated with dabigatran etexilate) that creates an acidic microenvironment to improve dissolution and absorption independent of gastric pH
Dosing	CrCl >30 mL/min: 150 mg twice daily
	CrCl 15–30 mL/min: 75 mg twice daily
	CrCl <15 mL/min or on dialysis: not recommended
Hemodialysis	Removes a substantial amount of dabigatran (62% at 2 hr, 68% at 4 hr)
	May be considered in case of overdose
Missed dose instructions	Take on the same day as soon as possible; skip the missed dose if it cannot be taken at least 6 hr before the next scheduled dose; dosing should not be doubled to make up for a missed dose
Hepatic impairment	No adjustment
Elderly	No significant pharmacokinetic differences in healthy elderly individuals
Reversal	See Chapter 7
	Activated charcoal may decrease absorption if used within 1–2 hr of ingestion
	Hemodialysis (see above)
	Benefits of FFP, rFVIIa, and PCC are unknown
	(Vitamin K, protamine, and aminocaproic acid are not anticipated to have any effect)

(*continued*)

Table 9-11: (Continued)

US/FDA-Approved Indication	Stroke Prevention in Atrial Fibrillation
Converting dabigatran to warfarin	Adjust the starting time of warfarin based on creatinine clearance • <u>CrCl >50 mL/min:</u> start warfarin 3 days before stopping dabigatran • <u>CrCl 31–50 mL/min:</u> start warfarin 2 days before stopping dabigatran • <u>CrCl 15–30 mL/min:</u> start warfarin 1 day before stopping dabigatran • <u>CrCl <15 mL/min:</u> not recommended Note: dabigatran can elevate the INR; the INR will better reflect warfarin's effect after dabigatran has been stopped for at least 2 days
Converting warfarin to dabigatran	Discontinue warfarin and start dabigatran when the international normalized ratio (INR) is below 2
Converting to or from a parenteral anticoagulant	When a parenteral anticoagulant is in use, start dabigatran 0–2 hr before the time that the next SQ dose of parenteral drug was to have been administered or at the time of discontinuation of a continuously administered IV parenteral drug For patients currently taking dabigatran, wait 12 hr (CrCl ≥30 mL/min) or 24 hr (CrCl <30 mL/min) after the last dabigatran dose before initiating the parenteral (SQ or IV) anticoagulant
Surgery or invasive procedures	Discontinue dabigatran 1–2 days (CrCl ≥50 mL/min) or 3–5 days (CrCl <50 mL/min) before invasive or surgical procedures if possible to reduce the risk of bleeding Note: depending on the risk of bleeding, urgency of the procedure and thrombosis risk, holding a shorter period of time may be considered Longer holding periods to establish complete hemostasis may be considered for major surgery, spinal puncture, or placement of a spinal or epidural catheter or port If a delay in surgery is not possible, the increased risk of bleeding should be weighed against the urgency of intervention
Contraindications	Active bleeding History of serious hypersensitivity reaction to dabigatran CrCl <15 mL/min

(*continued*)

Table 9-11: (Continued)

US/FDA-Approved Indication	Stroke Prevention in Atrial Fibrillation
Warnings and precautions	<u>Risk of bleeding:</u> dabigatran can cause serious and sometimes fatal bleeding; promptly evaluate signs and symptoms of blood loss
	<u>Temporary discontinuation:</u> avoid lapses in therapy to minimize risk of stroke
	Clinical significance of the increased incidence of acute coronary syndrome seen in the dabigatran cohorts from the RELY trial is unclear
Adverse reactions	GI Side effects are the most common
	Nausea, vomiting, constipation, pyrexia, wound secretion, hypotension, insomnia, peripheral edema, anemia, and dizziness
Drug interactions	Administration of dabigatran >2 hr before a P-Gp inhibitor should minimize the effect of the inhibitor on dabigatran absorption
	The clinical significance of most of the agents that increase or decrease dabigatran concentrations is unclear, with the exception of rifampin
	↑ Dabigatran serum concentration
	• amiodarone
	• quinidine
	• ketoconazole
	• verapamil
	• clopidogrel
	↓ Dabigatran serum concentration
	• antacids
	• atorvastatin
	• proton pump inhibitors
	• rifampin (significant interaction to avoid)
	↑ anticoagulation effect
	• other anticoagulants
	• antiplatelet agents
	• salicylates

Sources: prescribing information for dabigatran. Pradaxa [package insert]. Ridgefield, CT: Boehringer Ingelheim Pharmaceuticals Inc; 2010.

REFERENCES AND KEY ARTICLES

1. Ginsberg JS, Davidson BL, Comp PC, et al. Oral thrombin inhibitor dabigatran etexilate vs North American enoxaparin regimen for prevention of venous thromboembolism after knee arthroplasty surgery. *J Arthroplasty*. 2009;24:1–9.

2. Erikkson BI, Dahl OE, Rosencher N, et al. Oral dabigatran etexilate vs subcutaneous enoxaparin for the prevention of venous thromboembolism after total knee replacement: the RE-MODEL randomized trial. *J Thromb Haemost*. 2007;5:2178–2185.

3. Erikkson B, Dahl OE, Rosencher N, et al. Dabigatran etexilate versus enoxaparin for the prevention of venous thromboembolism after total hip replacement: a randomized, double-blind non-inferiority trial. *Lancet*. 2007;370:949–956.

4. Eriksson BI, Borris LC, Friedman RJ, et al. Rivaroxaban versus enoxaparin for thromboprophylaxis after hip arthroplasty. *New Engl J Med*. 2008;358:2765–2775.

5. Kakkar AK, Brenner B, Dahl OE, et al. Extended duration rivaroxaban versus short term enoxaparin for the prevention of venous thromboembolism after total hip arthroplasty: a double-blind, randomised controlled trial. *Lancet*. 2008;372:31–39.

6. Lassen MR, Ageno W, Borris LC, et al. Rivaroxaban vs enoxaparin for thromboprophylaxis after total knee arthroplasty. *New Engl J Med*. 2009;358:2776–2786.

7. Turpie AGG, Lassen MR, Davidson BL, et al. Rivaroxaban versus enoxaparin for thromboprophylaxis after total knee replacement arthroplasty (RECORD 4): a randomized trial. *Lancet*. 2009;373:1673–1680.

8. Lassen MR, Raskob GE, Gallus A, et al. Apixaban or enoxaparin for thromboprophylaxis after knee replacement. *New Engl J Med*. 2009;361:594–604.

9. Lassen AS, Gallus GF, Pineo GF, et al. The ADVANCE-2 Study: a randomized, double-blind trial comparing apixaban with enoxaparin for thromboprophylaxis after total knee replacement. *J Thromb Haemost*. 2009;7(suppl 2):abstract LB-MO-005.

10. Connolly SJ, Ezekowitz MB, Yusuf S, et al. Dabigatran versus warfarin in patients with atrial fibrillation. *New Engl J Med*. 2009;361:1139–1151.

11. Eriksson BI, Quinlan DJ, Weitz JI. Comparative pharmacodynamics and pharmacokinetics of oral direct thrombin and factor Xa inhibitors in development. *Clin Pharmacokinetics*. 2009;38:1–22.

12. EMEA CHMP Assessment Report for Xarelto. Available at: http://www.emea.europa.eu/humandocs/PDFs/EPAR/xarlelto/H-944-en6.pdf. Accessed August 2009.

13. EMEA CHMP Assessment Report for Pradaxa. Available at: http://www.emea.europa.eu/humandocs/PDFs/EPAR/pradaxa/H-829-en6.pdf. Accessed August 2009.

14. Wittkowsky AK. New oral anticoagulants: a practical guide for clinicians. *J Thromb Thrombolysis*. 2010;29:182–191.

PART II: Conditions Requiring Anticoagulation Therapy

Venous Thromboembolism Prevention

10

Paul P. Dobesh, Zachary A. Stacy

INTRODUCTION

Venous thromboembolism (VTE), which encompasses both deep vein thrombosis (DVT) and pulmonary embolism (PE), is a significant healthcare problem, producing considerable morbidity, mortality, and resource utilization. In the US alone, there are well over a million DVT events and more than 100,000 deaths per year from PE. These events occur in a wide range of both surgical and medical patients. With appropriate prophylaxis, many of these VTE events can be prevented. Despite over 30 years of demonstrated efficacy and safety of VTE prophylaxis, it is substantially underutilized. This underutilization has led to the recent involvement of government and other regulatory agencies in an attempt to improve VTE prophylaxis for both surgical and medical patients in US hospitals. The existence of numerous pharmacologic agents, abundance of major clinical trials, limited data in special populations, and a number of nationally recognized clinical guidelines can provide challenges to having an understanding of what constitutes appropriate VTE prophylaxis.

Table 10-1: Venous Thromboembolism Prevention Guidelines and Resources

Guideline/Resource	Web Link
American College of Chest Physicians (CHEST Guidelines)	http://www.chestjournal.org/content/133/6_suppl/381S.full.pdf+html
Surgical Care Improvement Project (SCIP)	https://www.qualitynet.org/dcs/ContentServer?c=MQParents&pagename=Medqic%2FContent%2FParentShellTemplate&cid=1228694349383&parentName=Category
Agency for Healthcare Research and Quality (AHRQ)	http://www.ahrq.gov/qual/vtguide/
Joint Commission	http://www.jointcommission.org/PerformanceMeasurement/PerformanceMeasurement/VTE.htm
Deep Vein Thrombosis Coalition	http://www.preventdvt.org/home.aspx

RATES AND RISK FACTORS FOR VENOUS THROMBOEMBOLISM

Table 10-2: Approximate Risk of DVT[a] in Different Hospitalized Patient Populations[1]

Patient Group	DVT Prevalence Without Prophylaxis
Medically ill patients	10% to 20%
Heart failure	
Chronic obstructive pulmonary disease	
Infection	
General surgery	15% to 40%
Major gynecologic surgery	15% to 40%
Major urologic surgery	15% to 40%
Neurosurgery	15% to 20%
Stroke	20% to 50%

(continued)

Table 10-2: (Continued)

Patient Group	DVT Prevalence Without Prophylaxis
Major orthopedic surgery	40% to 60%
Total hip replacement surgery	57%
Hip fracture surgery	60%
Total knee replacement surgery	84%
Major trauma	40% to 80%
Spinal cord injury patients	60% to 80%
Critical care patients	10% to 80%

[a]Rates of DVT are determined by venography.

Table 10-3: Levels of Thromboembolic Risk as Classified by ACCP[1]

Level of Risk	Approximate DVT Risk Without Prophylaxis
Low-risk Minor surgery in mobile patients Medical patients that are fully mobile	<10%
Moderate-risk Most general, open gynecologic or urologic surgery patients Medical patients, bed rest or sick	10% to 40%
High-risk Hip or knee replacement surgery, hip fracture surgery Major trauma, spinal cord injury	40% to 80%

Table 10-4: Venous Thromboembolism Risk Factors

Age greater than 40 years	Acute medical illness
Surgery	Heart failure
Major trauma or lower-extremity injury	Respiratory disease
Immobility, lower extremity paresis	Infection
Cancer (active or occult)	Stroke
Cancer therapy	Central venous catheterization
Hormonal therapy	Smoking
Chemotherapy	Varicose veins
Angiogenesis inhibitors	Medications
Radiation therapy	Estrogen-containing oral contraceptives
Pregnancy and the postpartum period	Hormone replacement therapy
Paroxysmal nocturnal hemoglobinuria	Selective estrogen receptor modulators
Myeloproliferative disorders	Erythropoiesis-stimulating agents
Inflammatory bowel disease	Inherited or acquired thrombophilia
Nephrotic syndrome	Previous/history of venous thromboembolism
	Venous compression (tumor, hematoma, arterial abnormality)

ACQUIRED AND INHERITED HYPERCOAGULABILITY DISORDERS (SEE CHAPTER 19)

Table 10-5: Hypercoagulability Risk of Cancer and Cancer Therapy[2]

Cancer	1-Year Incidence of VTE	Other VTE Risk Considerations in Cancer Management	Examples
Brain	6.9%	Chemotherapy	Anthracyclines, platinum-based Nitrogen mustard analogues
Pancreas	5.3%	Hormonal therapy	Tamoxifen, anastrozole, Exemestane, letrozole
Stomach	4.5%	Anti-angiogenic therapy	Thalidomide, lenalidomide
Leukemia	3.7%	Erythropoiesis-stimulating therapy	Erythropoietin, darbepoetin
Esophagus	3.6%	Central venous catheter placement	
Renal cell	3.5%		
Ovary	3.3%		
Lymphoma	2.8%		
Lung	2.4%		
Colon	2.3%		
Liver	1.7%		
Uterus	1.6%		
Bladder	1.5%		
Prostate	0.9%		
Breast	0.9%		

Table 10-6: Validated Risk Score for Prediction of Cancer-Associated Thromboembolism[3]

Predictive Variables		Risk Score
Site of Cancer	Very high risk (stomach, pancreas)	2
	High risk (lung, lymphoma, gynecologic)	1
Prechemotherapy platelet count ≥350,000/mm³		1
Hemoglobin <10 g/dL or use of red cell growth factors		1
Prechemotherapy leukocyte count >11,000/mm³		1
Body mass index ≥35 kg/m²		1

Risk Score	Risk Level	Estimated Rate of VTE at 2.5 Months
0	Lower risk	0.5%
1–2	Intermediate risk	2%
>3	High risk	7%

Clinical Pearls

- The incidence of VTE increases as the cancer stage advances (local, regional, and remote).

- The incidence of VTE is higher within 3–6 months of the diagnosis of cancer.

Table 10-7: Venous Thromboembolism Systematic Prophylaxis Strategies

Tool	Description
Risk scoring forms	Match risk level with appropriate prophylactic strategy
Electronic alerts	Electronic medical record requires response to prophylactic screening before proceeding

(continued)

Table 10-7: (Continued)

Tool	Description
Default prophylaxis strategy	All patients receive prophylaxis with efforts placed on identifying contraindications rather than indications
Opt-out approach	May be considered in the following clinical scenarios:
	Healthy, fully ambulatory, <40 yr
	Immobility/length of stay estimated at less than 2 days
	Warfarin with INR >1.4 or on therapeutic anticoagulation
	Imminent invasive procedure
	Recent intraocular or intracranial surgery
	Spinal tap or epidural anesthesia within 12 hr
	Thrombocytopenia
	History of HIT/hypersensitivity to UFH or LMWH
	Active bleeding
	Active or chronic severe liver disease
	Comfort care/hospice

NONPHARMACOLOGIC PROPHYLAXIS OPTIONS

Table 10-8: Nonpharmacological Prophylaxis Options

Option	Description
TED hose	Stocking without a compression gradient
Graduated compression stocking	Stockings with a gradual decline in pressure from the distal to the proximal end
Intermittent pneumatic compression device	A microprocessor directs pressurized air into segmental diaphragms secured around the leg for a fixed period of time; the compression is delivered in a sequential manner up the leg, producing a wavelike milking effect to evacuate leg veins
IVC filter	Medical device implanted into the inferior vena cava to catch emboli

SIZE	ANKLE	CALF	THIGH	HIP
S	7″– 8¼″ (18–21 cm)	11″– 15″ (28–38 cm)	15¾″– 24⅜″ (40–62 cm)	28″– 46″ (71–117 cm)
M	8⅜″– 9⅞″ (21–25 cm)	11⅞″– 16½″ (30–42 cm)	18⅛″– 27½″ (46–70 cm)	30″– 50″ (76–127 cm)
L	10″– 11⅜″ (25–29 cm)	12½″– 18⅛″ (32–46 cm)	21¼″– 30¾″ (54–78 cm)	32″– 54″ (81–137 cm)
XL	11½″– 13″ (29–33 cm)	13⅜″– 19⅝″ (34–50 cm)	23⅝″– 32″ (60–81 cm)	40″– 65″ (102–166 cm)

Figure 10-1: Custom Fit, Graduated Stocking Measurements

(Source: figure used with permission from JOBST, Inc.)

Clinical Pearls

- It may be easier to apply the stockings if the patient lies down and elevated each leg above the heart for several minutes to reduce swelling.

- Graduated stockings should be placed first thing in the morning.

- Rubber gloves may be used to help get a better grip on the stocking fabric.

- Cornstarch or grease-free talcum can be used in patients with moist skin to pull stocking up.

- Never fold or roll the graduated stocking down—the garment becomes a tourniquet.

- Stocking may not fit after (1) weight loss or gain or (2) changes in leg swelling. A stocking that falls or wrinkles on its own is too large and should be refitted.

- Stockings should be replaced every 3–6 months as the stocking may lose its elasticity over time. Followup is very important in patients prescribed graduated stockings.

- Monitoring the proper use of the stocking should occur daily for the inpatient setting and at each office visit for the outpatient setting.

Firm Support- 30–40 mm Hg

Moderate Support- 20–30 mm Hg

Mild Support- 15–20 mm Hg

Light Support- 8–15 mm Hg

Compression Guide

Light Support- 8–15 mm Hg

Recommended for minor ankle and leg swelling, minor
varicosities, pregnancy, and general leg fatigue. A
light energizing compression.

Mild Support- 15–20 mm Hg

Mild support is frequently recommended for minor ankle
and leg swelling, minor varicosities, and leg fatigue.
Great for traveling and those who sit or stand for long
periods of time.

Moderate Support- 20–30 mm Hg

Recommended for moderate ankle and leg swelling,
moderate varicosities, venous stasis ulcerations,
postschlerotherapy, and preventing DVT.

Firm Support- 30–40 mm Hg

Recommended for severe ankle and leg swelling,
severe varicosities, PTS, venous stasis ulcerations,
lymphadema, and preventing DVT.

Figure 10-2: Compression Guide

(Source: figure used with permission from JOBST, Inc.)

Table 10-9: Inferior Vena Cava Filters[a]

Indications	Contraindications	Complications
• Pulmonary embolism when anticoagulant therapy is contraindicated	• Chronically thrombosed inferior vena cava	• Migration of the filter (slippage) to the heart
• Failure of anticoagulant therapy in thromboembolic disease	• Inaccessible inferior vena cava	• Penetration of vena cava wall into vascular or gastrointestinal systems
• Emergency treatment following massive pulmonary embolism where anticipated benefits of conventional therapy are reduced	• Patients at risk for septic embolism	• Caval occlusion/IVC thrombosis
• Chronic, recurrent PE where anticoagulant therapy has failed or is contraindicated		• Puncture site bleeding
		• Thrombosis at the insertion site
		• Thrombosis on the top of the filter
• Massive trauma (including a GCS score <8, incomplete spinal cord injury with paraplegia or quadriplegia, complex pelvic fractures associated with long bones, or multiple long bone fractures)		• Tilting of fracture of the filter
		• ↑ rates of DVT recurrence[a]
		• Guidewire entrapment

[a]The PREPIC trial, an 8-year, followup study, was designed to assess the long-term safety and efficacy of permanent vena cava filter insertion in patients with a diagnosis of acute proximal DVT and considered high risk for the development of pulmonary embolism.[4] Filter insertion resulted in a number needed to treat of 12 to prevent one PE but was offset by a number needed to harm of 10 for causing one DVT (it increased the rate of DVT). No difference in post-thrombotic syndrome or mortality was observed between patients with or without a permanent filter.

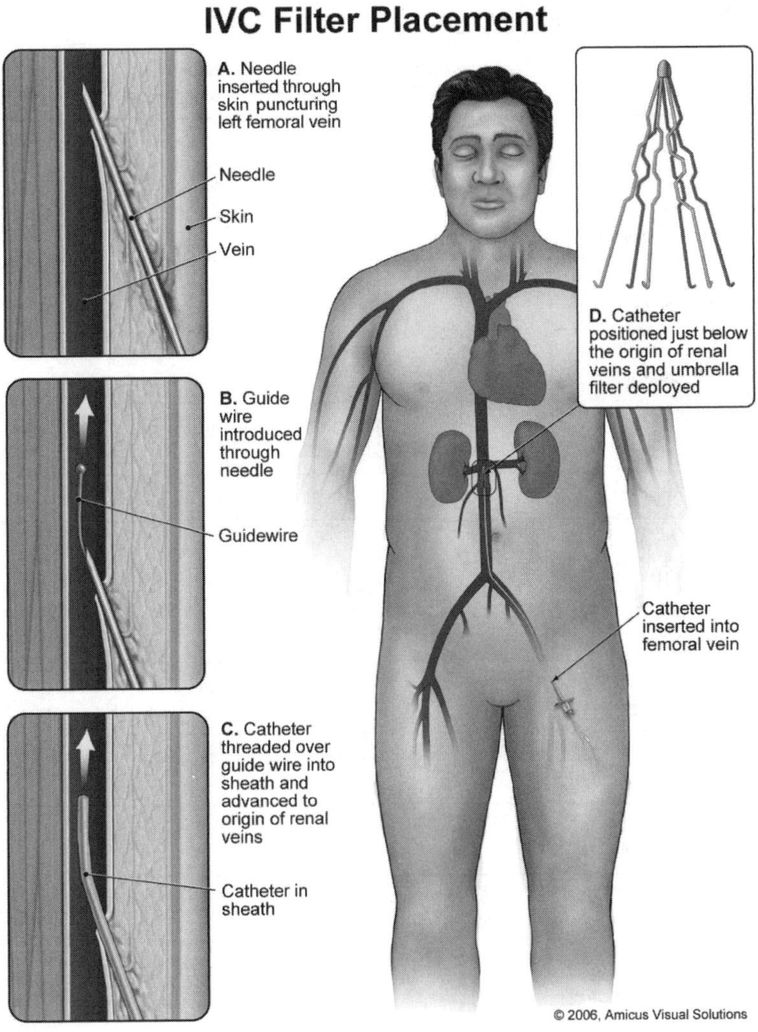

IVC Filter Placement

A. Needle inserted through skin puncturing left femoral vein

Needle

Skin

Vein

B. Guide wire introduced through needle

Guidewire

C. Catheter threaded over guide wire into sheath and advanced to origin of renal veins

Catheter in sheath

D. Catheter positioned just below the origin of renal veins and umbrella filter deployed

Catheter inserted into femoral vein

© 2006, Amicus Visual Solutions

Figure 10-3: IVC Filter Placement

(Source: image used with permission from Amicus Visual Solutions.)

Table 10-10: Inferior Vena Cava Filter Comparisons

Types	Permanent (P) or Retrievable (R)	Maximum IVC Diameter	MRI Compatible	Alloy
Bird's Nest Filter (Cook Medical)	P	40 mm	Yes[a]	Stainless steel
VenaTech Low Profile Filter (B. Braun Vena Tech)	P	35 mm	Yes	Phynox
Nitinol TrapEase Filter (Cordis Endovascular)	P	30 mm	Yes	Nitinol
OptEase (Cordis Endovascular)	R	30 mm	Yes	Nitinol
Gunther Tulip Filter (Cook Medical)	R	30 mm	Yes	Conichrome
Celect (Cook Medical)	P	30 mm	Yes	Conichrome
VenaTech LGM Filter (B. Braun Vena Tech)	P	28 mm	Yes	Phynox
Simon Nitinol Filter (C. R. Bard)	P	28 mm	Yes	Nitinol
Titanium Greenfield Filter (Boston Scientific)	P	28 mm	Yes	Titanium
Recovery/G2 (Bard Peripheral Vascular)	P	28 mm	Yes	Nitinol
Stainless-Steel Greenfield Filter (Boston Scientific)	P	28 mm	Yes[a]	Stainless steel

[a]No displacement due to the magnetic field has been demonstrated with MRI, but the metallic component causes an imaging artifact.

Clinical Pearls

- Retrievable filters must be rotated or removed within 2 weeks or they become permanently affixed to the IVC wall.

- The presence of a clot within a temporary filter, at the time of retrieval, may result in permanent placement.

- Once the contraindication for anticoagulation has been resolved, concomitant use of warfarin should be considered in patients with permanent filters.

- Filter retrieval does not require interruption of anticoagulation.

- MRI procedures should be postponed for 6 weeks following implantation to ensure incorporation into vessel wall.

VTE PROPHYLAXIS IN MEDICALLY ILL PATIENTS

Table 10-11: VTE Prophylaxis in Medically Ill Patients

UFH	Enoxaparin	Dalteparin	Tinzaparin	Fondaparinux	Warfarin
5,000 units SC q 8 hr or 5,000 units SC q 12 hr	40 mg SC q 24 hr	5,000 International Units SC q 24 hr	Insufficient evidence	2.5 mg SC q 24 hr[a]	Insufficient evidence

[a]Not approved by the US FDA.

Clinical Pearls

- A number of clinical trials have not demonstrated efficacy with the use of UFH 5,000 units every 12 hours; therefore, UFH 5,000 units every 8 hours would be the preferred UFH regimen.[5] While not evidence-based, UFH 5,000 units every 12 hours may be considered in individuals of advanced age and low weight (i.e., TBW <50 kg) or elevated baseline aPTT (>1.3 or 1.4 times baseline).

- Enoxaparin 20 mg once daily has been evaluated and is not more effective compared to placebo.[5]

- Enoxaparin 20 mg once daily has demonstrated equal efficacy compared to UFH 5,000 units every 12 hours.[5]

- In head-to-head trials between UFH 5,000 units every 8 hours and enoxaparin 40 mg daily, the regimens have demonstrated similar efficacy, except for higher-risk medically ill patients (heart failure and ischemic stroke) in which enoxaparin may have demonstrated greater protection against VTE. In these same trials, enoxaparin has demonstrated significantly less hematoma (>5 cm) compared to UFH. While some data suggest a lower bleeding rate with the use of LMWH in medically ill patients, these findings are not consistent across trials.

VTE PROPHYLAXIS IN NONORTHOPEDIC SURGERY PATIENTS

Table 10-12: VTE Prophylaxis in General Surgery

Surgical Indication	UFH	Enoxaparin	Dalteparin	Tinzaparin	Fondaparinux
General surgery	5,000 units SC q 8 hr or 5,000 units SC q 12 hr	40 mg SC q 24 hr	5,000 International Units SC q 24 hr[a]	3,500 International Units SC q 24 hr	2.5 mg SC q 24 hr
Neurosurgery	5,000 units SC q 8 hr	Enoxaparin 40 mg SC q 24 hr	Insufficient evidence	Insufficient evidence	Insufficient evidence
Vascular surgery	5,000 units SC q 8 hr or 5,000 units SC q 12 hr	40 mg SC q 24 hr	5,000 International Units SC q 24 hr[a]	3,500 International Units SC q 24 hr	2.5 mg SC q 24 hr
Gynecologic	5,000 units SC q 8 hr or 5,000 units SC q 12 hr	40 mg SC q 24 hr	5,000 International Units U SC q 24 hr[a]	3,500 International Units SC q 24 hr	2.5 mg SC q 24 hr

(continued)

Table 10-12: (Continued)

Surgical Indication	UFH	Enoxaparin	Dalteparin	Tinzaparin	Fondaparinux
Urologic	5,000 units SC q 8 hr or 5,000 units SC q 12 hr	40 mg SC q 24 hr	5,000 International Units SC q 24 hr[a]	3,500 International Units SC q 24 hr	2.5 mg SC q 24 hr
Laparoscopic	Patients undergoing laparoscopic procedures without additional VTE risk factors do not require prophylaxis beyond early ambulation				
Bariatric	5,000 units SC q 8 hr	40 mg SC q 12 hr	7,500 International Units SC q 24 hr	Insufficient evidence	2.5 mg SC q 24 hr
Thoracic	5,000 units SC q 8 hr or 5,000 units SC q 12 hr	40 mg SC q 24 hr	5,000 International Units SC q 24 hr[a]	3,500 International Units SC q 24 hr	2.5 mg SC q 24 hr
Coronary bypass surgery	5,000 units SC q 8 hr or 5,000 units SC q 12 hr	40 mg SC q 24 hr	5,000 International Units SC q 24 hr[a]	3,500 International Units SC q 24 hr	Not discussed in current guidelines

[a]Different strategies on when to initiate dalteparin after surgery have been studied. Please see the dalteparin package labeling for more details.

Clinical Pearls

- **General surgery**—Meta-analysis comparisons between UFH and LMWHs demonstrate comparative efficacy in preventing DVT, but a greater reduction in the incidence of PE when LMWH is used. Mechanical prophylaxis is sometimes inappropriately selected over pharmacologic prophylaxis due to concerns of bleeding in surgical patients. A meta-analysis of almost 34,000 surgical patients demonstrated that the most common bleeding complications occur are injection site bruising (6.9%) and wound hematomas (5.7%); major bleeding complications occur in less than 1% of patients (gastrointestinal bleeding: 0.2%, retroperitoneal bleeding: 0.08%, and surgery needed for bleeding: 0.7%).[6]

- **Neurosurgery**—Pharmacologic prophylaxis is typically given with mechanical prophylaxis and the combination has been demonstrated to be equally safe and more effective compared to mechanical prophylaxis alone. Pharmacologic prophylaxis is typically started 18–24 hours after neurosurgery.

- **Vascular surgery**—Routine prophylaxis is recommended for patients with additional risk factors such as advanced age, limb ischemia, long duration of surgery, and intra-operative local trauma. Due to the limited number of trials in patients with vascular surgery, dosing recommendations are based on evidence of pharmacologic agents in general surgery.

- **Gynecologic surgery**—Low-risk gynecologic surgery procedures (laparoscopic procedures or procedures lasting <30 minutes) do not require prophylaxis beyond early ambulation. Major surgery without malignancy should receive UFH or LMWH.

- **Gynecologic cancer surgery**—UFH three times daily is more effective than twice daily. UFH three times daily and LMWH seem to have similar efficacy and safety. In a subgroup analysis of a general surgery trial, fondaparinux was more effective than dalteparin in patients undergoing surgery for cancer.[7]

- **Urologic surgery**—Patients undergoing transurethral or laparoscopic urologic procedure do not require prophylaxis beyond early ambulation. Due to the limited number of trials in patients undergoing urologic surgery, dosing recommendations are based on evidence of pharmacologic agents in general surgery.

- **Bariatric surgery**—Higher than recommended doses of LMWH and UFH are suggested. UFH three times daily and enoxaparin 40 mg twice daily have been evaluated.[4] Dalteparin 7,500 units daily has been evaluated in a retrospective study using anti-Factor Xa levels. While not prospectively evaluated, a dose of LMWH can be administered about 4 hours preoperatively.

- **Thoracic surgery**—Due to the limited number of trials in patients undergoing thoracic surgery, dosing recommendations are based on evidence of pharmacologic agents in general surgery.

- **Coronary bypass surgery**—Due to the limited number of trials in patients undergoing coronary artery bypass surgery, dosing recommendations are based on evidence of pharmacologic agents in general surgery. Due to concerns about higher incidence of HIT in cardiac surgery patients, LMWH may be preferred over UFH for prophylaxis.

VTE PROPHYLAXIS IN ORTHOPEDIC SURGERY

Table 10-13: VTE Prophylaxis in Orthopedic Surgery

Orthopedic Indication	Enoxaparin	Dalteparin	Tinzaparin	Fondaparinux	Warfarin
Knee replacement surgery	30 mg SC q 12 hr initiated 12–24 hr after surgery	2,500 International Units SC given 6–8 hr after surgery, then 5,000 International Units SC q 24 hr[a]	75 units/kg SC q 24 hr initiated the evening prior to surgery or 12–24 hr after surgery[a]	2.5 mg SC q 24 hr initiated 6–8 hr after surgery	Initiated preoperatively or the evening of the surgical day with adjusted-dosing to achieve a target INR of 2.5 ± 0.5
Hip replacement surgery	30 mg SC q 12 hr initiated 12–24 hr after surgery or 40 mg SC q 24 hr initiated 10–12 hr prior to surgery	2,500 International Units SC given 6–8 hr after surgery, then 5,000 International Units SC q 24 hr or 5,000 International Units SC q 24 hr initiated the evening prior to surgery	75 units/kg SC q 24 hr initiated the evening prior to surgery or 12–24 hr after surgery[a] or 4,500 International Units SC q 24 hr initiated 12 hr prior to surgery[a]	2.5 mg SC q 24 hr initiated 6–8 hr after surgery	Initiated preoperatively or the evening of the surgical day with adjusted-dosing to achieve a target INR of 2.5 ± 0.5

(continued)

Table 10-13: (Continued)

Orthopedic Indication	Enoxaparin	Dalteparin	Tinzaparin	Fondaparinux	Warfarin
Hip fracture surgery	30 mg SC q 12 hr initiated 12–24 hr after surgery[a]	Insufficient evidence	Insufficient evidence	2.5 mg SC q 24 hr initiated 6–8 hr after surgery	Initiated preoperatively or the evening of the surgical day with adjusted-dosing to achieve a target INR of 2.5 ± 0.5
Spine surgery	Pharmacologic prophylaxis is generally not recommended unless patients have additional risk factors of advanced age, malignancy, neurologic deficit, previous VTE, or an anterior surgical approach; based on the lack of clinical trials, pharmacologic prophylaxis recommendations are general and include SC UFH or LMWH				

[a]Not approved by the US FDA.

Clinical Pearls

- UFH has consistently demonstrated insufficient protection against VTE in patients undergoing orthopedic surgery, and therefore should not be considered an acceptable alternative to the options listed above.

- Aspirin has consistently demonstrated insufficient protection against VTE in patients undergoing orthopedic surgery, and therefore should not be considered an acceptable alternative to the options listed above.

- Patients placed on mechanical prophylaxis after surgery due to high-risk of bleeding should have their risk of bleeding consistently re-assessed, with pharmacologic prophylaxis started as soon as the bleeding risk is decreased.

- Patients undergoing knee arthroscopy typically do not need VTE prophylaxis beyond early mobilization unless they have additional VTE risk factors or a complicated procedure. In those cases, patients should receive VTE prophylaxis with LMWH.

- Dalteparin has not been evaluated in a published prospective trial for VTE prophylaxis in knee replacement surgery.

- Timing of initiation of VTE prophylaxis after surgery is an important and complicated issue. The risk of thromboembolic events begins immediately after surgery; therefore, VTE prophylaxis is generally more effective when started earlier rather than later. The challenge comes in that early VTE prophylaxis is also associated with increased bleeding compared to VTE prophylaxis started later.

- Initiation of VTE prophylaxis after elective spinal surgery can typically start 12–24 hours postoperatively. Prophylaxis may need to be delayed if the surgical site remains open.

- The frequency and severity of complications using non-neuraxial techniques (plexus or peripheral delivery) are influenced by the size of the catheter and degree of anticoagulation. The most serious complication from excessive anticoagulation using non-neuraxial techniques appears to be blood loss rather than loss of neural function.

- Guidelines for the prevention of VTE in hip or knee surgery are provided by the American College of Chest Physicians (ACCP) and the American Association of Orthopedic Surgeons (AAOS).[1,8]

- Major differences in recommendations are the AAOS support for aspirin and warfarin at a lower INR (≤ 2), as well as a lack of appreciation for the correlation between a reduction in DVT events and prevention of PE.

- The AAOS guideline recommendations are not linked to all available clinical evidence and are consensus-based instead of evidence-based. Based on these limitations of the AAOS guidelines, the ACCP guidelines should be utilized for VTE prevention in hip or knee surgery.

Table 10-14: VTE Prophylaxis in Critically Ill Patients

Critical Care Setting	UFH	LMWH	Fondaparinux
Trauma	Insufficient evidence	Dalteparin 5,000 International Units SC q 24 hr Enoxaparin 30 mg SC q 12 hr	Insufficient evidence
Acute spinal cord injury	5,000 units SC q 8 hr	Enoxaparin 30 mg SC q 12 hr or enoxaparin 40 mg SC q 24 hr	Insufficient evidence
Burns	5,000 units SC q 8 hr or 5,000 units SC q 12 hr	Dalteparin 5,000 International Units SC q 24 hr Enoxaparin 40 mg SC q 24 hr	Insufficient evidence
Critical care	5,000 units SC q 8 hr or 5,000 units SC q 12 hr	Dalteparin 5,000 International Units SC q 24 hr Enoxaparin 30 mg SC q 12 hr or enoxaparin 40 mg SC q 24 hr	Insufficient evidence

Clinical Pearls

- **Trauma**—Meta-analysis has demonstrated UFH to be no more effective than control.[9] Enoxaparin 30 mg twice daily has demonstrated better efficacy to UFH 5,000 units twice daily.[10] Evidence for dalteparin is based on observational data. Pharmacologic prophylaxis can be safely started within 24–36 hours. Patients with acute spinal cord injury may need to be delayed for 48–72 hours. Patients with severe trauma (injury severity score >23) may present with antithrombin deficiency; therefore,

SC prophylaxis may be insufficient.[11] While not prospectively evaluated, an option may be to use a UFH infusion while the patient is in the intensive care unit early in the course of events. Only a slight bump in the aPTT (35–45 seconds) would be targeted since VTE prevention is the goal.

- **Acute spinal cord injury**—UFH three times daily demonstrated similar rates of DVT and bleeding compared to enoxaparin twice daily, but there was a significant reduction in PE with enoxaparin.[12] While enoxaparin 30 mg twice daily should be used during the acute injury period (about 2–3 weeks), either regimen could be used during the rehabilitation period. In a retrospective case-control study, dalteparin 5,000 units daily failed to demonstrated noninferiority to enoxaparin 30 mg twice daily in prevention of VTE (9.7% vs. 1.6%).[13] Further investigations of dalteparin and tinzaparin are warranted.

- **Burns**—The current evidence in burn patients currently comes from only observational studies with UFH, enoxaparin, and dalteparin. The most commonly used regimen is UFH 5,000 units SC every 12 hours.

- **Critical care**—In medically ill or postoperative general surgery patients UFH or LMWH can be used. In orthopedic surgery or trauma, LMWH is preferred. If mechanical prophylaxis is selected due to high-risk of bleeding, the patient should be frequently re-evaluated and switched to pharmacologic prophylaxis when the bleeding risk decreases. Some pharmacodynamic studies suggest that critical care patients with significant edema or receiving vasopressors may not achieve detectable anti-Factor Xa levels with LMWH. Dalteparin has shown to not have significant accumulation in critical care patients with renal insufficiency.[14] A retrievable IVC filter may be considered for PE prophylaxis, but it should be noted that this practice has limited evidence and is controversial. See the IVC discussion earlier in this chapter.

TRAVEL PROPHYLAXIS STRATEGIES

Table 10-15: Travel Prophylaxis Strategies

Indications	Patients at Low-to-Moderate Thrombosis Risk and a Travel Time of 8 Hours or Longer Patients at High Thrombosis Risk and a Travel Time of 6 Hours or Longer
Nonpharmacological	Hydration
	In-route exercises
	Foot lifts: place your heels on the floor and bring your toes up as high as you can; then put both feet back flat on the floor; then pull your heels up while keeping the balls of your feet on the floor
	Ankle turns: lift your feet off the floor and move your toes in a circle, one foot moving clockwise and the other foot moving counterclockwise; then change direction and repeat direction
	Frequent travel breaks every 1–2 hr
	Avoid restrictive clothing (tight clothes, belts, etc.)
	Avoid or limit alcohol and caffeine prior to travel
	Airline or bus aisle seating
	Graduated compression devices
Pharmacological	LMWH before take-off on the outgoing and return flights

Clinical Pearls

- Below knee compression devices with ≥15–20 mm Hg graduated pressure are recommended.

- Compression devices should be placed 3–4 hours before departure and removed upon arrival.

- Pharmacological therapy should be administered 2–4 hours prior to departure.

- The ACCP provides a recommendation (Grade 2C) for a single prophylactic dose of LMWH to be given prior to departure. Contrary to this recommendation, the only trial mentioned in the ACCP guidelines that used LMWH gave SC enoxaparin 1 mg/kg.

- Aspirin has been shown to be ineffective in this setting.

DURATION OF VTE PROPHYLAXIS

Table 10-16: Duration of VTE Prophylaxis

Indication	Duration
General medically ill patients	6–14 days as long as immobile during acute illness
Major general surgery	Until hospital discharge
Major general surgery in patients with previous venous thromboembolism	Beyond hospital discharge for up to 28 days
Surgery for gastrointestinal, genitourinary, or gynecologic cancer	Beyond hospital discharge for up to 28 days
Total knee replacement surgery	At least 10 days
Total hip replacement surgery	4–6 weeks[a]
Hip fracture surgery	4–6 weeks[a]
Critical care patients	For the duration of the intensive care unit stay with re-evaluation when the patient is transferred to the general medical ward
Major trauma	Until hospital discharge and continued prophylaxis in patients with impaired mobility who undergo inpatient rehabilitation (up to 8 weeks)
Spinal cord injury patients	Until hospital discharge in patients with incomplete injuries; for 8 weeks in patients with uncomplicated complete motor injury; for 12 weeks or discharge from rehabilitation in patients with complete motor injury and other risk factors

[a]While the average time from surgery to VTE in knee replacement surgery is 7 days, the average time to VTE with hip procedures is delayed to 17 days.[15] Therefore, extended prophylaxis is considered a Grade 1A recommendation from ACCP for patients undergoing hip procedures.[1]

PHARMACOLOGICAL PROPHYLAXIS IN SPECIAL POPULATIONS

Severe renal insufficiency

- Patients with renal insufficiency are at higher risk of bleeding regardless of the anticoagulant used.
- Patients with a serum creatinine >2.5 mg/dL have been excluded from most clinical trials.
- Enoxaparin should be dosed at 30 mg SC once daily regardless of the indication.
- Dalteparin and tinzaparin do not seem to significantly accumulate in patients with severe renal insufficiency when prophylaxis doses are used.
- Fondaparinux is contraindicated in patients with a CrCl <30 mL/min.
- Patients on hemodialysis (renal failure) should receive SC UFH.

Obesity

- ACCP guidelines recommend possible weight-adjusted dosing in obese patients, but the guidelines do not provide insight on what weight this should be considered or what the "adjusted" dosing should be. Obese patients are at considerable risk of PE, but data from clinical trials on drug dosing is limited.
- Enoxaparin 40 mg SC twice daily has demonstrated better efficacy than 30 mg SC twice daily in bariatric surgery patients.[16]
- Injections of enoxaparin into the thigh in obese patients have a lower bioavailability compared to injections into the abdomen.
- One study suggests that the typical dose of LMWH may have to be higher in patients with a body mass index ≥40.[17]

Pregnancy

- Warfarin has been associated with congenital abnormalities when used during the 1st trimester and is, therefore, contraindicated. While warfarin could be used during the 2nd trimester, it is typically avoided throughout pregnancy.
- LMWH or UFH can be used throughout pregnancy.
- LMWHs (or fondaparinux) are not contraindicated in the 3rd trimester of pregnancy and can be used in the early 3rd trimester. During the peripartum period, many prefer to use UFH due to the shorter half-life and decreased risk of bleeding during delivery.

HIT (see Chapter 15 for more information)

- A meta-analysis has demonstrated that the risk of HIT is 2.6% for UFH and 0.2% for LMWH when prophylactic doses are used.[18]

- Due to a cross reactivity of 80% to 90%, LMWH cannot be used as a substitute for UFH in patients who develop HIT.

- While fondaparinux may be an option in patients with a history of HIT due to low cross-reactivity, case reports of HIT with fondaparinux have been noted. (For information on neuraxial anesthesia/analgesia, see Chapter 4.)

QUALITY IMPROVEMENT

Table 10-17: Quality Improvement Strategies

Strategy	Description
Educational initiatives	Peer-led presentations and in-services
	Mailings
Decision support tools	Electronic alerts and reminders
	Risk assessment models and prophylaxis reminders in admission charts
Audit and feedback process	Quality indicators and reports
	Benchmarking against outcomes from highest performing provider
Organizational changes	Integrated care pathways
	Changing from paper to computer-held patient records
Standardized dosing times	Utilize pharmacologic prophylaxis options that require less frequent dosing to avoid possible missed doses.
	Utilize a standard dosing time in the evening (i.e., 2100) to avoid missing morning dosing due to patients being off the floor
Regulations and policy changes	Reimbursement schemes including fee-for-service
	Required assessment policy

Table 10-18: Quality Improvement Metrics

Joint Commission and National Quality Forum Venous Thromboembolism Core Measures	Surgical Care Improvement Project
• **Population** Medically ill • **Measure** VTE-1 venous thromboembolism prophylaxis rates VTE-2 venous thromboembolism prophylaxis rates in the intensive care unit VTE-6 incidence of potentially-preventable VTE	• **Population** Surgical • **History** National quality partnership of organizations interested in improving surgical care; the commitment and collaboration of surgeons, anesthesiologists, perioperative nurses, pharmacists, infection control professionals, and hospital executives is expected to significantly reduce surgical complications; the project focuses on preventing complications in four areas that comprise 40% of the most common complications after major inpatient surgery including infection, blood clots, and adverse cardiac and respiratory events • **Measure** SCIP VTE-1: venous thromboembolism prophylaxis ordered for surgery patients SCIP VTE-2: appropriate VTE prophylaxis received within 24 hr prior to surgical incision time to 24 hr after surgery end time

REFERENCES

*Key articles

1. Geerts WH, Bergqvist D, Pineo GF, et al. Prevention of venous thromboembolism. *Chest*. 2008;133:381S–453S.

2. Wun T, White RH. Epidemiology of cancer-related venous thromboembolism. *Best Pract Clin Haematol Res*. 2009;22(1):9–23.

3. Khorana AA, Kuderer NM, Culakova E, et al. Development and validation of a predictive model for chemotherapy-associated thrombosis. *Blood*. 2008;111(10):4902–4907.

4. The PREPIC Study Group. Eight-year follow-up of patients with permanent vena cava filters in the prevention of pulmonary embolism: the PREPIC (prevention du risque d'embolie pulmonaire par interruption cave) randomized study. *Circulation*. 2005;112:416–422.

5. Enders JM, Burke JM, Dobesh PP. Prevention of venous thromboembolism in acute medical illness. *Pharmacotherapy*. 2002;22:1564–1578.

* **6. Leonardi MJ, McGory ML, Ko CY. The rate of bleeding complications after pharmacologic deep venous thrombosis prophylaxis. A systematic review of 33 randomized controlled trials. *Arch Surg*. 2006;141:790–799.**

7. Agnelli G, Bergqvist D, Cohen AT, et al. Randomized clinical trial of postoperative fondaparinux versus perioperative dalteparin for prevention of venous thromboembolism in high-risk abdominal surgery. *Br J Surg*. 2005;92:1212–1220.

8. American Academy of Orthopaedic Surgeons Clinical Guideline on Prevention of Symptomatic Pulmonary Embolism in Patients Undergoing Total Hip or Knee Arthroplasty. Adopted by the American Academy of Orthopedic Surgeons Board of Directors May 2007. Available at www.aaos.org/Research/guidelines/PE_guideline.pdf. Accessed January 22, 2010.

9. Upchurch GR, Demling RH, Davies J, et al. Efficacy of subcutaneous heparin in prevention of venous thromboembolic events in trauma patients. *Am Surg*. 1995;61:749–755.

10. Geerts WH, Jay RM, Code KI, et al. A comparison of low-dose heparin with low-molecular-weight heparin as prophylaxis against venous thromboembolism after major trauma. *N Engl J Med*. 1996;335:701–707.

11. Owings J, Bagley M, Gosselin R, et al. Effect of critical injury on plasma antithrombin activity: low antithrombin levels are associated with thromboembolic complications. *J Trauma*. 1996;41:396–406.

12. Spinal Cord Injury Thromboprophylaxis Investigators. Prevention of venous thromboembolism in the acute treatment phase after spinal cord injury: a randomized, multicenter trial comparing low-dose heparin plus intermittent pneumatic compression with enoxaparin. *J Trauma*. 2003;54:1116–1124.

13. Slavik RS, Chan E, Gorman SK, et al. Dalteparin versus enoxaparin for venous thromboembolism prophylaxis in acute spinal cord injury and major orthopedic trauma patients: DETECT trial. *J Trauma*. 2007;62:1075–1081.

14. Prophylaxis of thromboembolism in critical care (PROTECT) trial: a pilot study. *J Crit Care*. 2005;20:364–372.

* **15. White RH, Romano PS, Zhou H, et al. Incidence and time course of thromboembolic outcomes following total hip or knee arthroplasty. *Arch Intern Med*. 1998;158:1525–1531.**

16. Scholten DJ, Hoedema RM, Scholten DE. A comparison of two different prophylactic dose regimens of low molecular weight heparin in bariatric surgery. *Obes Surg.* 2002;12:19–24.

17. Kucher N, Leizorovicz A, Vaikus PT, et al., for the PREVENT Medical Thromboprophylaxis Study Group. Efficacy and safety of fixed low-dose dalteparin in preventing venous thromboembolism among obese or elderly hospitalized patients. A subgroup analysis of the PREVENT trial. *Arch Intern Med.* 2005;165:341–345.

18. Martel N, Lee J, Wells PS. Risk for heparin-induced thrombocytopenia with unfractionated and low-molecular-weight heparin thromboprophylaxis: a meta-analysis. *Blood.* 2005;106:2710–2715.

Note: the following key articles are not cited in the text.

Bates SM, Greer IA, Pabinger I, et al. Venous thromboembolism, thrombophilia, antithrombotic therapy, and pregnancy: American College of Chest Physicians Evidence-Based Clinical Practice Guidelines (8th ed.). *Chest.* 2008;133:844S–886S.

Consortium for Spinal Cord Medicine: Prevention of Thromboembolism in Spinal Cord Injury: Clinical Practice Guidelines for Spinal Cord Medicine. Washington, DC: Paralyzed Veterans of America; 1997. Available at www.guideline.gov/summary/pdf.aspx?doc_id=2965&stat=1&string=. Accessed January 22, 2010.

Crowther MA, Kelton JG. Congenital thrombophilic states associated with venous thrombosis: a qualitative overview and proposed classification system. *Ann Intern Med.* 2003;138:128–134.

Dobesh PP, Wittkowsky AK, Stacy ZA, et al. Key articles and guidelines for the prevention of venous thromboembolism. *Pharmacotherapy.* 2009;29:410–458.

Haines ST, Witt DA, Nutescu EA. Venous thromboembolism. In: Dipiro JT, Talbert RL, Yee GC, et al., eds. *Pharmacology.* 7th ed. New York, NY: McGraw Hill Medical; 2008.

Leonardi MJ, McGory ML, Ko CY. A systematic review of deep venous thrombosis prophylaxis in cancer patients: Implications for improving quality. *Ann Surg Oncol.* 2007;14:929–936.

Lyman GH, Khorana AA, Falanga A, et al. American Society of Clinical Oncology guideline: Recommendations for Venous Thromboembolism Prophylaxis and Treatment in Patients with Cancer. *J Clin Oncol.* 2007;25:5490–5505.

Mismetti P, Laporte S, Darmon JY, et al. Meta-analysis of low molecular weight heparin in the prevention of venous thromboembolism in general surgery. *Br J Surg.* 2001;88:913–930.

Wein L, Wein S, Haas SJ, et al. Pharmacological venous thromboembolism prophylaxis in hospitalized medical patients: a meta-analysis of randomized controlled trials. *Arch Intern Med.* 2007;167:1476–1486.

ELEVEN

Chapter

11

Venous Thromboembolism Treatment

Michael P. Gulseth, Gregory J. Peitz

INTRODUCTION

Up to 350,000–600,000 patients suffer from deep vein thrombosis (DVT) and pulmonary embolism (PE) each year. In addition, it has been estimated that up to 100,000 patients directly or indirectly die of this disease process.[1] The optimal treatment of venous thromboembolism is critical to prevent death and future recurrence.

VENOUS THROMBOEMBOLISM OVERVIEW

Common areas for venous thrombosis

- Lower extremity DVT
- Lower extremity superficial vein thrombosis
- Upper extremity DVT

Table 11-1: Lower Extremity Venous Anatomy

Deep Veins of the Lower Leg	Superficial Lower Limb Veins
Femoral vein	Long saphenous vein
Deep femoral vein	External pudendal veins
Medial and lateral circumflex femoral veins	Superficial circumflex iliac vein
Popliteal vein	Superficial epigastric vein

(continued)

Table 11-1: (Continued)

Deep Veins of the Lower Leg	Superficial Lower Limb Veins
Sural veins	Accessory saphenous vein
Genicular veins	Posterior arch vein
Anterior and posterior tibial veins	Short saphenous vein
Fibular veins	Femoropopliteal vein
Dorsal and plantar metatarsal veins	Dorsal venous network
Plantar digital veins	Dorsal venous arch
	Plantar venous network
	Plantar venous arch

See Figure 11–1.

Clinical Pearls

- DVT can embolize; superficial vein thrombi do not (unless they extend into a deep vein).

- Isolated calf DVTs are less likely to embolize than proximal DVTs.

- "Proximal" DVTs are any DVTs that occur above the level of the knee (popliteal vein) and higher.

- Patients can often present with nonspecific symptoms.

See Figure 11-2 for the pathophysiology of DVT/PE.

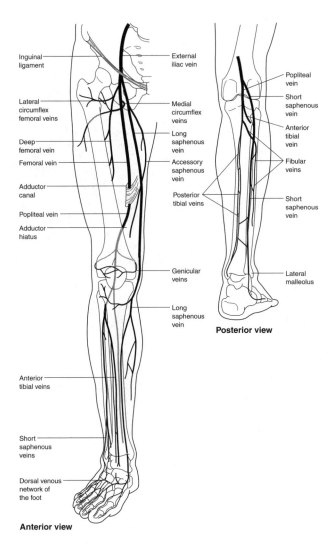

Figure 11-1: Lower Extremity Venous Anatomy

PATHOPHYSIOLOGY OF DVT/PE

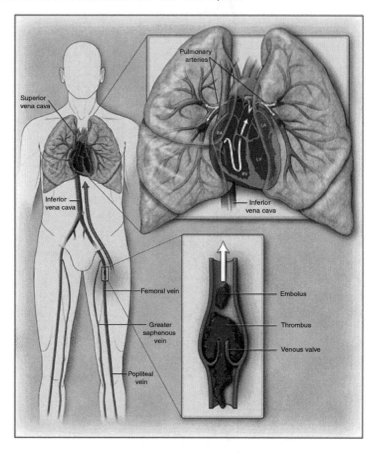

Figure 11-2: Pathophysiology of DVT and PE[2]

Pulmonary emboli usually originate in the deep veins of the leg. The thrombus typically originates around the venous valves and other areas of stasis. Clots that extend above the knee or originate above knee are at a higher risk of embolization. Pulmonary emboli travel through the venous system, into the right side of the heart, to the lungs. (Source: used with permission from reference 2. ©2008. Massachusetts Medical Society. All rights reserved.)

Table 11-2: Upper Extremity Venous Anatomy

Deep Veins of the Upper Extremity	Superficial Upper Extremity Veins
Subclavian vein	Cephalic vein
Axillary vein	Accessory cephalic vein
Brachial veins	Basilic vein
Ulnar veins	Median cubital vein
Radial veins	Median antebrachial vein
Anterior interosseous veins	Median cephalic vein
Posterior interosseous veins	Median basilica vein
Deep palmar venous arch	Dorsal venous network of the hand
Palmar metacarpal veins	Superficial palmar venous arch

Clinical Pearl

- Most upper extremity DVTs are related to central lines.

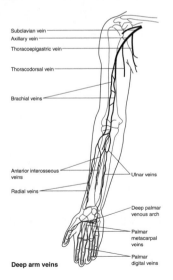

Figure 11-3: Upper Extremity Venous Anatomy

Paroxysmal embolism

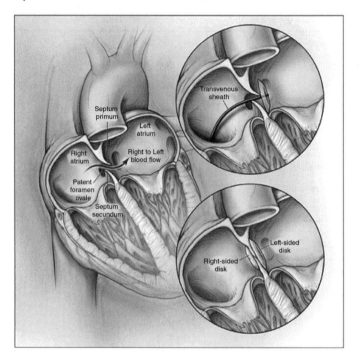

Figure 11-4: Paroxysmal Embolism[3]

In some patients with atrial septal defects (i.e., a patent foramen ovale [PFO]) of the heart, DVT that embolize can cross over to the arterial system. These patients have right-to-left blood flow, in the heart, as depicted. Also shown is a technique that can be used to mechanically close a PFO. (Source: used with permission from reference 3. ©2005. Massachusetts Medical Society. All rights reserved.)

DIAGNOSIS OF DEEP VEIN THROMBOSIS

DVT signs/symptoms*

- Leg swelling
- Pain in the leg

- Calf tenderness
- Increased leg warmth
- Erythema
- Palpable superficial veins
- Pain in the back of the knee when the foot is dorsiflexed (Homans' sign)

*Key point: these are very nonspecific signs/symptoms; objective testing is needed to confirm the diagnosis.

DVT DIAGNOSTIC TESTING

Role of D-dimer testing in establishing the diagnosis of DVT

- D-dimer is a degradation product that is produced from the breakdown of a fibrin blood clot.
- D-dimer is elevated during acute venous thromboembolism, but other conditions can also cause elevation.
- D-dimer is an effective "rule out" of venous thromboembolism in the setting of low clinical pretest probability, but a positive result requires further diagnostic verification (other common causes of elevated D-dimer include recent surgery/trauma, pregnancy, and cancer).
- The sensitivity of D-dimer is dependent on the assay method and no universal "cutoff" level exists.
- Sensitivity of D-dimer may be reduced if the duration of signs and symptoms of venous thromboembolism exceed 2–3 days or if the patient has received heparin therapy.

Role of duplex ultrasonography (with compression) in establishing the diagnosis of DVT

- Preferred to venography since it is noninvasive and does not carry the side effects of venography (i.e., hypotension, cardiac arrhythmias, vessel wall irritation, and nephrotoxicity due to the contrast medium).

- Positive duplex ultrasound in combination with moderate-to-high pretest probability scoring or a positive D-dimer can be used to confirm the diagnosis.
- Negative testing does not exclude DVT, particularly in calf veins.
- The ability to diagnose new DVT can be difficult in patients with previous history of DVT.

Table 11-3: Wells Pretest Probability Scoring for Deep Vein Thrombosis[4]

Clinical Features	Score
Tenderness along entire deep vein system	1
Swelling of the entire leg	1
Greater than 3-cm difference in calf circumference	1
Pitting edema	1
Collateral superficial veins	1
Risk factors:	
Active cancer	1
Prolonged immobility or paralysis	1
Recent surgery or major medical illness	1
Alternative diagnosis likely	−2
Total	

≥ 3 = high probability; 1–2 = moderate probability; ≤ 0 = low probability.

Clinical Pearl

- Further diagnostic testing is not necessary in patients with low pretest probability score for DVT and a negative D-dimer.

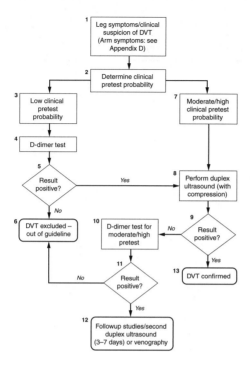

Figure 11-5: Diagnosis Algorithm from the Institute on Clinical Systems Improvement[5]

(Source: used with permission from reference 5. ©2009. Institute for Clinical Systems Improvement. All rights reserved.)

DIAGNOSIS OF PULMONARY EMBOLISM

Table 11-4: Diagnosis of Pulmonary Embolism

PE Signs/Symptoms—Three Most Common Signs/Symptoms

Dyspnea

Pleuritic chest pain with clear x-ray

Tachypnea

(*continued*)

Table 11-4: (Continued)

PE Signs/Symptoms—Less Frequent Signs/Symptoms

Cough

Hemoptysis

Fever

Syncope

Diaphoresis

Nonpleuritic chest pain

Apprehension

Rales

Increased pulmonic component (P2) of the second heart sound

Systolic murmur (tricuspid regurgitation)

ECG findings: right bundle branch block, $S_I Q_{III} T_{III}$, and T wave inversions in leads V1-V4

Wheezing

Hypotension

Tachycardia

Cyanosis

Pleural rub

Elevated neck veins

PE Signs/Symptoms—Massive PE

Hemodynamic instability

Cardiac arrest

Cyanosis

Hypoxia

Oliguria

(*continued*)

Table 11-4: (Continued)

PE Signs/Symptoms—Massive PE

Greater than 50% or more absent perfusion of the lung on angiography or ventilation/perfusion scanning

Right ventricular strain on echocardiogram

Elevated pulmonary artery pressure

Elevated B-type natriuretic peptide

Elevated troponin

Clinical Pearl

- Similar to patients with DVT, patients with PE often present with atypical symptoms or can also present with asymptomatic disease.

PULMONARY EMBOLISM DIAGNOSTIC TESTING

Computed tomographic (CT) pulmonary angiography

- Considered first-line choice for use in diagnosis unless contraindications exist

- Contrast dye is typically used, which can make the test unsuitable for patients with poor renal function.

- Positive scan results for a PE have good specificity and generally confirms the diagnosis.

- Negative scans lack sensitivity and may require further diagnostic studies if PE seems likely due to pretest probability scoring and/or D-dimer results.

- Both sensitivity and specificity of the scan is improved with central clots as to those that are more peripheral.

- Scan must be technically performed well including appropriate timing from contrast injection, patient holding their breath about 20 seconds, and optimized spatial resolution parameter settings.

- False positives are more common for segmental/subsegmental embolism and followup testing may be needed

Table 11-5: Wells Pretest Probability Scoring for Pulmonary Embolism[6]

Clinical Features	Score
DVT signs and symptoms	3
PE as likely or more likely than alternative diagnosis	3
Heart rate greater than 100 beats/min	1.5
Immobilization or surgery in the previous 4 weeks	1.5
Previous DVT or PE	1.5
Hemoptysis	1
Cancer	1
Total	

>6 = high probability; 2–6 = moderate probability; <2 = low probability.

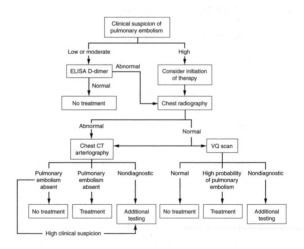

Figure 11-6: Pulmonary Embolism Diagnosis Algorithm[2]

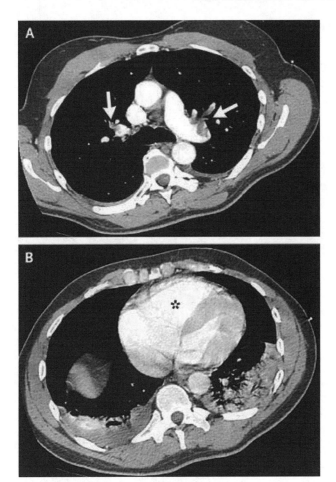

Figure 11-7: CT of a Pulmonary Embolism[2]

Panel A shows bilateral PE (arrows). Note that newer CTs are capable of higher resolution and detect smaller, peripheral emboli as depicted in Panel A. Panel B shows an enlarged right ventricle (asterisk), caused by acute PE. Note that the right ventricle can dilate reducing left ventricular filling volumes and compromising hemodynamic effects. (Source: used with permission from reference 2. ©2008. Massachusetts Medical Society. All rights reserved.)

Ventilation/Perfusion (V/Q) lung scan

- Highly positive scan results for a PE have good specificity and can help confirm the diagnosis.

- The specificity of the scan can be impaired by chronic obstructive pulmonary disease, asthma, and congestive heart failure.

- A negative scan has good specificity and generally rules out the diagnosis.

- A nondiagnostic (intermediate or low radiologic probability scan) result lacks sensitivity and requires further diagnostic studies if PE seems likely.

- V/Q scanning is often preferred in patients with renal insufficiency or with allergies to contrast dye.

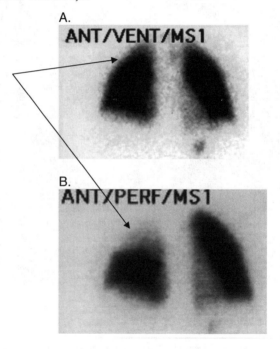

Figure 11-8: V/Q Lung Scan of a Pulmonary Embolism[7]

Panel A shows good ventilation of the lung, while panel B shows poor blood perfusion to the right upper lobe. This patient had a PE. (Source: used with permission from reference 7.)

VENOUS THROMBOEMBOLISM TREATMENT PRINCIPLES

Early and aggressive anticoagulation is the preferred treatment modality in patients with PE. Thrombolysis can be considered in selected high-risk cases as highlighted below.

When should systemic thrombolysis be considered for PE?

1. Sustained hypotension/cardiogenic shock
2. Patients without hemodynamic compromise who
   - are very ill in conjunction with severe dyspnea, anxiety, and poor oxygen saturation
   - have elevated troponin (indicative of right ventricular micro-infarction)
   - have right ventricular dysfunction demonstrated by an echocardiogram
   - have right ventricular enlargement on chest CT
   - are at low risk of bleeding (see Table 11-6)

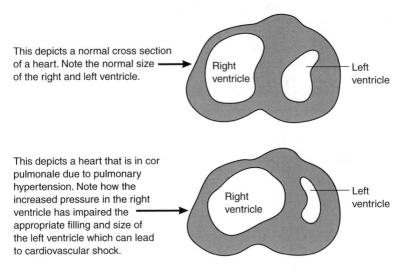

This depicts a normal cross section of a heart. Note the normal size of the right and left ventricle.

Right ventricle — Left ventricle

This depicts a heart that is in cor pulmonale due to pulmonary hypertension. Note how the increased pressure in the right ventricle has impaired the appropriate filling and size of the left ventricle which can lead to cardiovascular shock.

Right ventricle — Left ventricle

Figure 11-9: Right Ventricular Dysfunction in Acute Pulmonary Embolism

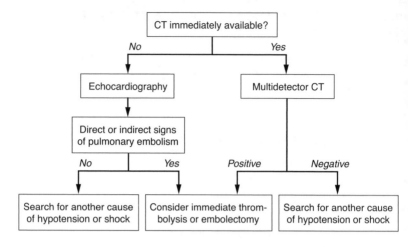

Figure 11-10: Proposed Diagnosis/Treatment Algorithm for PE Accompanied by Hypotension or Shock[8]

Direct sign of PE on an echocardiogram would include (1) thrombi in the right atrium, right ventricle, or pulmonary artery; and (2) thrombi that protrude into the left atrium through a patent foramen ovale. Indirect signs on an echocardiogram would include (1) right ventricular dysfunction (see Figure 11-10); (2) a systolic pressure gradient between the right ventricle and the right atrium of more than 30 mm Hg; and (3) pulmonary arterial flow acceleration time of less than 80 msec. (Source: used with permission from reference 8. ©2008. Massachusetts Medical Society. All rights reserved.)

Table 11-6: Absolute and Relative Contraindications to Systemic Thrombolysis

Absolute

Active internal bleeding or bleeding diathesis (not menses)

Previous intracranial hemorrhage

Ischemic (thrombotic) stroke within 3 mo

Intracranial neoplasm

Structural vascular lesion (i.e., arteriovenous malformation)

(continued)

Table 11-6: (Continued)

Suspected aortic dissection

Significant closed head or facial trauma within 3 mo

Relative

Severe, uncontrolled hypertension on presentation (BP >180/110 mm Hg)

History of prior ischemic (thrombotic) stroke >3 mo, dementia, or known intracranial pathology not covered in absolute contraindications

Traumatic or prolonged (>10 min) CPR

Major surgery (<3 weeks)

Recent internal bleeding (2–4 weeks)

Noncompressible vascular puncture (i.e., recent liver biopsy or carotid artery puncture)

Pregnancy

Active peptic ulcer

Current anticoagulant use

History of severe, chronic poorly controlled hypertension

If streptokinase, prior use (5 days to 2 yr) or known allergic response

Table 11-7: Thrombolytic Dosing When Given Systemically for the Treatment of Pulmonary Embolism

The 2008 American College of Chest Physician (ACCP) guidelines[9] recommend that, "In patients with acute PE, with administration of thrombolytic therapy, we recommend use of regimens with short infusion times (e.g., a 2-hour infusion) over those with prolonged infusion times (e.g., a 24-hour infusion)." Below, are commonly utilized infusion regimens that meet this standard that have been studied in clinical trials.

Alteplase 100 mg IV given over 2 hr (some trials gave a 10-mg bolus followed by another 90 mg over 2 hr) (FDA approved, and the most peer-reviewed patient data)

Urokinase 3,000,000 units IV over 2 hr (1,000,000 units as a bolus over 10 min, then 2,000,000 units over the remaining time)

Streptokinase 1,500,000 units IV over 2 hr

Reteplase[a] 10 units bolus injection; repeat, X 1 in 30 min (two bolus doses)

Tenecteplase[a] bolus dose given over 5–10 sec X 1 (less than 60 kg = 30 mg; 60 less than 70 kg = 35 mg; 70 less than 80 kg = 40 mg; 80 less than 90 kg = 45 mg; 90 kg and above = 50 mg)

[a]Data is limited for these agents.

Table 11-8: Heparin Dosing Considerations When Given with Systemic Thrombolysis for Pulmonary Embolism Treatment

Anticoagulation with intravenous heparin therapy should not be delayed when making the decision whether to utilize thrombolytic therapy. Initial recommended dosing is 80 units/kg (max 10,000 units) followed by an infusion of 18 units/kg/hr (max 1500 units/hr).

Once the decision is made to use thrombolytic therapy, it is important to note that some of the clinical trials that utilized thrombolytic therapy for PE continued heparin therapy, while others suspended therapy while the thrombolytic was infusing

Concurrent heparin use should be specifically avoided if using streptokinase or urokinase for thrombolysis

The FDA recommends suspending the heparin infusion while the thrombolytic is infusing

If this option is chosen:

- Check an aPTT at the end of the infusion
- If less than 2 times normal (some authorities recommend less than roughly 80 seconds), restart the heparin *without* a bolus at the same dose
- If greater than 2 times normal, recheck in another 4 hr, and if acceptable, start the heparin at that time *without* a bolus

Heparin dosing considerations when given with catheter directed thrombolysis for DVT treatment

- Catheter directed thrombolysis is often utilized for massive iliofemoral DVT to help prevent the development of post-thrombotic syndrome.
- The heparin dosing is not standardized for this indication and often lower intensities were used in reported studies than standard DVT therapy (often 1,000 units/hr or less).

Clinical Pearl

- Caution must be exercised whenever using anticoagulants with, or in close proximity to thrombolytics. See Chapter 6 for more details and dosing considerations.

Use of inferior vena cava (IVC) filters

- Inferior vena cava filters come in two types: permanent and retrievable.
- Retrievable filters can be removed when the need for the filter has dissipated.
    - Removal can be difficult if the filter has become imbedded in the wall of the IVC or if a large amount of clot is present in the filter; the filter then becomes permanent.
    - To help prevent imbedding in the wall, filters can be rotated periodically.
    - Warfarin therapy may not be initiated until the filter is removed in some cases.
- Only one randomized study has assessed the efficacy and safety of IVC filters and found that while filters decrease PE rates, they also increase DVT rates with no mortality benefit.[10]

Standard indications for IVC filter placement

- Known VTE with a contraindication to anticoagulation therapy
- Known VTE with complications of anticoagulation therapy
- Recurrent VTE despite anticoagulation treatment (anticoagulation failure)
- Chronic thromboembolic hypertension patients who will undergo thromboendarterectomy

Evolving indications for IVC filter placement*

- Recurrent PE leading to pulmonary hypertension
- DVT patients with limited cardiopulmonary reserve capacity or COPD patients
- Patients who have large, free-floating iliofemoral thrombus
- Patients who have had thrombectomy, embolectomy, or thrombolysis of DVT
- High-risk trauma patients (spinal cord injury, pelvic, or lower extremity fractures) who cannot be safely anticoagulated
- High-risk surgical patients who are contraindicated for anticoagulation
- DVT patients who are pregnant, or have burns or cancer
- Treatment of acute DVT organ transplant patients

*Many of these indications are controversial with little high quality evidence to support their use.

Table 11-9: Potential IVC Filter Use Complications

Filter Use Complications

Thrombosis at the insertion site	Tilting or fracture of the filter (filter fragments can embolize)
IVC thrombosis	Penetration of the IVC
Filter thrombosis (can be on top of the filter)	DVT recurrence
Filter migration	Post-thrombotic syndrome
Vena caval obstruction	Guidewire entrapment

Clinical Pearl

- When IVC filters should be used is a very controversial topic. Clinicians who routinely work in anticoagulation should be familiar with the data regarding their use. Warfarin anticoagulation generally should be used long term in patients with permanent (including those with retrievable filters that are not removed) IVC filters *provided* they are appropriate for long-term anticoagulation.

Use of anticoagulants to treat VTE

General principles of therapy

- For patients with a high clinical suspicion of DVT/PE, parenteral anticoagulation therapy should be started even if diagnostic tests are pending.

- Parenteral anticoagulation therapy should be overlapped with warfarin for at least 5 days and until the INR is >2 and stable to allow the vitamin K antagonist enough time to reach its full anticoagulant effect (new Joint Commission Core Measure).

- Warfarin can be started on the first day along with the parenteral anticoagulation.

- Anticoagulants should be combined with the use of an elastic compression stocking with and ankle pressure of 30–40 mm Hg to help prevent post-thrombotic syndrome if possible; therapy should continue at least 2 years.

- Upper extremities DVTs are generally treated in a similar fashion to lower extremity DVTs, but this is based on limited data.

Clinical Pearls

Use of UFH for treatment of VTE (more detailed information can be found in Chapter 3):

- Preferred agent when thrombolytics would be used (systemic thrombolytic treatment of PE, catheter directed therapies, etc.)

- May also be preferred in patients with severe renal insufficiency

- Both IV infusions and subcutaneous therapy are acceptable options for VTE treatment.

- When IV infusions are utilized, achieving a therapeutic aPTT in the first 24 hours has been linked to decreased VTE recurrence rates.

- Targeted aPTTs should be regularly correlated to therapeutic heparin levels of 0.3–0.7 units/mL anti-Factor Xa activity (see Chapter 18).

- IV route is the preferred option whenever there are concerns over subcutaneous absorption.

Use of LMWH/fondaparinux for treatment of VTE (detailed information can be found in Chapter 4):

- Best studied therapies to facilitate home treatment of VTE

- Patients who were initially treated with IV UFH can have a single injection at discharge to complete a full 5 days of heparin therapy.

- Routine measurements of anti-Factor Xa activity levels are not needed.

- Can be utilized long term, alone, for the treatment of VTE; recommended initial approach to the treatment of VTE in the setting of cancer (see Clinical Pearls below)

LMWH/fondaparinux for treatment of VTE in cancer:

- The ACCP guidelines, the National Comprehensive Cancer Network (NCCN), and the American Society of Clinical Oncology (ASCO) recommend LMWH therapy alone for the initial treatment of venous thromboembolism.

- This is recommended for the first 3–6 months of therapy of the total duration of therapy; longer term therapy, if needed, should be continued with warfarin or LMWH depending on the patient specific scenario.

- Dalteparin is FDA indicated for this use, but other agents are also used in practice despite weaker evidence.[11]

Use of LMWH/fondaparinux at home:

- Assure the patient/caregiver is fully educated on administering the injection and willing to comply.

- Assure the followup appointments have been made for anticoagulation monitoring.

- Assure the outpatient provider clearly understands the treatment plan and the importance of making sure the patient follows up.

- Assure the patient can pay for the drug before a final decision on treatment is made.

- Assure that the pharmacy the patient will obtain the medication from has it in stock.

- Assure the patient has phone numbers to call if they have any question/concerns about therapy when at home and that the care providers have the patient's contact information if needed.

Use of warfarin for treatment of VTE (detailed warfarin dosing/titration information can be found in Chapter 2):

- Typical warfarin initiation doses are between 5–10 mg; lower doses are needed in some populations who are sensitive to warfarin (see Chapter 2).

- Higher initial treatment doses (e.g., 10 mg) have been associated with obtaining a more rapid therapeutic INR in outpatients being treated for DVT.

- Delay in obtaining therapeutic INRs has the potential to prolong costly hospitalization or LMWH therapy.

- Assure that all transitional care issues are addressed if initial therapy is given in the inpatient setting (followup INR scheduled, provider is aware of discharge and transition plans, duration of therapy is communicated).

- Make sure the patient receives warfarin education and venous thromboembolism education (Joint Commission National Patient Safety Goal requirement and part of the VTE Core Measures).

- Desired goal INR range is 2–3; higher INR targets have been linked to more bleeding events and lower INR targets (1.5–2) were not as effective with no clear benefit on bleeding outcomes.[9,12]

- A lower INR range of 1.5–2.0 has been found to be superior to placebo after an initial 6 months of conventional goal therapy (2–3 target INR) and may be an option to help decrease the number of needed INR tests (INR measurements were 8 weeks apart if INR 1.3–3.0).[13]

Duration of anticoagulation for VTE

Clinical Pearls

Determining the duration of therapy:

- The length and duration of anticoagulation should be tailored to each patient, considering that the risk for overall recurrent VTE at 10 years is 30%.

- In general, the long-term risks of anticoagulant use (bleeding) must be weighed against the risk of repeat thrombosis when deciding the optimal length of therapy.

- The role of thrombophilia assessment to help guide the length of therapy decision is controversial (see Table 11-10).

Table 11-10: Recommended Duration of Anticoagulation Therapy

Type of Venothromboembolism	Duration of Treatment
Provoked[a]	At least 3 mo of treatment
Idiopathic cause (unprovoked)	
1st event	At least 3 mo; consider indefinite therapy when bleeding risk is low after an initial 3 mo of therapy[b]

(continued)

Table 11-10: (Continued)

Type of Venothromboembolism	Duration of Treatment
2nd or more events	Indefinite therapy
Active cancer	3–6 mo with LMWH and continued anticoagulation until cancer has resolved (see above)
Upper extremity VTE	At least 3 mo of treatment[b]
Spontaneous superficial vein thrombosis	4 weeks[c]

[a]See Table 11-11 for common VTE-provoking factors.

[b]Risk/benefits of longer term anticoagulation should be considered.

[c]Using prophylactic or intermediate LMWH, intermediate heparin, or VKA with INR of 2–3 after 5-day overlap with heparin/LMWH.

Emerging options to determine optimal length of anticoagulation therapy

Evidence supports earlier discontinuation of VKA anticoagulation in patients with early response indicated by various procedures and labs.

Table 11-11: Evidence of Early Discontinuation of VKA

Indicating Factors Suggesting Shorter Duration of Therapy (3 mo)[a]

- Negative or nonabnormal D-dimer 1 mo after initial 3 mo VKA anticoagulation
  - Recurrent VTE rates similar to other trials with prolonged VKA anticoagulation (2.9% to 3.5%)[14,15]
- Residual venous thrombosis testing done following 3 mo VKA anticoagulation
  - Patients with negative findings had recurrent VTE rates of 1.9%[16]
  - An anticoagulation "flexible duration" strategy based on residual thrombosis finding and patient type led to a 11.9% recurrence rate[17]

[a]Evident in first-occurrence, nonprovoked VTE population.

Table 11-12: Common Provoking (reversible) Risk Factors for VTE

Common Provoking Risk Factors
Major risk (all within 1 mo of event)
Surgery
Hospitalization
Plaster cast immobilization
Minor risk
Estrogen therapy
Pregnancy
Prolonged travel (>8 hr)
Any major factor within 1–3 mo

Table 11-13: Positive and Negative Risk Factors for Recurrent VTE to Help Determine Length of Therapy to Prevent Recurrent VTE

Risk Factor	RR
Antiphospholipid antibody syndrome	2
Male gender	1.6
Hereditary thrombophilia	1.5
Residual thrombosis in proximal veins	1.5
Two or more prior VTE	1.5
Asian descent	0.8
Isolated calf thrombosis (vs. proximal DVT)	0.5
Negative D-Dimer 1 mo after VKA discontinuation	0.4

Patients with risk factors for bleeding complications to aid in determining risk/benefit of long-term warfarin therapy

- Patient >75 years old
- History of GI bleed (especially if nonprovoked)
- History of noncardioembolic stroke
- Chronic renal or hepatic disease
- Concurrent antiplatelet therapy
- Poor anticoagulation control
- Suboptimal monitoring of anticoagulation therapy
- Current serious or acute illness

Thrombophilia testing

Indications when hereditary hypercoagulability tests may be useful to guide therapy*

- VTE before the age of 40
- Strong family history of VTE
- Thrombosis at an atypical anatomical site
- Large PE
- Neonatal purpura fulminans or warfarin skin necrosis
- Multiple VTEs
- Recurrent pregnancy losses, stillbirth

*These tests can be deferred until after 3–6 months after primary event, as initial anticoagulation management is unlikely to change in regard to results.

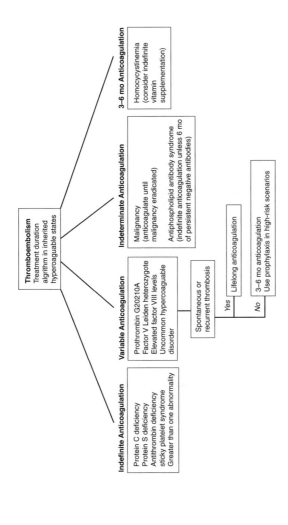

Figure 11-11: Proposed Treatment Algorithm When Thrombophilia Information is Known[18]

(Source: adapted from reference 18.)

REFERENCES

*Key articles

1. Unknown. The surgeon general's call to action to prevent deep vein thrombosis and pulmonary embolism. Available at: http://www.surgeongeneral.gov/topics/deepvein/calltoaction/call-to-action-on-dvt-2008.pdf. Accessed July 13, 2010.

* 2. **Tapson VF. Acute pulmonary embolism. *N Engl J Med*. 2008;358(10):1037–1052.**

3. Kizer JR, Devereux RB. Clinical practice. Patent foramen ovale in young adults with unexplained stroke. *N Engl J Med*. 2005;353(22):2361–2372.

4. Wells PS, Anderson DR, Bormanis J, et al. Value of assessment of pretest probability of deep-vein thrombosis in clinical management. *Lancet*. 1997;350(9094):1795–1798.

* 5. **Burnett B. Venous thromboembolism diagnosis and treatment (guideline; 9th ed.). March 2009. Available at: http://www.icsi.org/guidelines_and_more/gl_os_prot/cardiovascular/venous_thromboembolism/venous_thromboembolism_6.html. Accessed May 9, 2009.**

6. Wells PS, Anderson DR, Rodger M, et al. Derivation of a simple clinical model to categorize patients probability of pulmonary embolism: increasing the models utility with the SimpliRED D-dimer. *Thromb Haemost*. 2000;83(3):416–420.

7. Unknown. Case twenty seven—pulmonary embolism (PE). Available at: http://www.uhrad.com/spectarc/nucs027.htm. Accessed May 9, 2009.

8. Konstantinides S. Clinical practice. Acute pulmonary embolism. *N Engl J Med*. 2008;359(26):2804–2813.

* 9. **Kearon C, Kahn SR, Agnelli G, et al. Antithrombotic therapy for venous thromboembolic disease: American College of Chest Physicians Evidence-Based Clinical Practice Guidelines (8th ed.). *Chest*. 2008;133(6 Suppl):454S–545S.**

10. Eight-year follow-up of patients with permanent vena cava filters in the prevention of pulmonary embolism: the PREPIC (Prevention du Risque d'Embolie Pulmonaire par Interruption Cave) randomized study. *Circulation*. 2005;112(3):416–422.

11. Lee AY, Levine MN, Baker RI, et al. Low-molecular-weight heparin versus a coumarin for the prevention of recurrent venous thromboembolism in patients with cancer. *N Engl J Med*. 2003;349(2):146–153.

12. Kearon C, Ginsberg JS, Kovacs MJ, et al. Comparison of low-intensity warfarin therapy with conventional-intensity warfarin therapy for long-term prevention of recurrent venous thromboembolism. *N Engl J Med*. 2003;349(7):631–639.

13. Ridker PM, Goldhaber SZ, Danielson E, et al. Long-term, low-intensity warfarin therapy for the prevention of recurrent venous thromboembolism. *N Engl J Med*. Apr 10 2003;348(15):1425–1434.

14. Palareti G, Cosmi B, Legnani C, et al. D-dimer testing to determine the duration of anticoagulation therapy. *N Engl J Med*. 2006;355(17):1780–1789.

15. Verhovsek M, Douketis JD, Yi Q, et al. Systematic review: D-dimer to predict recurrent disease after stopping anticoagulant therapy for unprovoked venous thromboembolism. *Ann Intern Med.* 2008;149(7):481–490, W494.

16. Siragusa S, Malato A, Anastasio R, et al. Residual vein thrombosis to establish duration of anticoagulation after a first episode of deep vein thrombosis: the duration of anticoagulation based on compression ultrasonography (DACUS) study. *Blood.* 2008;112(3):511–515.

17. Prandoni P, Prins MH, Lensing AW, et al. Residual thrombosis on ultrasonography to guide the duration of anticoagulation in patients with deep venous thrombosis: a randomized trial. *Ann Intern Med.* 2009;150(9):577–585.

18. **Thomas RH. Hypercoagulability syndromes. *Arch Intern Med.* 2001;161(20): 2433–2439.**

Note: the following key articles are not cited in the text.

Baglin T, Luddington R, Brown K, et al. Incidence of recurrent venous thromboembolism in relation to clinical and thrombophilic risk factors: prospective cohort study. *Lancet.* 2003;362:523–526.

Crowther MA. Inferior vena cava filters in the management of venous thromboembolism. *Am J Med.* 2007;120(10 Suppl 2):S13–S17.

Haines ST, Witt DA, Nutescu EA. Venous thromboembolism. In: Dipiro JT, Talbert RL, Yee GC, et al., eds. *Pharmacotherapy.* 7th ed. New York, NY: McGraw Hill Medical; 2008.

Ho WK, Hankey GJ, Quinlan DJ, et al. Risk of recurrent venous thromboembolism in patients with common thrombophilia: a systematic review. *Arch Intern Med.* 2006;166:729–736.

Snow V, Qaseem A, Barry P, et al. Management of venous thromboembolism: a clinical practice guideline from the American College of Physicians and the American Academy of Family Physicians. *Ann Intern Med.* 2007;146(3):204–210.

Atrial Fibrillation

12

Daniel M. Witt

INTRODUCTION

Atrial fibrillation (AF) is a common cardiac rhythm disorder. While AF rarely causes life-threatening hemodynamic compromise, it is an important independent risk factor for cardiogenic embolic stroke and systemic arterial thromboembolism.[1] Approximately 90% of AF thromboembolic complications are stroke related while the remaining 10% are systemic.

The following contribute to thromboembolic risk associated with AF[2]:

- Stasis or turbulence of blood flow within the left atrial appendage leads to thrombus formation.

- Dysfunction of vascular endothelium predisposes to local or systemic hypercoagulability.

- Conversion to normal sinus rhythm (NSR)—spontaneous or intentional— may dislodge any existing left atrial thrombi.

MORBIDITY AND MORTALITY ASSOCIATED WITH AF[1,3]

- 15% of all strokes occur in people with AF.
- The annual stroke risk in untreated AF patients varies between 3% and 8% (average 4.5%) depending on concurrent individual risk factors.
- Attributable stroke risk in AF increases with age.
    - 1.5% in 50–59 year age group
    - 23.5% in 80–89 year age group
- The 30-day case fatality rate of AF stroke is 24%.

Data from high-quality, randomized controlled clinical trials overwhelmingly demonstrates that long-term, adjusted-dose anticoagulation therapy with vitamin K-antagonists like warfarin virtually eliminates the stroke risk associated with AF.[1,2] Despite the proven efficacy of warfarin therapy in preventing AF-related stroke, only about half of patients who could benefit receive anticoagulation therapy.[1] Increasing age, perceived bleeding risk, and the innate complexity of managing anticoagulation therapy are negative predictors of warfarin use in AF.

Table 12-1: Classification of Atrial Fibrillation

Acute AF	Onset within previous 48 hr
Paroxysmal AF	Terminates spontaneously within 7 days (may recur)
Recurrent AF	More than one episode
Persistent AF	Duration for more than 7 days without spontaneous termination
Permanent AF	Persistence of AF despite electrical or pharmacologic cardioversion attempts

TREATMENT OVERVIEW

Rate vs. rhythm control

- Two landmark randomized trials, Atrial Fibrillation Follow-up Investigation of Rhythm Management (AFFIRM) and Rate Control vs. Electrical cardioversion for persistent atrial fibrillation (RACE) provide evidence that cardioversion of AF to normal sinus rhythm (rhythm control) is not necessary nor preferable to allowing AF to continue while controlling ventricular response rate with AV node blockade (rate control).[4–6]

  - AFFIRM found no difference in mortality or stroke rate between patients assigned to one strategy or the other.

  - RACE found rate control not inferior to rhythm control for prevention of death and morbidity.

  - Rate- or rhythm-control strategies do not seem to affect quality of life significantly or differently.

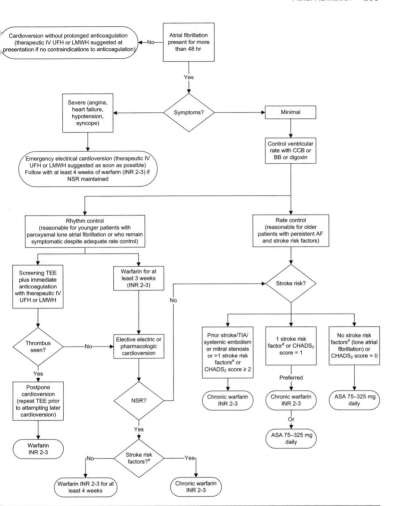

IV = intravenous; UFH = unfractionated heparin; LMWH = low-molecular-weight heparin; NSR = normal sinus rhythm; CCB = calcium channel blocker; BB = beta blocker; TEE = transesophageal echocardiogram; INR = international normalized ratio; TIA = transient ischemic attack; ASA = aspirin.

[a]Stroke risk factors include age >75 years; history of hypertension; diabetes mellitus; moderately or severely impaired left ventricular systolic function and/or heart failure.

Figure 12-1: Stroke Prevention in Atrial Fibrillation Treatment Algorithm

- Ischemic events occurred with similar frequency with either a rhythm or rate control strategy, especially when warfarin was discontinued o when anticoagulation was subtherapeutic.

- In younger individuals a combined rate and rhythm approach ma minimize the risk of related heart failure.

- Whether a rate or rhythm control strategy is employed, AF patients with *thromboembolic risk factors* should probably receive chronic dose-adjusted warfarin anticoagulation.[1,2]

Adjusted-dose warfarin vs. daily aspirin (ASA) therapy for stroke prevention in AF

- ASA provides little protection against stroke in AF and is markedly inferio to adjusted-dose (INR 2–3) warfarin therapy.[1]

- Pooled analysis of trials comparing ASA to placebo yield a relative risk reduc tion (RRR) estimate of 21% with a 95% confidence interval (CI) of 0% t 38%—compared to a RRR of 68% (95% CI 50% to 79%) with warfarin.[1]

- Compared with ASA alone, the combination of clopidogrel and ASA sig nificantly reduces the rate of major vascular events (mainly stroke) bu increases the risk of serious bleeding including ICH[7]—thus, the net effec of the combination is comparable to ASA alone.

- A randomized comparison of warfarin vs. clopidogrel plus ASA was termi nated early after showing the superiority of warfarin.[8]

- Adding ASA to warfarin therapy increases the risk of major bleeding and does not provide further protection against ischemic stroke in patient with AF (possible exception is patients with AF and prosthetic heart valve replacement).[9,10]

- **The key decision in AF stroke risk reduction is warfarin, yes or no?**—ASA should only be considered when the answer this question is "warfarin, no" due to either very low stroke risk or contraindications to warfarin therapy (e.g., bleeding risk, inability to comply with the requirements of warfarin therapy).[1]

AF stroke risk stratification tools

- Based on warfarin's superiority over any comparator in preventing stroke in AF, *it is not unreasonable to recommend warfarin therapy for all patient with AF.*[1]

- However, warfarin therapy is associated with bleeding risk, most importantly the risk for intracranial hemorrhage.
- Therefore, various risk stratification schemes have evolved with the following goals[1]:
  - Identifying AF patients at such low risk of stroke that warfarin-associated bleeding risk may outweigh stroke prevention benefit.
  - Encouraging warfarin use in patients at high risk for AF stroke where warfarin's benefit has been clearly demonstrated.
- The CHADS$_2$ score, which is well validated and easy to use, is the most popular AF stroke risk stratification tool.[11]

Risk factor	Points
Congestive heart failure	= 1
Hypertension	= 1
Age ≥75 years of age	= 1
Diabetes	= 1
Prior **S**troke/TIA/systemic embolus	= 2

Example: an 82-year-old male with hypertension and prior stroke would have a CHADS$_2$ score = 4.

Higher CHADS$_2$ score = higher AF stroke risk[1,11]:

CHADS$_2$ Score	Stroke Rate (%/year)	Recommended Therapy
0	1.9 (1.2–3.0)	Daily ASA
1	2.8 (2.0–3.8)	Warfarin (INR 2–3) or daily ASA
2	4.0 (3.1–5.1)	Warfarin (INR 2–3)
3	5.9 (4.6–7.3)	
4	8.5 (6.3–11.1)	
5	12.5 (8.2–17.5)	
6	18.2 (10.5–27.4)	

- A revised scoring approach (CHA_2DS_2VASc) has been proposed[12]:

Stroke Risk Factor	Points
Congestive heart failure	= 1
Hypertension	= 1
Age ≥75 years of age	= 2
Diabetes	= 1
Prior **S**troke/TIA/systemic embolus	= 2
Vascular disease (prior MI, PAD, or aortic plaque)	= 1
Age 65–74	= 1
Sex category (female)	= 1
Recommended antithrombotic therapy	
Score >1: oral anticoagulation (VKA INR 2–3)	
Score = 1: either oral antithrombotic therapy (INR 2–3)—preferred, or aspirin 75–325 mg/day	
Score = 0: no anticoagulation therapy (preferred), or aspirin 75–325 mg daily	
The CHA_2DS_2VASc identifies a lower risk population; the impact of the approach over the $CHADS_2$ has not been determined	

Table 12-2: Risk-Stratified Treatment Recommendations of The American College of Chest Physicians Evidence-Based Clinical Practice Guidelines (8th ed.)[1]

Risk Category	Prior ischemic stroke, TIA, systemic embolism, or history of mitral stenosis (valvular AF) or prosthetic heart valve[a]	≥2 stroke risk factors[b]	Only 1 stroke risk factor[b]	Age ≤75 years and no other stroke risk factors[b]
Recommended Therapy	Warfarin (INR 2–3)	Warfarin (INR 2–3)	Warfarin (INR 2–3) or daily ASA 75–325 mg	Daily ASA 75–325 mg

[a]INR target may be higher than 2–3 for patients with prosthetic heart valves.

[b]Stroke risk factors: age >75 years, history of hypertension, diabetes mellitus, and moderately or severely impaired left ventricular systolic function and/or heart failure.

Table 12-3: Risk-Stratified Treatment Recommendations of The American College of Cardiology/American Heart Association/European Society of Cardiology 2006 Guidelines for the Management of Patients with Atrial Fibrillation[2]

Risk Category	Any high-risk factor[a] or more than 1 moderate-risk factor[b]	One moderate-risk factor[b]	No risk factors
Recommended Therapy	Warfarin (INR 2–3)	Warfarin (INR 2–3) or daily ASA 81–325 mg	Daily ASA 81–325 mg

[a]High-risk factors: previous stroke/TIA/embolism, mitral stenosis, prosthetic heart valve (INR target may be higher than 2–3).

[b]Moderate-risk factors: age ≥75 years, hypertension, heart failure, left ventricular ejection fraction ≤35%, diabetes mellitus.

- *Echocardiography* is often used in treatment decision making but has limited proven value in determining the need for chronic warfarin therapy.
  - Echocardiography can detect the presence of features associated with thromboembolism. Anticoagulation therapy in patients with these features has been shown to reduce stroke risk (e.g., impaired left ventricular systolic function, left atrial thrombus, dense spontaneous echo contrast, "smoke," or reduced velocity of blood flow in the left atrial appendage); however, the absence of these echocardiographic abnormalities has not been established as identifying a low-risk group of AF patients who could safely forgo warfarin therapy.[2]
  - Echocardiography is valuable for detecting rheumatic mitral valve disease (there is universal agreement that these patients should receive warfarin therapy).[2]
  - Detection of left atrial thrombus is a contraindication for cardioversion of AF (see below).
  - Transesophageal echocardiography (TEE) far surpasses transthoracic echocardiography (TTE) in the evaluation of cardiogenic risk factors in patients with AF.[2]
- Risk stratification caveats
  - No published risk stratification tool is ideal and all can frequently underestimate stroke risk.[9]

- Risk stratification tools perform less well when limited to patients without prior history of stroke/transient ischemic attack (TIA)/systemic embolism.[1]

- While risk stratification tools identify AF patients who will benefit most and least from warfarin therapy, the stroke vs. bleeding risk tipping point for anticoagulation therapy use is controversial, especially for those at intermediate risk for stroke.[2]

- No tool can incorporate all potential AF stroke risk factors. Risk stratification tools can therefore best be described as "rough guides" to help inform clinicians.[9]

- Validated bleeding risk stratification tools are lacking.

- Patient perspectives and preferences should also factor into clinical decision making.[1]

Optimal intensity of anticoagulation for AF[2]

- Optimal anticoagulation therapy intensity involves a careful balancing between maximizing protection against thromboembolism while minimizing bleeding risk (ICH in particular rivals ischemic stroke in terms of clinical importance).
  - The risk of ischemic stroke is low at INR levels ≥2.0.[1]
  - The risk of ICH increases at INR levels of 3.5–4.0 and above, particularly in the elderly.[1]
  - An INR of <2.0 at admission for a new stroke substantially increases the likelihood of death and severe disability from AF-related stroke.[13]
  - There is no decreased risk of ICH at INR levels <2.0.[1]
- Strong evidence supports the recommended INR target of 2.5 (range 2–3).
  - The American College of Cardiology/American Heart Association/European Society of Cardiology 2006 Guidelines' suggestion that a lower target INR (1.6–2.5) may be considered in patients unable to tolerate standard intensity warfarin therapy is *not* evidence based.
  - Narrower target ranges have been suggested in certain situations (e.g., INR 2.0–2.5 has been recommended in patients requiring warfarin, ASA, and clopidogrel following percutaneous coronary intervention).[14] Such

narrow ranges are not supported by good evidence, make achieving therapeutic INRs more difficult, and usually result in the need for more frequent INR testing.

– Target INR range 2–3 should be used for most patients with AF.

Stroke prevention considerations during cardioversion

- Systemic embolism is the most serious complication of cardioversion whether NSR is reestablished by electrical, pharmacologic, or spontaneous means.[1]
- Conversion of AF to NSR, regardless of method, results in transient mechanical dysfunction of the left atrium ("stunning").[2]
    - Recovery of mechanical function occurs over a period of days to weeks (depending in part on duration of AF prior to conversion).
    - Thrombus formed prior to conversion to NSR or during the period of atrial stunning can be expelled after the return of mechanical functioning resulting in stroke or systemic embolism.
- There is no evidence that cardioversion followed by prolonged maintenance of NSR effectively reduces thromboembolism in AF.[2]
    - Although at least 4 weeks of warfarin therapy (INR 2–3) is recommended following successful cardioversion, patients with risk factors for thromboembolism should continue anticoagulation beyond 4 weeks unless there is convincing evidence that NRS is maintained.[1]
- There are no published data to guide anticoagulation for emergency cardioversion. Expert opinion suggests that hemodynamically unstable patients requiring emergency cardioversion should receive therapeutic anticoagulation with either IV UFH or LMWH started as soon as possible, followed by at least 4 weeks of warfarin therapy (INR 2–3).[1]
    - The optimal strategy for initiating warfarin once patients are hemodynamically stable is not known. Most stable patients do not require cross-coverage with parenteral anticoagulants ("bridge therapy").[1]
    - Some providers are more comfortable bridging more worrisome AF patients with UFH/LMWH during warfarin initiation. Examples include patients with echocardiographic evidence of left atrial thrombus or those with advanced heart failure.

– Limited data comparing UFH (infusion targeting aPTT ratio 1.5–2.5 times control) to LMWH (enoxaparin 1 mg/kg SC q 12 hr) as a bridge to warfarin with transesophageal echocardiography (TEE) prior to cardioversion (if no thrombus detected) found no differences between strategies.[15]

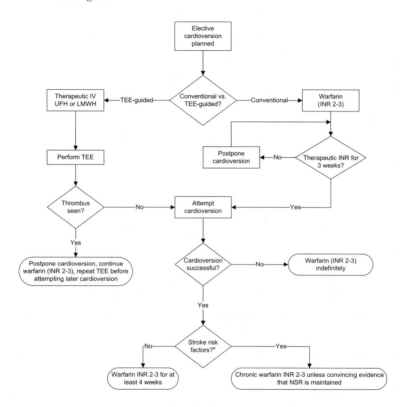

IV = intravenous; UFH = unfractionated heparin; LMWH = low-molecular-weight heparin; TEE = transesophageal echocardiogram; INR = international normalized ratio; NSR = normal sinus rhythm.

[a]Stroke risk factors include age >75 years; history of hypertension; diabetes mellitus; moderately or severely impaired left ventricular systolic function and/or heart failure.

Figure 12-2: Anticoagulation Therapy for Elective Cardioversion Treatment Algorithm

Electrical vs. pharmacologic cardioversion, implications for anticoagulation therapy

- Anticoagulation therapy recommendations are similar for electrical and pharmacologic cardioversion.
- Amiodarone is commonly used to maintain NSR in AF patients following successful cardioversion and presents unique challenges for patients on warfarin therapy.[16]
  - Amiodarone inhibits the metabolism of warfarin leading to the potential for excessive anticoagulation and increased bleeding risk.
  - Amiodarone may take hundreds of days to reach steady state due to its very long half-life. In addition, amiodarone can cause hypo- or hyperthyroidism that can also affect warfarin metabolism.
  - Co-administration of warfarin and amiodarone requires vigilant INR monitoring (at least weekly for several weeks and as needed thereafter). Some have advocated empiric warfarin dose reductions (between 35% and 65%) when amiodarone is added to ongoing warfarin thereapy.[16]

NONPHARMACOLOGIC PREVENTION OF AF STROKE

- Obliteration of the left atrial appendage by direct surgical truncation, amputation, or closure devices inserted into the left atrial appendage (e.g., the Watchman device) are emerging options for patients who cannot safely undergo anticoagulation therapy.[2]
  - These techniques should be considered investigational until more information is available to establish their efficacy and safety compared to available therapies. The use and duration of anticoagulation therapy with these techniques has yet to be determined.
  - In some cases, small pockets may still be present after the procedure creating a continued risk for thrombus formation.
- Other nonpharmacologic measures aimed at restoring NSR, including the surgical Maze procedure and various catheter ablation techniques, are playing an increasing role in AF management.
  - The current version of the Maze procedure involves cryotherapy or bipolar radiofrequency ablation in the atria along with the amputation

of both atrial appendages to prevent the occurrence of AF and restores NSR in over 90% of patients.[2] The procedure can be done in conjunction with other surgical procedures, such as cardiac valve replacement or independently through a small incision to access the atria.

- Many less invasive alternatives, including thoracoscopic and catheter-based ablation techniques, are under investigation.[2] The primary indication for catheter AF ablation is the presence of symptomatic AF refractory to or intolerant of antiarrhythmic medication.[17]

- Ablation involves placing a catheter into the left atrium and either using a heating or freezing technique to tissues surrounding the pulmonary veins to disrupt their electrical conduction by blocking or destroying abnormal electrical pathways and/or ectopic foci.

  - AF recurrence rates with catheter ablation are high and may be asymptomatic, even among previously symptomatic patients.[1]

  - For this reason, AF patients with stroke risk factors should continue warfarin therapy for a prolonged period after surgery or ablation procedures.[1]

- Embolic stroke complicates from 0% to 5% of catheter-based ablation procedures. Various intravenous unfractionated heparin regimens have been proposed for use during the procedure with those prolonging the activated clotting time (ACT) above 300 seconds, reducing the risk of thrombus formation more than when the ACT was 250–300 seconds.[2]

- The Heart Rhythm Society/European Hearth Rhythm Association/European Cardiac Arrhythmia Society Expert Consensus Statement on Catheter and Surgical Ablation of Atrial Fibrillation makes the following recommendations regarding anticoagulation therapy during ablation procedures[17]:

  - Recommendations regarding anticoagulation at the time of cardioversion apply to patients who are in AF at the time of the ablation procedure.

  - Patients with persistent AF who are in AF at the time of ablation should have TEE to screen for thrombus even if warfarin anticoagulation was used prior to the procedure. When warfarin is discontinued for the ablation, some experts recommend 0.5—1 mg/kg of enoxaparin twice daily until the evening prior to the ablation (postprocedure anticoagulation plans may be in part driven by the procedure and potential complications).

- After catheter ablation, anticoagulation is interrupted briefly (e.g., 4–6 hours) to allow sheath removal followed by prompt resumption of warfarin. UFH or enoxaparin should be continued until therapeutic INR is achieved (some experts suggest 0.5 mg/kg enoxaparin twice daily to reduce the risk of postprocedure bleeding complications, such as groin hematoma and retroperitoneal bleeding).

- Warfarin is recommended for all patients for at least 2 months following an AF ablation procedure (consider prolonged therapy for $CHADS_2$ ≥2).

REFERENCES

*Key articles

1. **Singer DE, Albers GW, Dalen JE, et al. Antithrombotic therapy in atrial fibrillation: American College of Chest Physicians Evidence-Based Clinical Practice Guidelines (8th ed.). *Chest*. 2008;133:546S–592S.**

2. **Fuster V, Ryden LE, Cannom DS, et al. ACC/AHA/ESC 2006 Guidelines for the Management of Patients with Atrial Fibrillation: a report of the American College of Cardiology/American Heart Association Task Force on Practice Guidelines and the European Society of Cardiology Committee for Practice Guidelines. *Circulation*. 2006;114:e257–e354.**

3. Lloyd-Jones D, Adams R, Carnethon M, et al. Heart disease and stroke statistics—2009 update: a report from the American Heart Association Statistics Committee and Stroke Statistics Subcommittee. *Circulation*. 2009;119:e21–181.

4. Van GI, Hagens VE, Bosker HA, et al. A comparison of rate control and rhythm control in patients with recurrent persistent atrial fibrillation. *N Engl J Med*. 2002;347:1834–1840.

5. Wyse DG, Waldo AL, DiMarco JP, et al. A comparison of rate control and rhythm control in patients with atrial fibrillation. *N Engl J Med*. 2002;347:1825–1833.

6. Hagens VE, Ranchor AV, Van SE, et al. Effect of rate or rhythm control on quality of life in persistent atrial fibrillation. Results from the Rate Control Versus Electrical Cardioversion (RACE) Study. *J Am Coll Cardiol*. 2004;43:241–247.

7. Connolly SJ, Pogue J, Hart RG, et al. Effect of clopidogrel added to aspirin in patients with atrial fibrillation. *N Engl J Med*. 2009;360:2066–2078.

8. Connolly S, Pogue J, Hart R, et al. Clopidogrel plus aspirin versus oral anticoagulation for atrial fibrillation in the Atrial fibrillation Clopidogrel Trial with Irbesartan for prevention of Vascular Events (ACTIVE W): a randomised controlled trial. *Lancet*. 2006;367:1903–1912.

9. Lip GY. The balance between stroke prevention and bleeding risk in atrial fibrillation: a delicate balance revisited. *Stroke.* 2008;39:1406–1408.

10. Johnson SG, Rogers K, Delate T, et al. Outcomes associated with combined antiplatelet and anticoagulant therapy. *Chest.* 2008;133:948–954.

* **11. Gage BF, Waterman AD, Shannon W, et al. Validation of clinical classification schemes for predicting stroke: results from the National Registry of Atrial Fibrillation. *JAMA*. 2001;285:2864–2870.**

12. Lip GY, Nieuwlaat R, Pisters R, et al. Refining clinical risk stratification for predicting stroke and thromboembolism in atrial fibrillation using a novel risk factor-based approach: the euro heart survey on atrial fibrillation. *Chest.* 2010;137:263–272.

13. Hylek EM, Go AS, Chang Y, et al. Effect of intensity of oral anticoagulation on stroke severity and mortality in atrial fibrillation. *N Engl J Med.* 2003;349:1019–1026.

14. King SB III, Smith SC Jr., Hirshfeld JW Jr., et al. 2007 Focused Update of the ACC/AHA/SCAI 2005 Guideline Update for Percutaneous Coronary Intervention: a report of the American College of Cardiology/American Heart Association Task Force on Practice Guidelines. *Circulation.* 2008;117:261–295.

15. Klein AL, Jasper SE, Katz WE, et al. The use of enoxaparin compared with unfractionated heparin for short-term antithrombotic therapy in atrial fibrillation patients undergoing transoesophageal echocardiography-guided cardioversion: assessment of Cardioversion Using Transoesophageal Echocardiography (ACUTE) II randomized multicentre study. *Eur Heart J.* 2006;27:2858–2865.

16. Lu Y, Won KA, Nelson BJ, et al. Characteristics of the amiodarone-warfarin interaction during long-term follow-up. *Am J Health-Syst Pharm.* 2008;65:947–952.

* **17. Calkins H, Brugada J, Packer DL, et al. HRS/EHRA/ECAS expert Consensus Statement on catheter and surgical ablation of atrial fibrillation: recommendations for personnel, policy, procedures and follow-up. A report of the Heart Rhythm Society (HRS) Task Force on catheter and surgical ablation of atrial fibrillation. *Heart Rhythm*. 2007;4:816–861.**

Acute Coronary Syndromes

13

Sarah A. Spinler

INTRODUCTION

It is estimated that more than 1.2 million patients experience an acute coronary syndrome (ACS) each year with 935,000 diagnosed with myocardial infarction (MI).[1] Of patients presenting with suspected ACS, recent international registry data indicate that approximately 31% have ST segment elevation (STE) MI, 32% non-ST segment elevation (NSTE) MI, 26% unstable angina, 8% another cardiac diagnosis, and 4% a noncardiac final diagnosis. During hospitalization, approximately 70% of patients undergo cardiac catheterization and angiography, 66% percutaneous coronary intervention (PCI), commonly known as angioplasty, and less than 5% coronary artery bypass graft (CABG) surgery. Recurrent ischemia occurs in approximately 20% of patients (Table 13-1).[2]

Table 13-1: In-hospital Outcomes of ACS with MI[2]

Estimated In-hospital Outcomes	STE MI	NSTE MI	Unstable Angina
Death (%)	6.2	2.9	1.7
Reinfarction (%)	12	10	1.2
Heart failure (%)	15	10	6
Stroke (%)	1	0.5	0.2
Major bleeding (%)	1.4	1.2	0.5

PATHOPHYSIOLOGY AND EPIDEMIOLOGY OF ACS

ACSs, (MI, or myocardial ischemia) are caused by partial or complete thrombotic occlusion of a coronary artery due to plaque rupture, erosion, fissuring, or dissection (Figure 13-1).

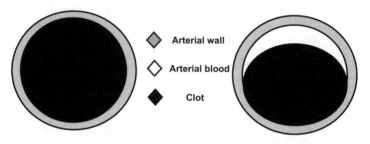

Cross Section of a Coronary Artery

◇ Arterial wall

◇ Arterial blood

◆ Clot

Myocardial infarction: complete occlusion

Unstable angina: partial occlusion

Figure 13-1: Pathophysiology of ACS

SIGNS AND SYMPTOMS OF ACS

Signs

- ECG changes: ST-segment elevation, ST-segment depression, T-wave inversion, new left bundle branch block, Q waves (Figure 13-2A & B)
- Elevated biochemical markers: elevated troponin T or I*, elevated creatine kinase MB
- Acute heart failure or cardiogenic shock: rales, S3, hypoxia, hypotension, pulmonary edema on chest x-ray
- Ventricular arrhythmias

*Negative biomarkers measured within 6 hours of symptom onset should be remeasured 8–12 hours after symptom onset; positive biomarkers may be remeasured at 6–8-hour intervals until a peak is observed.

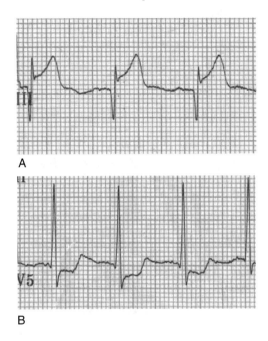

Figure 13-2: Electrocardiographic Findings in ACS

A. ST-segment elevation; B. ST-segment depression.

Symptoms

- Anterior medial chest pain, pressure, tightness, or squeezing occurring at rest
- Radiation of chest discomfort to left arm, shoulder, back, or jaw
- Increasing frequency, severity, or duration of angina
- Nausea, vomiting
- Acute heart failure: dyspnea

DIAGNOSTIC CRITERIA FOR ACS

Universal criteria for acute myocardial infarction[3]

Any one of the following criteria:

- Detection of a rise or fall in biochemical markers (troponin preferred) with at least one value above the 99th percentile of a normal reference population (upper reference limit) together with at least one of the following:
  - Symptoms of ischemia
  - ECG changes
  - A new regional wall motion abnormality (akinesis, dyskinesis) on echocardiogram
- Sudden, unexplained cardiac death involving cardiac arrest (often preceded by signs and symptoms suggesting ACS) and/or evidence of fresh thrombus at coronary angiography or autopsy
- For patients undergoing PCI:
  - If preprocedure troponin negative—elevated troponin level above the 99th percentile of the upper reference limit
  - If preprocedure positive—elevated troponin level greater than 3 times the 99th percentile of the upper reference limit

RISK STRATIFICATION FOR NSTE ACS

An early invasive approach with coronary angiography and revascularization with either PCI or CABG is recommended for high-risk patients with NSTE ACS defined as either TIMI risk score of ≥5 (Table 13-2) or GRACE risk score >140 (Figure 13-3).

Table 13-2: TIMI Risk Score for NSTE ACS[4,5]

One point is assigned for each of the seven medical history and clinical presentation findings. The point total is calculated and the patient is assigned a risk for experiencing the composite endpoint of death, myocardial infarction, or urgent need for revascularization as follows:

- Age ≥65 yr

- Three or more CHD risk factors: smoking, hypercholesterolemia, hypertension, diabetes mellitus, family history of premature CHD death/events

- Known CAD (≥50% stenosis of at least one major coronary artery on coronary angiogram)

- Aspirin use within the past 7 days

- Two or more episodes of chest discomfort within the past 24 hr

- ST-segment depression ≥0.5 mm

- Positive biochemical marker for infarction

High-Risk	Medium-Risk	Low-Risk
TIMI risk score	TIMI risk score	TIMI risk score
5–7 points	3–4 points	0–2 points

TIMI Risk Score	Mortality, MI, or Severe Recurrent Ischemic Requiring Urgent Target Vessel Revascularization
0/1	4.7%
2	8.3%
3	13.2%
4	19.9%
5	26.2%
6/7	40.9%

1. Find the number of points that most closely matches each characteristic. If your value falls between two listed, extrapolate to the closest point. Write the number of points at the bottom of each column.

Killip Class	Points	Systolic BP	Points	Heart Rate	Points	Age	Points	Creatinine	Points
I	0	≤70	66	≤70	10	≤30	0	0–0.39	3
II	17	70–89	53	70–89	15	30–49	10	0.4–0.9	9
III	34	90–109	40	90–109	26	50–69	29	1.0–1.9	32
IV	51	110–129	27	110–129	32	70–79	56	≥2	51
		≥130	19	130–149	24	80–89	73		
				150–169	16	≥90	91		
				170–199	8				
				≥200	0				
____		+ ____		+ ____		+ ____		+ ____	

Baseline Risk Factors	Points
Cardiac arrest at admission	38
ST-segment deviation	18
Positive cardiac markers	14
STEMI	14
Total from clinical evaluation	

2. Sum points for all predictive factors:

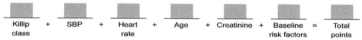

Killip class + SBP + Heart rate + Age + Creatinine + Baseline risk factors = Total points

3. Look up risk corresponding to total points:

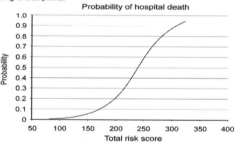

Probability of hospital death

Probability of hospital death	0.2%	0.9%	4.6%	21%	58%	88%	97%	99%

Figure 13-3: Updated GRACE Risk Score[6]

(Reprinted with permission from KS Pieper, JM Gore, G FitzGerald, et al. Validity of a risk-prediction tool for hospital mortality: the Global Registry of Acute Coronary Events. *Am Heart J.* 2009;157:1097–1105.)

Clinical Pearl

- A TIMI risk score calculator is available from http://www.mdcalc. com/timi-risk-score-for-uanstemi. Accessed October 20, 2009.[5]

ANTICOAGULATION CONSIDERATIONS IN PATIENTS WITH ACS

Relationship between aPTT for unfractionated heparin and outcomes

- Recent clinical trials have targeted a therapeutic range of 50–70 seconds without calibration to anti-Factor Xa activity to account for reagent variability.

- Data evaluating bleeding and thrombotic risk with unfractionated heparin (UFH) in ACS are sparse and consist of post hoc analysis of large, randomized trials.

- Data supporting the therapeutic range of 50–70 seconds is strongest from early fibrinolytic trials.[7–10]

  - In the GUSTO-1 trial of patients with STE MI treated with fibrinolytics, an aPTT of 50–70 seconds was associated with the lowest rates of 30-day mortality, stroke, and bleeding. There was no evidence of increased thrombotic risk with aPTTs below 50 seconds. Unexpectedly, there was an increased mortality and reinfarction risk, as well as bleeding, in patients with aPTTs greater than 70 seconds.[7]

  - In GUSTO-IIb, another STE MI fibrinolytic trial, weight was the strongest predictor of a therapeutic aPTT and a simulated bolus dose of 60 units/kg and initial infusion of 12 units/kg/hr resulted in the highest proportion of therapeutic aPTTs. An aPTT of approximately 70 seconds and an initial infusion dose of 12 units/kg/hr were associated with the lowest mortality rate.[8]

  - This dosing scheme and target aPTT range of 50–70 seconds using weight-based heparin dosing nomograms was tested prospectively in the GUSTO-V trial of patients with STE MI treated with reteplase and heparin with or without abciximab. Higher aPTTs greater than 70 seconds were associated with bleeding, but there was no association between peak aPTT and mortality. Lower aPTTs <50 seconds were also associated with worse outcomes (the authors speculated that this was because heparin was discontinued in patients with bleeding complications).[9]

- In the EXTRACT-TIMI 25 trial, markedly high aPTTs ≥2.75 times control were associated with increased bleeding risk while low aPTTs <1.25 times control tended to be associated with increased risk of MI at 48 hours.[10]

- The data supporting a heparin therapeutic range in patients with NSTE ACS is less robust.

  - In the OASIS-2 trial, a target aPTT of 60–100 seconds was suggested for investigators. Patients with aPTTs <60 seconds had higher rates of recurrent ischemic events while those with aPTTs higher than 100 seconds had an increased risk of bleeding.[11]

  - In PARAGON-A, there was no statistically significant association between aPTT and either death, reinfarction, or bleeding.[12]

  - In TIMI-IIIB, a large randomized trial in patients with NSTE ACS treated with fibrinolytics or placebo, neither heparin anti-Factor Xa activity levels nor aPTT were predictive of recurrent ischemia, reinfarction, or death.[13]

- While aPTT calibration to a heparin anti-Factor Xa activity level of 0.3–0.7 International Units/mL from which to develop a weight-based heparin nomogram is recommended by both the ACCP and the American College of Pathologists, no data from ACS clinical trials support this target heparin anti-Factor Xa activity range, which was originally developed from a single study of venous thromboembolism treatment.[14,15]

Relationship between anti-Factor Xa activity with low-molecular-weight heparin and outcomes

The best predictor of bleeding in patients treated with low-molecular-weight heparins (LMWHs) is dose (mg) per kg.

- A desired therapeutic range for anti-Factor Xa activity with LMWHs in patients with ACS has not been determined.[14]

- In the TIMI-11A trial of patients with NSTE ACS, enoxaparin doses of 1.25 mg/kg every 12 hours had a higher rate of major hemorrhage than patients receiving a dose of 1 mg/kg every 12 hours. In the subgroup treated with the higher dose of enoxaparin, patients who experienced a major bleeding event had peak anti-Factor Xa levels of 1.8 International Units/mL compared to 1.4 International Units/mL in patients without major bleeding. Peak levels in patients treated with the 1-mg/kg dose were 1.0 International Units/mL, and only two patients experienced bleeding.[16]

- In the STEEPLE trial, patients undergoing elective PCI for stable coronary heart disease (CAD) received a single IV dose of either 0.5 mg or 0.75 mg, and those with anti-Factor Xa levels >0.9 International Units/mL had increased non-CABG major or minor bleeding but not major bleeding alone in multivariate analysis.[17]

- Results from a third smaller prospective study in patients with NSTE ACS suggested that anti-Factor Xa levels <0.5 International Units/mL were an independent predictor of 30-day mortality. However, the mean dose of enoxaparin dose administered to patients with low anti-Factor Xa levels was only 0.66 mg/kg.[18]

- Overall, there are no strong data to suggest routine monitoring of anti-Factor Xa levels to achieve a target anti-Factor Xa therapeutic range with LMWHs if dosing according to body weight is adhered to.

CRUSADE BLEEDING RISK SCORE[19]

The CRUSADE bleeding risk score can give practitioners an estimate of the likelihood of major bleed in patients with NSTE ACS. In patients with a higher CRUSADE bleeding risk score, anticoagulants with lower bleeding risk, such as bivalirudin or fondaparinux, may be considered. Glycoprotein IIb/IIIa inhibitors should be avoided in patients estimated to be at high risk of bleeding.

Table 13-3: CRUSADE Bleeding Risk Score

Predictor	Score
Baseline hematocrit (%)	
<31	9
31.0–33.9	7
34.0–36.9	3
37.0–39.9	2
≥40	0
Creatinine clearance (mL/min, Cockcroft-Gault formula, total body weight)	
≤15	39
>15–30	35
>30–60	28
>60–90	17
>90–120	7
>120	0
Heart rate (beats per minute)	
≤70	0
71–80	1
81–90	3
91–100	6
101–110	8
111–120	10
≥121	11
Sex	
Male	0
Female	8
Signs of heart failure at presentation	
No	0
Yes	7
Prior PAD or stroke	
No	0
Yes	6
Diabetes mellitus	
No	0
Yes	6
Systolic blood pressure (mm Hg)	
≤90	10
91–100	8
101–120	5
121–180	1
181–200	3
≥200	5

Abbreviation: PAD = peripheral arterial disease.

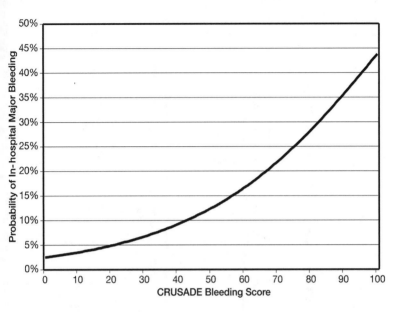

Figure 13-4: Predicted Probability of CRUSADE In-hospital Major Bleeding According to CRUSADE Bleeding Risk Score

Add up point total from each section. Minimum score 1, maximum score 96. (Reprinted with permission from S Subherwal, RG Bach, AY Chen, et al. Baseline risk of major bleeding in non-ST-segment-elevation myocardial infarction: the CRUSADE [Can Rapid risk stratification of Unstable angina patients Suppress ADverse outcomes with Early implementation of the ACC/AHA Guidelines] Bleeding Score. *Circulation*. 2009;119(14):1873–1882. Copyright 2009 Wolters Kluwer Health.)

Clinical Pearl

- On-line calculator available from http://www.crusadebleedingscore. org/. Accessed October 16, 2009.[20]

GUIDELINE-BASED SELECTION OF ANTICOAGULANT THERAPY

Table 13-4: Primary PCI for STE MI[21-24]

Agent	2004 ACC/AHA STE MI Full Guidelines, 2005 ACC/AHA PCI Guidelines, 2007 ACC/AHA PCI Guideline Update, or 2009 STE MI/PCI Update Class Recommendation	Contraindications	Dose (class recommendation)	Duration	Comments (class recommendation)
UFH	IA (2004)	Active bleeding, HIT	Primary PCI (without GP IIb/IIIa inhibitor): 70–100 units/kg (max 100 units/kg) (2009 IC) Primary PCI (with GP IIb/IIIa inhibitor): 50–70 units/kg (max 70 units/kg) (2009 IC)	Discontinue at end of procedure	Primary PCI without GP IIb/IIIa inhibitor: ACT 250–300 sec with HemoTec and 300–350 sec with Hemochron (2009 IC) Primary PCI with GP IIb/IIIa inhibitor: ACT of 200–250 sec (2009 IC)

Table 13-4: (Continued)

Agent	2004 ACC/AHA STE MI Full Guidelines, 2005 ACC/AHA PCI Guidelines, 2007 ACC/AHA PCI Guideline Update, or 2009 STE MI/PCI Update Class Recommendation	Contraindications	Dose (class recommendation)	Duration	Comments (class recommendation)
Dalteparin[a]	No recommendation				
Enoxaparin[a]	IIB (2005)	Active bleeding, HIT	IV dose not known, not studied for primary PCI; single IV doses of 0.5 mg/kg and 0.75 mg/kg used in elective PCI	Single dose	Avoid in patients previously treated with UFH
Fondaparinux[a]	III alone, IC in combination with UFH (2007)	Active bleeding, CrCl <30 mL/min	2.5 mg IV (with GP IIb/IIIa inhibitor) 5 mg IV (without GP IIb/IIIa inhibitor) At time of PCI, administer additional 50–60 units/kg UFH	Single dose	Similar death or MI rate and similar bleeding rate compared to UFH

(continued)

Table 13-4: (Continued)

Agent	2004 ACC/AHA STE MI Full Guidelines, 2005 ACC/AHA PCI Guidelines, 2007 ACC/AHA PCI Guideline Update, or 2009 STE MI/PCI Update Class Recommendation	Contraindications	Dose (class recommendation)	Duration	Comments (class recommendation)
Bivalirudin	IB for primary PCI and IB for PCI in patients with renal dysfunction (2009)	Active bleeding	0.75-mg/kg IV bolus followed by 1.75 mg/kg/hr (for patients receiving UFH; discontinue UFH and wait 30 min prior to starting bivalirudin)	Until end of PCI procedure (preferred); option to continue at same IV infusion dose for 4 hr postprocedure; option to continue lower dose 0.2 mg/kg/hr for an additional 20 hr postprocedure	No dose reduction for renal dysfunction used in clinical trials; may consider reduction in infusion to 1 mg/kg/hr for patients with CrCl <30 mL/min and to 0.25 mg/kg/hr for patients receiving dialysis; may also be used in patients previously treated with UFH; preferred for patients with history of HIT; pretreatment with thienopyridine preferred; lower rate of bleeding and mortality reduction compared to UFH

ᵃNot FDA approved.

Table 13-5: STE MI with Fibrinolytics[25]

Agent	2007 ACC/AHA STE MI Guideline Update Class Recommendation	Contraindications	Dose	Duration	Comments
UFH	IC	Active bleeding, HIT	60-units/kg (max 4,000 units) IV bolus followed by 12 units/kg/hr IV infusion (max 1,000 units/hr)	48 hr (IA)	aPTT 1.5–2.0 times control (50–70 sec); for secondary PCI following administration of fibrinolytics, administer additional IV bolus doses to PCI ACT targets (IC)
Dalteparin[a]	No recommendation				
Enoxaparin	IA	Active bleeding, HIT; serum creatinine ≥2.5 mg/dL in men or ≥2.0 mg/dL in women	For patients <75 yr old: 30-mg IV bolus followed by 1 mg/kg SC q 12 hr For patients ≥75 yr old: 0.75 mg/kg SC q 12 hr (omit IV bolus) For patients weighing >100 kg and <75 yr old: cap first two doses at 100 mg For patients weighing ≥100 kg and ≥75 yr old: cap first two doses at 75 mg If during therapy CrCl <30 mL/min: decrease dose to 1 mg/kg SC once daily	Minimum of 48 hr and up to 8 days (IA)	Avoid in patients previously treated with UFH; for secondary PCI during hospitalization following fibrinolytics, if the last SC dose was administered at least 8–12 hr earlier, administer an IV dose of 0.3 mg/kg; if the last SC dose was administered within the prior 8 hr, no additional enoxaparin should be given (IB); lower rate of death or MI but higher bleeding rate compared to UFH

(continued)

Table 13-5: (Continued)

Agent	2007 ACC/AHA STE MI Guideline Update Class Recommendation	Contraindications	Dose	Duration	Comments
Fondaparinux[a]	IB	Active bleeding, serum creatinine >3.0 mg/dL	2.5 mg IV followed by 2.5 mg SC daily starting day 2	Minimum of 48 hr and up to 8 days (IA)	Similar death or MI rate and similar bleeding rate compared to UFH; for secondary PCI during hospitalization, administer with additional UFH as for primary PCI (IC)
Bivalirudin[a]	No recommendation				Avoid with fibrinolytics (is associated with excess bleeding compared to UFH); for secondary PCI during hospitalization following fibrinolytics, may be administered in patients previously treated with UFH or bivalirudin at same dose as primary PCI (IC)

[a]Not FDA approved.

Agent	2007 ACC/AHA UA/NSTE MI Guideline Update Recommendation	Contraindications	Dose	Duration	Comments
UFH	For initial invasive strategy (high-risk patients): IA For initial conservative strategy (low-risk patients): IA	Active bleeding, HIT	60-units/kg (max 4,000 units) IV bolus followed by 12 units/kg/hr IV infusion (max 1,000 units/hr)	At least 48 hr or until hospital discharge, discontinue after PCI	aPTT 1.5–2.0 times control (50–70 sec)
Dalteparin[a]	No recommendation	Active bleeding, HIT	120 International Units/kg SC q 12 hr (max 10,000 International Units/dose)	Treatment duration was 5–8 days in clinical trials	
Enoxaparin	For initial invasive strategy (high-risk patients): IA For initial conservative strategy (low-risk patients): IA, preferred over UFH unless CABG is planned IIA	Active bleeding, HIT	1 mg/kg SC q 12 hr; reduce dose to 1 mg/kg q 24 hr if CrCl <30 mL/min; consider dose cap of 120 mg (higher doses associated with bleeding risk in CRUSADE registry)[27]	Continue for the duration of hospitalization (up to 8 days); discontinued after PCI	For PCI, if the last SC dose was administered at least 8–12 hr earlier, administer an IV dose of 0.3 mg/kg; if the last SC dose was administered within the prior 8 hr, no additional enoxaparin should be given (IB); not studied in patients receiving dialysis; similar death or MI rate and higher bleeding risk compared to bivalirudin for high-risk patients treated with an early interventional strategy;

(continued)

Table 13-6: (Continued)

Agent	2007 ACC/AHA UA/NSTE MI Guideline Update Recommendation	Contraindications	Dose	Duration	Comments
					lower death, MI or urgent revascularization and higher bleeding risk compared to UFH for patients undergoing an early conservative strategy; similar death or MI risk and higher bleeding risk compared to fondaparinux for patients undergoing an early conservative strategy
Fondaparinux[b]	For initial invasive strategy (high-risk patients): IB For initial conservative strategy (low-risk patients): IB, preferred over UFH unless CABG planned IIA; preferred for patients with increased bleeding risk IB	Active bleeding, CrCl <30 mL/min	2.5 mg/kg SC daily	Continue for the duration of hospitalization (up to 8 days); discontinued after PCI	Increased risk of catheter thrombosis during PCI if used as sole anticoagulant; administer 50–60 units/kg IV heparin bolus during PCI; similar death or MI risk and lower bleeding risk compared to fondaparinux for patients undergoing an early conservative strategy

Table 13-6: (Continued)

Agent	2007 ACC/AHA UA/NSTE MI Guideline Update Recommendation	Contraindications	Dose	Duration	Comments
Bivalirudin[c]	For initial invasive strategy (high-risk patients): IB For initial conservative strategy (low-risk patients): no recommendation	Active bleeding	0.1-mg/kg IV bolus followed by 0.25-mg/kg/hr infusion; at time of PCI, administer additional IV bolus of 0.5 mg/kg and increase infusion rate to 1.75 mg/kg/hr	Until end of PCI procedure (preferred); option to continue at same IV infusion dose for 4 hr postprocedure; option to continue lower dose 0.2 mg/kg/hr for an additional 20 hr postprocedure	Not studied for initial conservative strategy; preferred for patients with PCI and initial invasive strategy; similar efficacy and lower bleeding rate compared to UFH or enoxaparin for early invasive strategy; no dose reduction for renal dysfunction used in clinical trials; may consider reduction in infusion to 1 mg/kg/hr for patients with CrCl <30 mL/min and to 0.25 mg/kg/hr for patients receiving dialysis; preferred for patients with history of HIT; pretreatment with thienopyridine preferred

[a] "…relative efficacy and safety…not well established"…in contemporary practice of early intervention and PCI.

[b] Not FDA approved.

[c] Not FDA approved for initial conservative strategy.

Table 13-7: Injectable Anticoagulant Monitoring

Agent	Monitoring
UFH	Daily weight, clinical signs and symptoms of bleeding, aPTT baseline and q 4–6 hr[a] until in desired range then daily thereafter, ACT during PCI; baseline and daily platelet count, baseline INR
Enoxaparin	Daily weight, clinical signs and symptoms of bleeding, baseline and daily CrCl, baseline platelet count, baseline and daily CBC, baseline INR
Fondaparinux	Daily weight, clinical signs and symptoms of bleeding, baseline and daily CrCl, baseline and daily CBC, baseline platelet count, baseline INR
Bivalirudin	Daily weight, clinical signs and symptoms of bleeding, baseline and daily CrCl, baseline and daily CBC, baseline platelet count, baseline INR

[a]Some institutions monitor heparin with anti-Factor Xa activity levels instead of aPTT to monitor UFH infusions for ACS. See the above literature discussion for more details.

Table 13-8: Interventional Issues: Arterial Femoral Sheath Management Following Cardiac Catheterization[22,28–30]

Agent	Recommended Sheath Management
UFH	ACT <180 sec[a]
Enoxaparin	1) 4 hr after last IV dose or 6–8 hr after last SC dose[a]
	2) Can consider immediate removal with arterial closure device if single 0.5 mg/kg IV dose used
	If continuing treatment, give next scheduled dose no sooner than 6 hr after sheath removed
Bivalirudin	1) Immediate removal using an arterial closure device, or
	2) Remove 2 hr after discontinuation without ACT monitoring[a]

[a]Follow with direct manual groin compression (preferred over mechanical compression device).

Table 13-9: Concomitant Aspirin Therapy[23,25,26,31]

ACS	Initial Dose	Subsequent Doses Starting Day 2 and Duration of Therapy
NSTE ACS medical management[26]	162–325 mg nonenteric coated formulation either oral or chewed	75–100 mg/day indefinitely
NSTE ACS PCI, bare metal stent[23,26,31]	300–325 mg nonenteric coated formulation either oral or chewed	1) 300–325 mg/day on days 2 to 30, then 75–100 mg/day indefinitely[23,26] or 2) 162–325 mg/day on days 2 to 30, then 75–162 mg/day indefinitely[31]
NSTE ACS PCI, drug-eluting stent[23,26,31]	300–325 mg nonenteric coated formulation either oral or chewed	1) 300–325 mg/day on days 2 to 30, then 75–100 mg/day indefinitely[23,26] or 2) 162–325 mg/day on days 2 to 3 mo for paclitaxel-eluting stent or days 2 to 6 mo for sirolimus-eluting stent, then 75–162 mg/day indefinitely[31]
STE MI medical management (including fibrinolysis)[21,25]	162–325 mg nonenteric coated formulation either oral or chewed	75–100 mg/day indefinitely
STE MI primary PCI bare metal stent[23,25,31]	300–325 mg nonenteric coated formulation either oral or chewed	1) 300–325 mg/day on days 2 to 30, then 75–100 mg/day indefinitely[23,25] or 2) 162–325 mg/day on days 2 to 30, then 75–162 mg/day indefinitely[31]
STE MI primary PCI drug-eluting stent[23,25,31]	300–325 mg nonenteric coated formulation either oral or chewed	1) 300–325 mg/day on days 2 to 30, then 75–100 mg/day indefinitely[23,25] or 2) 162–325 mg/day on days 2 to 3 mo for sirolimus-eluting stent or on days 2 to 6 mo for paclitaxel, then 75–162 mg/day indefinitely[31]

Table 13-10: Concomitant Thienopyridine Therapy[24–26,31,32]

ACS	Initial Dose	Subsequent Doses Starting Day 2 and Duration of Therapy (class recommendation)
NSTE ACS medical management[26]	Clopidogrel 300 mg	Clopidogrel 75 mg daily for at least 1 mo and ideally up to 1 yr (in patients who are not at high risk of bleeding)
NSTE ACS PCI, bare metal stent[24,31,32]	Clopidogrel 300–600 mg	1) Clopidogrel 75 mg daily for at least 1 mo and ideally up to 1 yr (with option to discontinue earlier if bleeding risk outweighs anticipated benefit—Class IC) or 2) Clopidogrel 150 mg daily on days 2–7 followed by 75 mg daily[31]
	Prasugrel 60 mg	Prasugrel 10 mg daily for 12 mo (with option to discontinue earlier if bleeding risk outweighs anticipated benefit—Class IC); consider dose reduction to 5 mg daily for patients weighing <60 kg[a]; contraindicated in patients with prior stroke/TIA
NSTE ACS, drug-eluting stent[24,31,32]	Clopidogrel 300–600 mg	1) Clopidogrel 75 mg daily for at least 1 yr (2009 IC) and for up to 15 mo (2009 IIB), (with option to discontinue earlier if bleeding risk outweighs anticipated benefit—2009 Class IC)[24] or 2) Clopidogrel 150 mg daily on days 2–7 followed by 75 mg daily[31]
	Prasugrel 60 mg	Prasugrel 10 mg daily for 12 mo (2009 IB) and for up to 15 mo (2009 IIB), with option to discontinue earlier if bleeding risk outweighs anticipated benefit (2009 IC); consider dose reduction to 5 mg daily for patients weighing <60 kg[a]; contraindicated in patients with prior stroke/TIA[24]

(continued)

Table 13-10: (Continued)

ACS	Initial Dose	Subsequent Doses Starting Day 2 and Duration of Therapy (class recommendation)
STE MI medical management (including fibrinolysis)[25]	For patients age >75 yr: 75 mg For patients age ≤75 yr: 300 mg	Clopidogrel 75 mg daily on days 2–14
STE MI primary PCI, bare metal stent[24,31,32]	Clopidogrel 300–600 mg	1) Clopidogrel 75 mg daily for at least 1 mo and ideally up to 1 yr (with option to discontinue earlier if bleeding risk outweighs anticipated benefit—Class IC)[24] or 2) Clopidogrel 150 mg daily on days 2–7 followed by 75 mg daily[31]
	Prasugrel 60 mg	Prasugrel 10 mg daily for 12 mo (with option to discontinue earlier if bleeding risk outweighs anticipated benefit—Class IC); consider dose reduction to 5 mg daily for patients weighing <60 kg; contraindicated in patients with prior stroke/TIA[24]
STE MI primary PCI, drug-eluting stent[24,31,32]	Clopidogrel 300–600 mg	1) Clopidogrel 75 mg daily for at least 1 yr (2009 IC) and for up to 15 mo (2009 IIB) (with option to discontinue earlier if bleeding risk outweighs anticipated benefit—2009 Class IC)[24] or 2) Clopidogrel 150 mg daily on days 2–7 followed by 75 mg daily[31]
	Prasugrel 60 mg	Prasugrel 10 mg daily for 12 mo (2009 IB) and for up to 15 mo (2009 IIB), with option to discontinue earlier if bleeding risk outweighs anticipated benefit (2009 IC); consider dose reduction to 5 mg daily for patients weighing <60 kg[a]; contraindicated in patients with prior stroke/TIA[24]

(continued)

Table 13-10: (Continued)

ACS	Initial Dose	Subsequent Doses Starting Day 2 and Duration of Therapy (class recommendation)
STE MI nonprimary PCI[24]	If fibrinolytic administered, continue clopidogrel if already initiated, otherwise administer 300–600 mg If fibrinolytic not administered, initiate clopidogrel or prasugrel as above for primary PCI	Same as primary PCI above
For patients undergoing CABG surgery[24]	Clopidogrel	Withhold for at least 5 days (2009 IB) unless the urgency for revascularization and/or need for thienopyridine outweighs the risks of excess bleeding (2009 IC)
	Prasugrel	Contraindicated; withhold for at least 7 days (2009 IC) unless the urgency for revascularization and/or need for thienopyridine outweighs the risks of excess bleeding (2009 IC)

[a]Prasugrel 5-mg dose not prospectively studied in clinical trials.

Table 13-11: Glycoprotein IIb/IIIA Inhibitors for PCI in ACS

Agent	2005 ACC/AHA PCI Guideline Recommendations[22]	Contraindications	Dose (started at time of PCI, i.e., "downstream")	Duration	Comments
Abciximab	NSTE ACS, class I without clopidogrel, class IIA with clopidogrel STE MI, class IIa	Active bleeding, thrombocytopenia, history of stroke	0.25-mg/kg IV bolus followed by 0.125 mcg/kg/min (maximum 10 mcg/min) started at time of angiography	12 hr after PCI	Agent with most data for STE MI primary PCI
Eptifibatide	NSTE ACS, class I without clopidogrel, class IIA with clopidogrel STE MI, class IIb	Active bleeding, thrombocytopenia, history of stroke, kidney dialysis	180-mcg/kg IV bolus times two, 10 min apart with an infusion of 2 mcg/kg/min	12–24 hr after PCI[33]	Early routine use prior to coronary angiography increases bleeding and not efficacy in high-risk patients with NSTE ACS[33]; dose adjusted to 1 mcg/kg/min in patients with CrCl <50 mL/min
Tirofiban	NSTE ACS, class I without clopidogrel, class IIA with clopidogrel STE MI, class IIa	Active bleeding, thrombocytopenia, history of stroke	High bolus dose, high maintenance dose regimen[34]: bolus of 25 mcg/kg administered over 3 min followed by an infusion of 0.15 mcg/kg/min		Not an FDA-approved dose; reduce maintenance infusion to 0.05 mcg/kg/min for patients with CrCl <30 mL/min

Table 13-12: Warfarin Following MI[21,25]

Indication for Warfarin Anticoagulation	Recommended INR	Duration of Warfarin Therapy
Chronic atrial fibrillation or atrial flutter[21,25]	2.0–3.0; 2.0–2.5 for patients receiving concomitant aspirin plus thienopyridine	Indefinitely
Left ventricular thrombus (noted on echocardiogram)[21,25]	2.0–3.0; 2.0–2.5 for patients receiving concomitant aspirin plus thienopyridine	At least 3 mo (repeat echocardiogram)
Extensive regional wall motion abnormality (akinetic segment) noted on echocardiogram[21]	2.0–3.0; 2.0–2.5 for patients receiving concomitant aspirin plus thienopyridine	At least 3 mo (repeat echocardiogram)
Patients unable to receive aspirin or a thienopyridine[21]	2.5–3.5	Indefinitely

Clinical Pearls

For using triple antithrombotic therapy (ASA, thienopyridine plus warfarin):

- Triple therapy is most commonly indicated for patients with chronic atrial fibrillation (CHADS$_2$ risk score 2 or higher necessitating chronic anticoagulation) undergoing intracoronary stent placement.

- For patients receiving a stent requiring long-term anticoagulation, bare metal stents are preferred as they necessitate the shortest period of dual antiplatelet therapy.

- Prasugrel has a higher risk of bleeding in studies of dual antiplatelet therapy and has not been studied as triple antithrombotic therapy so cannot be recommended. Clopidogrel is preferred in patients receiving warfarin.

- Use dual antiplatelet therapy for the shortest period of time based on the type of stent. For patients receiving bare metal stents, 1 month of clopidogrel is typically prescribed. For drug eluding stents, the length of therapy is at least 3 months with a sirolimus- or everolimus-eluting stent and 6 months with a paclitaxel-eluting stent.

- Use 81 mg aspirin daily to minimize bleeding risk.

- Monitor INR more often during triple antithrombotic therapy and maintain INR 2.0–2.5.

Table 13-13: Joint Commission Core Measures for Acute Myocardial Infarction[35,a]

Core Measure Name	Performance Measure
AMI-1	Aspirin administered before or within 24 hr after hospital arrival
AMI-2	Aspirin prescribed at hospital discharge
AMI-7	Median time from hospital arrival to administration of fibrinolytic therapy
AMI-7a	Fibrinolytic therapy received within 30 min of hospital arrival

[a]In addition, some hospitals are utilizing the AHA 2008 MI performance measures[36] and/or reporting outcomes to the ACC's NCDR® (National Cardiovascular Data Registry) Acute Coronary Treatment & Interventions Network (ACTION®)—Get with the Guidelines (GWTG™)[37] as part of quality improvement programs.

REFERENCES

*Key articles

1. Lloyd-Jones D, Adams R, Carnethon M, et al. Heart disease and stroke statistics—2009 update: a report from the American Heart Association Statistics Committee and Stroke Statistics Subcommittee. *Circulation.* 2009;119:480–486.

2. Rich JD, Cannon CP, Murphy SA, et al. Prior aspirin use and outcomes in acute coronary syndromes. *J Am Coll Cardiol.* 2010;56:1376–1385.

3. Thygesen K, Alpert JS, White HD, et al. Universal definition of myocardial infarction. *Circulation.* 2007;116:2634–2653.

4. **Antman EM, Cohen M, Bernink PJ, et al. The TIMI risk score for unstable angina/ non-ST elevation MI: A method for prognostication and therapeutic decision making. *JAMA.* 2000;284:835–842.**

5. TIMI Risk Score for UA/NSTEMI. Available at http://www.mdcalc.com/timi-risk-score-for-uanstemi. Accessed October 20, 2009.

6. Pieper KS, Gore JM, FitzGerald G, et al. Validity of a risk-prediction tool for hospital mortality: the Global Registry of Acute Coronary Events. *Am Heart J.* 2009;157:1097–1105.

7. Granger CB, Hirsch J, Califf RM, et al. Activated partial thromboplastin time and outcome after thrombolytic therapy for acute myocardial infarction: results from the GUSTO-I trial. *Circulation.*1996;93:870–878.

8. Gilchrist IC, Berkowitz SD, Thompson TD, et al. Heparin dosing and outcome in acute coronary syndromes: the GUSTO-IIb experience. Global use of strategies to open occluded coronary arteries. *Am Heart J.* 2002;144:73–80.

9. Nallamothu BK, Bates ER, Hochman JS, et al. Prognostic implication of activated partial thromboplastin time after reteplase or half-dose reteplase plus abciximab: results from the GUSTO-V trial. *Eur Heart J.* 2005;26:1506–1512.

10. Cheng S, Morrow DA, Sloan S, et al. Predictors of initial nontherapeutic anticoagulation with unfractionated heparin in ST-segment elevation myocardial infarction. *Circulation.* 2009;119:1195–1202.

11. Anand SS, Yusuf S, Pogue J, et al. Relationship of activated partial thromboplastin time to coronary events and bleeding in patients with acute coronary syndromes who receive heparin. *Circulation.* 2003;107:2884–2888.

12. Newby LK, Harrington RA, Bhapkar MV, et al. An automated strategy for bedside aPTT determination and unfractionated heparin infusion adjustment in acute coronary syndromes: insights from PARAGON A. *J Thromb Thrombolysis.* 2002;14:33–42.

13. Becker RC, Cannon CP, Tracy RP, et al. Relation between systemic anticoagulation as determined by activated partial thromboplastin time and heparin measurements and in-hospital clinical events in unstable angina and non-Q wave myocardial infarction. Thrombolysis in Myocardial Ischemia III B Investigators. *Am Heart J.* 1996;131:421–433.

* 14. **Harrington RA, Becker RC, Cannon CP, et al. Antithrombotic therapy for non-ST-segment elevation acute coronary syndromes: American College of Chest Physicians Evidence-Based Clinical Practice Guidelines (8th ed.). *Chest.* 2008;133 (6 Suppl):670S–707S.**

15. Goodman SG, Menon V, Cannon CP, et al. Acute ST-segment elevation myocardial infarction: American College of Chest Physicians Evidence-Based Clinical Practice Guidelines (8th ed.). *Chest.* 2008;133(6 Suppl):708S–775S.

16. TIMI 11A Investigators. Dose-ranging trial of enoxaparin for unstable angina: results of TIMI 11A. The Thrombolysis in Myocardial Infarction (TIMI) 11A Trial Investigators. *J Am Coll Cardiol.* 1997;29:1474–1482.

17. Montalescot G, Cohen M, Salette G, et al. Impact of anticoagulation levels on outcomes in patients undergoing elective percutaneous coronary intervention: insights from the STEEPLE trial. *Eur Heart J.* 2008;29:462–471.

18. Montalescot G, Collet JP, Tanguy A, et al. Anti-Xa activity related to survival and efficacy in unselected acute coronary syndrome patients treated with enoxaparin. *Circulation.* 2004;110:392–398.

19. Subherwal S, Bach RG, Chen AY, et al. Baseline risk of major bleeding in non-ST-segment-elevation myocardial infarction: the CRUSADE (Can Rapid risk stratification of Unstable angina patients Suppress ADverse outcomes with Early implementation of the ACC/AHA Guidelines) Bleeding Score. *Circulation.* 2009;119(14):1873–1882.

20. CRUSADE Bleeding Score Calculator. Available at http://www.crusadebleedingscore. org/. Accessed October 20, 2009.

21. Antman EM, Anbe DT, Armstrong PW, et al. ACC/AHA guidelines for the management of patients with ST-elevation myocardial infarction—executive summary: a report of the American College of Cardiology/American Heart Association Task Force on Practice Guidelines (Writing Committee to Revise the 1999 Guidelines for the Management of Patients With Acute Myocardial Infarction). *Circulation.* 2004;110:588–636.

22. Smith SC Jr, Feldman TE, Hirshfeld JW Jr, et al. ACC/AHA/SCAI 2005 guideline update for percutaneous coronary intervention: a report of the American College of Cardiology/American Heart Association Task Force on Practice Guidelines (ACC/AHA/SCAI Writing Committee to Update the 2001 Guidelines for Percutaneous Coronary Intervention). *J Am Coll Cardiol.* 2006;47(1):e1–e121.

23. King SB 3rd, Smith SC Jr, Hirshfeld JW Jr, et al. 2007 Focused Update of the ACC/ AHA/SCAI 2005 Guideline Update for Percutaneous Coronary Intervention: a report of the American College of Cardiology/American Heart Association Task Force on Practice Guidelines: 2007 Writing Group to Review New Evidence and Update the ACC/AHA/SCAI 2005 Guideline Update for Percutaneous Coronary Intervention, Writing on Behalf of the 2005 Writing Committee. *Circulation.* 2008;117(2):261–295.

24. Kushner FG, Hand M, Smith SC Jr, et al. 2009 Focused Updates: ACC/AHA Guidelines for the Management of Patients With ST-Elevation Myocardial Infarction (updating the 2004 Guideline and 2007 Focused Update) and ACC/ AHA/SCAI Guidelines on Percutaneous Coronary Intervention (updating the 2005 Guideline and 2007 Focused Update): a report of the American College of Cardiology Foundation/American Heart Association Task Force on Practice Guidelines. *Circulation.* 2009;120(22):2271–2306.

25. Antman EM, Hand M, Armstrong PW, et al. 2007 Focused Update of the ACC/AHA 2004 Guidelines for the Management of Patients With ST-Elevation Myocardial Infarction: a report of the American College of Cardiology/American Heart Association Task Force on Practice Guidelines: developed in collaboration With the Canadian Cardiovascular Society endorsed by the American Academy of

Family Physicians: 2007 Writing Group to Review New Evidence and Update the ACC/AHA 2004 Guidelines for the Management of Patients With ST-Elevation Myocardial Infarction, Writing on Behalf of the 2004 Writing Committee. *Circulation*. 2008;117(2):296–329.

* 26. Anderson JL, Adams CD, Antman EM, et al. ACC/AHA 2007 guidelines for the management of patients with unstable angina/non ST-elevation myocardial infarction: a report of the American College of Cardiology/American Heart Association Task Force on Practice Guidelines (Writing Committee to Revise the 2002 Guidelines for the Management of Patients with Unstable Angina/Non ST-Elevation Myocardial Infarction): developed in collaboration with the American College of Emergency Physicians, the Society for Cardiovascular Angiography and Interventions, and the Society of Thoracic Surgeons: endorsed by the American Association of Cardiovascular and Pulmonary Rehabilitation and the Society for Academic Emergency Medicine). *Circulation*. 2007;116:e148–e304.

27. Spinler SA, Ou FS, Roe MT, et al. Weight-based dosing of enoxaparin in obese patients with non-ST-segment elevation acute coronary syndromes: results from the CRUSADE initiative. *Pharmacotherapy*. 2009;29:631–638.

28. Gallo R, Steinhubl SR, White HD, et al. Impact of anticoagulation regimens on sheath management and bleeding in patients undergoing elective percutaneous coronary intervention in the STEEPLE trial. *Catheter Cardiovasc Interv*. 2009;73:319–325.

29. Cantor WJ, Mahaffey KW, Huang Z, et al. Bleeding complications in patients with acute coronary syndrome undergoing early invasive management can be reduced with radial access, smaller sheath sizes, and timely sheath removal. *Catheter Cardiovasc Interv*. 2007;69:73–83.

30. Angiomax (bivalirudin) for injection. Removal of the femoral artery catheter. Available at http://www.angiomax.com/Catheter/Default.aspx. Accessed October 20, 2009.

* 31. Mehta SR, Tanguay JF, Eikelboom JW, et al. Double-dose versus standard-dose clopidogrel and high-dose versus low-dose aspirin in individuals undergoing percutaneous coronary intervention for acute coronary syndromes (CURRENT-OASIS 7): a randomised factorial trial. *Lancet*. 2010;376:1233–1243.

32. Wiviott SD, Braunwald E, McCabe CH, et al. Prasugrel versus clopidogrel in patients with acute coronary syndromes. *N Engl J Med*. 2007;357:2001–2015.

33. Giugliano RP, White JA, Bode C. Early versus delayed, provisional eptifibatide in acute coronary syndromes. *N Engl J Med*. 2009;360:2176–2190.

34. Juwana YB, Suryapranata H, Ottervanger JP, et al. Tirofiban for myocardial infarction. *Expert Opin Pharmacother*. 2010.11:861–866.

35. The Joint Commission. Acute myocardial infarction core measure set. Available at http://www.jointcommission.org/PerformanceMeasurement/PerformanceMeasurement/Acute+Myocardial+Infarction+Core+Measure+Set.htm. Accessed March 8, 2010.

36. Krumholz HM, Anderson JL, Bachelder BL, et al. ACC/AHA 2008 performance measures for adults with ST-elevation and non-ST-elevation myocardial infarction: a report of the American College of Cardiology/American Heart Association Task Force on Performance Measures (Writing Committee to develop performance measures for ST-elevation and non-ST-elevation myocardial infarction): developed in collaboration with the American Academy of Family Physicians and the American College of Emergency Physicians: endorsed by the American Association of Cardiovascular and Pulmonary Rehabilitation, Society for Cardiovascular Angiography and Interventions, and Society of Hospital Medicine. *Circulation*. 2008;118:2596–2648.

37. National Cardiovascular Data Registry (NCDR®) ACTION® Get with the Guidelines (GWTG)™. Available at http://www.ncdr.com/webncdr/ACTION/Default.aspx. Accessed March 9, 2010.

FOURTEEN

Chapter

14

Prosthetic Heart Valves

Douglas C. Anderson, Jr.

INTRODUCTION

Patients with mechanical prosthetic heart valves (MPHVs) are at high risk for thromboembolic complications including cerebrovascular accident (CVA), and all MPHVs require antithrombotic prophylaxis. An ideal valve, which would be infinitely durable and nonthrombogenic, does not exist.

- Prosthetic valves are made of a broad range of materials that differ in their thrombogenicity.[1]

  - Newer materials reduce the thrombogenicity, and future materials such as polymerics may reduce thrombogenicity even more.[2]

- Valve prosthetics alter cardiac hemodynamics causing turbulence and other flow anomalies.[3]

  - MPHVs in particular create high sheer stresses, which destroy blood elements leading to activation of platelets, endothelial cells, and some coagulation proteins, thus resulting in a very high level of thrombogenicity.

  - Bioprosthetic valves are less thrombogenic, but not as durable as MPHVs and are thus more prone to failure requiring replacement.

Clinical Pearls

- Since valve position, type, and materials affect thrombogenicity, it is important to determine exactly *which* valve has been repaired and the *type* of prosthesis was used in order to avoid mistakes in anticoagulation.

- In clinical practice, "MVR" can be a confusing abbreviation. It could mean "mechanical valve replacement," "mitral valve repair" (often with an annuloplasty ring), or "mitral valve replacement." Any time this abbreviation is encountered, it is critical for the clinician to specifically determine what type of prosthetic device has been inserted in a patient for the same reasons as listed in the above clinical pearl.

- Thromboembolic events include valve thrombosis, systemic embolism, and stroke. Prosthetic valve thrombosis may necessitate treatment with fibrinolytics or valve replacement.

- There are only a finite number of times a valve can be replaced. After two replacements, careful oversight of anticoagulation is critical to avoid any future thrombotic complications.

RISK FACTORS FOR THROMBOSIS

- Annual risk for thromboembolism (TE) ranges from 4% to 23% without prophylaxis.[6,7]

- Prophylaxis reduces the risk of TE to 1% to 2% per year.[4]

- Risk of TE is highest in the early postsurgical period (approximately 3 months) until the valve is fully endothelialized.[8]

Clinical Pearl

- Transesophageal echocardiography (TEE) is the gold standard for imaging heart valves for thrombosis and is preferred over transthoracic echocardiogram (TTE) because of higher sensitivity of TEE in detecting thrombi.[9]

TYPES OF VALVES

Mechanical prostheses

- Three basic types of mechanical valves: caged ball/disk, tilting disk, and bileaflet

- Older caged ball and tilting disk valves are more thrombogenic than bileaflet valves

- Annual TE event rate in patients anticoagulated to an INR 2.5–4.9[10]
    - Bileaflet 0.5% per year
    - Tilting disk 0.7% per year
    - Caged ball 2.5% per year

Table 14-1: Types and Models of Mechanical Valves

Type	Models	Example
Caged-ball	Starr-Edwards	Starr-Edwards (see Figure 14-1)
Tilting disc	Björk-Shiley Monostrut	Björk-Shiley (see Figure 14-2)
	Medtronic Hall Omniscience Omnicarbon Ultracor	Medtronic Hall valve (see Figure 14-3)
Bileaflet	St. Jude On-X Carbomedics Baxter TEKNA Duromedics Sorin Bicarbon	On-X (see Figure 14-4)

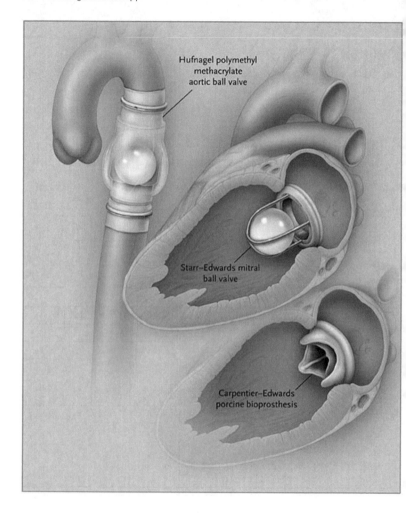

Figure 14-1: Evolution of Mechanical Valve Prostheses

The Hufnagel aortic ball valve implanted in the descending thoracic aorta; the Starr-Edwards caged-ball valve in the mitral position; and the Carpentier-Edwards porcine bioprosthesis in the mitral position. (Source: used with permission from Chaikoff EL. The development of prosthetic heart valves: lessons in form and function. *N Engl J Med.* 2007;357(14):1368-1371. ©2007. Massachusetts Medical Society. All rights reserved.)

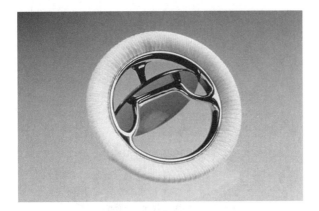

Figure 14-2: Björk-Shiley Tilting Disc Valve

(Source: used with permission from Sorin Group.)

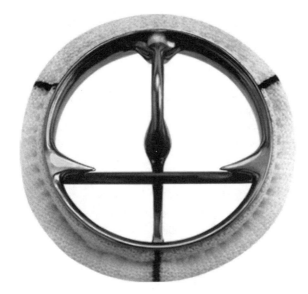

Figure 14-3: Medtronic-Hall Tilting Disc Valve

(Source: used with permission from Medtronic, Inc.)

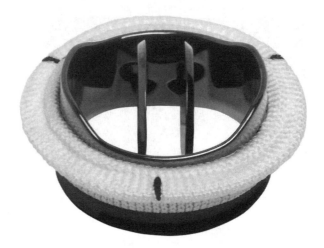

Figure 14-4: On-X ConformX Bileaflet Aortic Valve

(Source: photo(s) reproduced with permission from Austin, TX: On-X Life Technologies; 2009.)

Bioprostheses

- Bioprosthetic valves use a ring of material to which valves from an animal source (e.g., porcine, bovine).
  - Porcine valves use the tissue valve from pig hearts (usually aortic valves) (see Figure 14-1).
  - Pericardial valves use tissue from the bovine pericardium to make the valve leaflets, which are supported by a synthetic frame.
- Bioprosthetics are less thrombogenic than MPHVs.
  - Less disturbance in hemodynamics
  - Less damage to cellular components of blood
- Bioprosthetics are less durable than MPHVs and are more likely to require replacement for valve failure.
- Homografts involve replacing aortic or pulmonary valves with donated human valves.

Table 14-2: Types and Models of Bioprosthetic Valves

Type	Models	Example
Porcine	Hancock I Hancock II Intact Carpentier-Edwards Freestyle Bicor	Hancock II porcine valve (see Figure 14-5) Carpentier-Edwards (see Figure 14-1)
Pericardial (bovine)	Carpentier-Edwards Perimount Ionescu-Shiley Mitroflow	

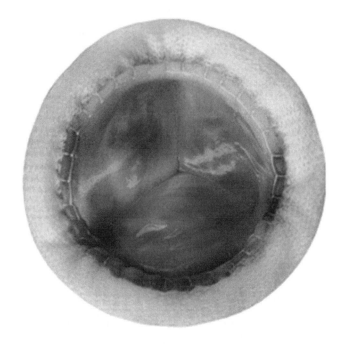

Figure 14-5: Hancock II Porcine Bioprosthetic Valve

(Source: printed with permission from Medtronic, Inc.)

Valve position

- Valve position influences thrombogenicity
    - MPHVs in mitral position appear to be more thrombogenic than MPHVs in the aortic position.
        - Annual TE rate with St. Jude Medical bileaflet valves without antithrombotic prophylaxis[11]:
            - Aortic position: 12%
            - Mitral position: 22%
        - 5-year TE event rate with Starr-Edwards valves[12]
            - Aortic: 35%
            - Mitral: 70%

Table 14-3: Other Risk Factors for Thrombosis and/or Total Morbidity/Mortality

Comorbid Condition	Effect(s) on Morbidity/Mortality
Aortic + mitral valve replacement	TE rate 2.4 times higher than aortic valve replacement alone and 1.33 times higher than mitral valve replacement alone[10]
	Early mortality rate 3 times higher than aortic valve replacement alone and 1.4 times higher than mitral valve replacement alone[13]
Atrial fibrillation	TE rate 1.6 times higher than patients with aortic valve replacement in sinus rhythm, and long-term mortality rate 2.2 times higher[14]
Poor LV function/heart failure	Patients with NYHA IV heart failure were 10.7 times more likely to die within 5 yr of aortic valve replacement with an MPHV compared with NYHA I-II[14]
Left atrial enlargement	3 times higher incidence of systemic embolism for patients with left atrial dimension ≥4 cm compared with patients with left atrial dimension <4 cm[15]

(*continued*)

Table 14-3: (Continued)

Comorbid Condition	Effect(s) on Morbidity/Mortality
Age >70 yr[a]	1.9 times higher incidence of stroke compared to patients <70 yr[16]
	Higher risk of perioperative mortality[17,18]
	Higher incidence of valve-related reoperation[18]
History of prior TE	Patients with history of preoperative TE had 3.2 times risk for TE and 5.4 times risk for repeated TE after aortic valve replacement[14]

[a]While increased age does increase the risk of thrombosis, neither Chest or AHA guidelines recommend to treat patients age >70 years as "high risk."

ANTITHROMBOTIC PROPHYLAXIS

* IV adjusted dose UFH or LMWH can be used postoperatively after valve insertion, provided bleeding has been controlled, until INR is therapeutic for two consecutive days.

* All MPHVs should receive VKA adjusted to recommended INR range.

* Patients should be considered "high risk" if they meet one or more of the criteria in Table 14-3 (excluding age).

    – Example: if a patient with concurrent atrial fibrillation was having a native aortic valve replaced with a bileaflet MPHV, then the VKA should be titrated to an INR of 2.5–3.5 in conjunction with low dose ASA (see below for recommended ASA dosage ranges).

* Patients who have systemic embolism despite a therapeutic INR

    – If patient was not previously on ASA, then add ASA 50–100 mg daily, and

    – Titrate VKA to a higher INR range

Previous INR Range	Postsystemic Embolism INR Range
2–3	2.5–3.5
2.5–3.5	3.0–4.5[a]

[a]Chest recommends INR 3–4 and ACC/AHA recommend 3.5–4.5.

Table 14-4: Level of Anticoagulation by Risk of Thromboembolism

	Caged Ball/Disk	Tilting Disk (except Medtronic Hall tilting disk)	Bileaflet (and Medtronic Hall tilting disk)	Bioprosthesis
Aortic Valve Replacement				
Low risk	INR 2.5–3.5[a]	INR 2.5–3.5[a]	INR 2–3[a]	ASA[b]
High risk	INR 2.5–3.5 + ASA	INR 2.5–3.5 + ASA	INR 2.5–3.5 + ASA	INR 2–3[c]
Mitral Valve Replacement				
Low risk	INR 2.5–3.5[a]	INR 2.5–3.5[a]	INR 2.5–3.5[a]	INR 2–3 for first 3 mo, then ASA
High risk	INR 2.5–3.5 + ASA	INR 2.5–3.5 + ASA	INR 2.5–3.5 + ASA	INR 2–3 ± ASA
Either Position				
Hx of systemic embolism				INR 2–3 for first 3 mo, then reassess
Left atrial thrombus present at surgery				INR 2–3 until documented resolution

[a]ACC/AHA recommends adding ASA for all patients with an MPHV.

[b]Dosage recommendations for all indications: ACC/AHA 75–100 mg/day[4]; Chest 50–100 mg/day.[5] Both recommend against giving ASA to patients at high risk of bleeding (e.g., hx of GI bleed, age >80 years). For high-risk patients who cannot take ASA, ACC/AHA suggests clopidogrel 75 mg/day or INR 3.5–4.5.[4]

[c]ACC/AHA recommends INR 2.5–3.5 for first 3 months.[4]

SUMMARY

- Patients with an MPHV need lifelong anticoagulation with a VKA ± ASA.
- Highest risk of TE is in the early postoperative period.
- Thrombogenic potential is influenced by valve design, materials, and placement

- Multiple valve replacement, atrial fibrillation, poor LV function/heart failure, left atrial enlargement, age >70 years, and history of prior TE increase the risk of TE and other morbidity/mortality.

REFERENCES

1. Vongpatanasin W, Hillis LD, Lange RA. Prosthetic heart valves. *N Engl J Med.* 1996;335(6):407–416.

2. Ghanbari H, Viatge H, Kidane AG, et al. Polymeric heart valves: new materials, emerging hopes. *Trends Biotechnol.* 2009;27(6):359–367.

3. Schoen FJ. Evolving concepts of cardiac valve dynamics: the continuum of development, functional structure, pathobiology, and tissue engineering. *Circulation.* 2008;118(18):1864–1880.

4. Bonow RO, Carabello BA, Chatterjee K, et al. 2008 focused update incorporated into the ACC/AHA 2006 guidelines for the management of patients with valvular heart disease: a report of the American College of Cardiology/American Heart Association Task Force on Practice Guidelines (Writing Committee to Revise the 1998 Guidelines for the Management of Patients with Valvular Heart Disease): endorsed by the Society of Cardiovascular Anesthesiologists, Society for Cardiovascular Angiography and Interventions, and Society of Thoracic Surgeons. *Circulation.* 2008;118(15):e523–e661.

5. Salem DN, O'Gara PT, Madias C, et al. Valvular and structural heart disease. *Chest.* 2008;133(6 suppl):593S–629S.

6. Björk VO, Henze A. Management of thrombo-embolism after aortic valve replacement with the Björk-Shiley tilting disc valve. Medicamental prevention with dicumarol in comparison with dipyridamole - acetylsalicylic acid. Surgical treatment of prosthetic thrombosis. *Scand J Thorac Cardiovasc Surg.* 1975;9(3):183–191.

7. Cannegieter S, Rosendaal F, Briet E. Thromboembolic and bleeding complications in patients with mechanical heart valve prostheses. *Circulation.* 1994;89(2):635–641.

8. Benussi S, Verzini A, Alfieri O. Mitral valve replacement and thromboembolic risk. *J Heart Valve Dis.* 2004;13(Suppl 1):S81–S83.

9. Roudaut R, Serri K, Lafitte S. Thrombosis of prosthetic heart valves: diagnosis and therapeutic considerations. *Heart* 2007;93(1):137–142.

9. Cannegieter SC, Rosendaal FR, Wintzen AR, et al. Optimal oral anticoagulant therapy in patients with mechanical heart valves. *N Engl J Med.* 1995;333(1):11–17.

10. Baudet EM, Puel V, McBride JT, et al. Long-term results of valve replacement with the St. Jude Medical prosthesis. *J Thorac Cardiovasc Surg.* 1995;109(5):858–870.

11. Macmanus Q, Grunkemeier G, Thomas D, et al. The Starr-Edwards model 6000 valve. A fifteen-year follow-up of the first successful mitral prosthesis. *Circulation.* 1977;56(4):623–625.

12. Horstkotte D, Schulte H, Bircks W, et al. Unexpected findings concerning thromboembolic complications and anticoagulation after complete 10 year follow up of patients with St. Jude Medical prostheses. *J Heart Valve Dis.* 1993;2(3):291–301.

13. Kvidal P, Bergström R, Malm T, et al. Long-term follow-up of morbidity and mortality after aortic valve replacement with a mechanical valve prosthesis. *Eur Heart J.* 2000;21(13):1099–1111.

14. Burchfiel C, Hammermeister K, Krause-Steinrauf H, et al. Left atrial dimension and risk of systemic embolism in patients with a prosthetic heart valve. Department of Veterans Affairs Cooperative Study on Valvular Heart Disease. *J Am Coll Cardiol.* 1990;15(1):32–41.

15. Arom K, Nicoloff D, Lindsay W, et al. Should valve replacement and related procedures be performed in elderly patients? *Ann Thorac Surg.* 1984;38(5):466–472.

16. Lawrie GM, Earle EA, Earle NR. Abstract 2308: conventional aortic valve replacement in very elderly patients. *Circulation.* 2008;118:S_703.

17. Jebara VA, Dervanian P, Acar C, et al. Mitral valve repair using Carpentier techniques in patients more than 70 years old. Early and late results. *Circulation.* 1992;86 (5 Suppl):1153–1159.

18. Chan V, Jamieson WRE, Germann E, et al. Performance of bioprostheses and mechanical prostheses assessed by composites of valve-related complications to 15 years after aortic valve replacement. *J Thorac Cardiovasc Surg.* 2006;131(6):1267–1273.

KEY ARTICLES

Chan WS, Anand S, Ginsberg JS. Anticoagulation of pregnant women with mechanical heart valves: a systematic review of the literature. *Arch Intern Med.* 2000;160(2):191–196.

Gohlke-Barwolf C, Acar J, Oakley C, et al. Guidelines for prevention of thromboembolic events in valvular heart disease. *Eur Heart J.* 1995;16(10):1320–1330.

Little SH, Massel DR. Antiplatelet and anticoagulation for patients with prosthetic heart valves. *Cochran Database Syst Rev.* javascript:AL_get(this, 'jour', 'Cochrane Database Syst Rev.'); 2003;(4):CD003464.

Wittkowski AK. Thrombosis. In: Koda-Kimble MA, Young LY, Kradjan WA, et al., eds. *Applied Therapeutics: The Clinical Use of Drugs.* Baltimore, MD: Lippincott Williams & Wilkins; 2005:16-23–16-25.

FIFTEEN

Chapter

Heparin-Induced Thrombocytopenia

William E. Dager

INTRODUCTION

Heparin-induced thrombocytopenia (HIT) is an immune-mediated process triggered by exposure to unfractionated heparin (UFH) or low molecular weight heparin (LMWH) that can create the paradox of increased thrombosis risk with concurrent thrombocytopenia. It is important to recognize and promptly initiate appropriate management when present. No gold standard test currently exists; thus, diagnosis typically combines signs and symptoms with laboratory observations. Stopping the heparin agent alone will not prevent the potential risk for thrombosis, limb ischemia (which can lead to amputation), or death.

Identification of HIT[1]

Table 15-1: Characteristics of Heparin-Related Nonimmune and Immune Mediated Thrombocytopenia

	Nonimmune Mediated Heparin Associated Thrombocytopenia (HAT)	Immune Mediated (HIT)
Frequency	10% to 30%	<1% to 3%
Timing of onset	1–4 days	Typical 5–10 days
		Acute: immediate if recent exposure
		Delayed: up to 40 days after last exposure to the heparin compound

(continued)

Table 15-1: (Continued)

	Nonimmune Mediated (HAT)	**Immune Mediated (HIT)**
Decrease in platelets	Slight	Moderate/large
Antibody mediated	No	Yes
Thrombosis	No	30% to 75%
Hemorrhage	None	Rare
Management	Observe	Discontinue all heparin/LMWH products, flushes, coated lines, and rinses Start alternate parenteral anticoagulant

Table 15-2: HIT Terminology[2]

Term	**Description**	**Treatment Duration**
Acute HIT	Period of thrombocytopenia associated with current or recent exposure to heparin prior to platelet count recovery	—
Isolated HIT	Presence of HIT that is not associated with thrombosis as a consequence	Continue anticoagulation until recovery of platelet counts to a stable plateau
HIT-related thrombosis syndrome (HITTS)	Presence of thrombosis that formed as a result of HIT	3–6 mo unless other factors require longer anticoagulation
History of HIT	Previous history of HIT, but not acute, or related thrombocytopenia	NA—long-term treatment of HIT is not needed; may receive anticoagulation for other reasons (i.e., DVT prophylaxis)

HIT-related disorders (not common)[2]

- Skin lesions at heparin injection sites
- Adrenal infarct
- Cardiovascular/anaphylactoid reactions on reexposure
- Venous limb gangrene (VLG) with warfarin exposure
- Warfarin-induced skin necrosis

Clinical Pearl

- Starting warfarin alone (no other alternative anticoagulant present), especially in higher doses potentially leading to INR values >4, can increase the risk for VLG due to protein C depletion.

Table 15-3: Pseudo-HIT Disorders That Can Mimic HIT Including Thrombocytopenia and Thrombosis[3]

Early Onset	Late Onset
GP IIb/IIIa inhibitors	Adenocarcinoma
Pulmonary embolism	Post-transfusion purpura
Thrombolytic therapy	Postsurgical thrombotic thrombocytopenic purpura
Antiphospholipid disorder	
Diabetic ketoacidosis	Pulmonary embolism
Infective endocarditis	Drug (nonheparin) induced thrombocytopenia
Septicemia-related purpura fulminans	
Paroxysmal nocturnal hemoglobinuria	
Postsurgical thrombotic thrombocytopenic purpura	

Table 15-4: Factors Associated with the Development of HIT[4-6]

Factor	Importance	Hierarchy
Type of heparin	Major	UFH >LMWH >fondaparinux Higher risk with more recent exposure
Duration of heparin	Major	11–14 days[a] >5–10 days >4 (or fewer) days
Type of patient	Moderate	Postsurgery >medical >pregnancy or neonate
Dose of heparin	Moderate	Therapeutic ≥ prophylaxis >"flushes"
Gender of patient	Minor	Female >male

Abbreviations: > = greater than; ≥ = greater than or similar to.

[a]Minimal additional risk if heparin continued beyond 14 days.

Table 15-5: ACCP Recommendations for Platelet Count Monitoring to Recognize HIT[4]

Situation	Concurrent HIT Patient Specific Risk Factors	Platelet Count Monitoring	ACCP Recommendation Grade
UFH or LMWH used at any dose	UFH exposure within 100 days	Baseline and within 24 hr	1C
UFH bolus given	Anaphylactoid reaction within 30 min of UFH bolus	Immediate and compare to prior count	1C
Therapeutic UFH administered		Every 2–3 days (days 4–14 or until D/C) Heparin	2C

(continued)

Table 15-5: (Continued)

Situation	Concurrent HIT Patient Specific Risk Factors	Platelet Count Monitoring	ACCP Recommendation Grade
Prophylactic UFH administered	Postoperative (HIT risk >1%)	Every other day (days 4–14 or until D/C) Heparin	2C
Prophylaxis with UFH or LMWH administered	UFH use in medical/obstetrics patients UFH flushes used in postoperative patients LMWH use in postoperative patients LMWH use in medical/obstetrics patient who previously received UFH (HIT risk 0.1 to 1.0%)	Every 2–3 days (days 4–14 or until D/C) Heparin	2C
Prophylaxis with UFH or LMWH administered	LMWH use in medical/obstetrics patients UFH catheter flushes in a medical patient (HIT risk 0.1% to 1.0%)	Not recommended	2C
Fondaparinux at any dose administered	All situations (HIT only reported in rare case reports)	Not recommended	1C

Table 15-6: Pretest Probability Scoring (4Ts) for HIT[2,a]

Indicator	2 Points	1 Point	No Points
Thrombocytopenia	>50% fall or platelet nadir 20–100 K/mm^2	30% to 50% fall, or platelet nadir 10–19 K/mm^2	<30% fall or platelet nadir <10 K/mm^2
Timing of platelet count fall or other sequelae	Clear onset 5–10 days after exposure; <1 day if reexposure within 100 days	Consistent with immunization but not clear (e.g., missing platelet counts) or onset after 10 days	Platelet count fall to early (without recent heparin exposure)
Thrombosis or other sequelae	New thrombosis, skin necrosis; acute systemic reactions postheparin bolus	Progressive or recurrent thrombosis; presence of erythematous skin lesions; suspected thrombosis not yet proven	No related thrombosis
Other causes of thrombocytopenia	No other cause for platelet count fall evident	Other possible causes evident	Definite other causes present

Pretest Probability

6–8 High

4–5 Intermediate

0–3[b] Low

[a]4 Ts = **T**hrombocytopenia, **T**iming, **T**hrombosis, O**t**her.

[b]Some facilities classify patients with a score of 3 as an intermediate risk.

Table 15-7: Post-HIT Probability Assessment Tool Proposed by Chong[7]

Indicator	Points
Onset of thrombocytopenia[a] (or a substantial decrease in platelet by >50% between 4–14 days after exposure)	3
If onset of thrombocytopenia is <4 days or >4 days	1
Exclusion of other causes of thrombocytopenia	2

(continued

Table 15-7: (Continued)

Indicator	Points
Thrombocytopenia resolves after stopping agent	2
Thrombocytopenia recurs on heparin reexposure	1
Thrombosis associated with thrombocytopenia	1
Laboratory tests	
— Immunoassay positive	2
— Functional assay: two-point system positive[b]	3
— Functional assay: non-two-point system[b]	2

>7 = definite; 5–6 = probable; 3–4 = possible; and <3 = unlikely.

[a]Thrombocytopenia defined as platelet count <150 K/mm^3 or drop $>50\%$.

[b]In the two-point system, there is the addition of a control using a high heparin concentration (100 units/mL), which characterizes the heparin antibody (suppresses the antibody reaction).

Clinical Pearl

- Both the 4Ts and the Chong post-HIT assessment tools are useful decision aids in the diagnosis and management of HIT. However, after adoption into clinical practice, neither tool has been prospectively validated to improve the treatment outcomes of patients who may or may not have HIT.

Table 15-8: Laboratory Assays for HIT Antibody[3]

- Platelet activation or functional assays detect platelet activation when the patient's serum is incubated with normal platelets and heparin

- Antigen or immunoassays detect presence of antiplatelet factor 4/heparin antibodies; these antibodies may or may not be pathogenic

- For patients receiving heparin agents, ACCP does not recommend (grade 1C) routine screen for HIT antibody in the absence of thrombocytopenia, thrombosis, heparin-induced skin lesions, or other signs of HIT

(continued)

Table 15-8: (Continued)

Platelet activation Washed platelet assays	Serotonin release assay (SRA) Heparin-induced platelet activation (HIPA) ATP release using luminography Platelet microparticle assay using flow cytometry
Platelet activation Platelets in citrated platelet-rich plasma	Platelet aggregation test (PAT) Annexin V-binding assay Serotonin release using flow cytometry
Antigen assays	Enzyme-linked immunosorbent assay (ELISA) Fluid phase immunoassays Rapid assays (particle gel immunoassay—PaGIA) Particle immunofiltration assay (PIFA)

Table 15-9: Differences Between Common Assays Used to Detect HIT[3,8,9]

	Serotonin Release Assay	Heparin/ ELISA	Heparin/PF4 Rapid Assay	Platelet Aggregation Assay
Measures	Serotonin release for aggregated platelets	Heparin dependent antibodies	Presence of PF4 antibodies	Platelet aggregation of IgG
Advantages	High sensitivity (99%); high specificity (95%)	Fast turnaround; low false-negative rate	Sensitive and specific; rapid turnaround time	Easy to perform >90% specificity
Disadvantages	Time consuming; expensive; radio isotopes involved; very long turnaround time	Low specificity; high (~25%) false-positive rate	No controls and limited experience with outcomes	Very low sensitivity (40%) leading to high false-negative rates
Comment	Consideration for long-term decisions where reexposure to heparin anticipated, and clinical diagnosis unclear	Commonly used; one product (GTI ELISA) has conformation step		Not routinely recommended given availability of SRA and ELISA

PRINCIPLES OF PHARMACOTHERAPY MANAGEMENT

Table 15-10: Initial Management of Suspected HIT[4,5,10]

Intervention	Comment
Remove all exposure to heparin-related agents where possible	Heparin or LMWH; consider all heparin-related sources including flushes, coated lines, dialysis rinses; LMWH should be avoided (ACCP grade 1B)
Reverse concurrent warfarin therapy	Vitamin K 10 mg PO, or 5–10 mg IV should be considered to reverse the effects of a VKA in acute HIT (ACCP grade 1C)
Initiate alternative anticoagulant	Stopping heparin agent alone does not stop the progression of HIT and may increase risk for thrombosis from loss of anticoagulant effects (see Table 15-11 for agent options); if significant bleeding concerns are present and alternative anticoagulant therapy poses a notable risk, consider frequent assessment for thrombosis (i.e., duplex ultrasonography with compression) and initiate alternative therapy as soon as possible
Platelet transfusions	Prophylactic transfusions of platelets in the absence of bleeding should be avoided (ACCP grade 2C)

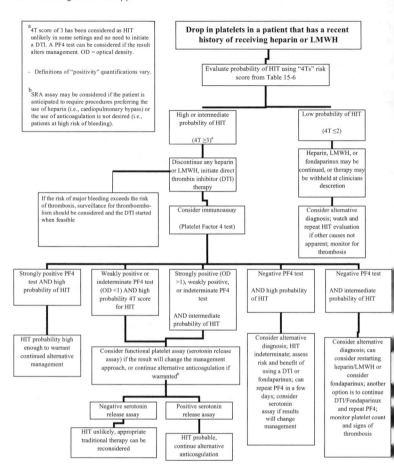

Figure 15-1: Flow Diagram

Diagram describes a generalized approach to decisions incorporating the use of the 4T scoring system, functional and immunoassays, and anticoagulation therapy decisions when HIT is suspected. (Source: adapted from reference 6.)

Table 15-11: Agents Used in the Management of HIT[3,4,10,11]

Agent (ACCP grade)	Chemistry	Route of Elimination	Half-life[a]	Assay (usual target range)[b]	Comments
Argatroban (1C)	DTI: L-arginine derivative	Hepato-biliary	40–50 min	aPTT: 1.5–3.0 x baseline	FDA-approved for HIT prophylaxis or treatment, including PCI; prolongs INR
Lepirudin (1C)	DTI: 65-amino acid peptide derived from leech anticoagulant (hirudin)	Renal	≥80 min	aPTT: 1.5–2.5 x baseline	FDA-approved for HIT complicated by thrombosis; immunogenic; IV or SC
Bivalirudin (2C)	DTI: 20-aa hirudin analogue	Enzymatic (80%); renal (20%)	25 min	aPTT: 1.5–2.5X baseline	Not approved for HIT (except during PCI)
Danaparoid (1B)	Mixture of GAGs with predominant anti-Xa activity	Renal; other	25 hr	Anti-Xa activity level (0.5–0.8 units/mL) Peak effect post-SC injection at 4–5 hr	Not marketed in US (approved for HIT in EU, Canada); no effect on INR; IV or SC
Fondaparinux	Sulfated penta-saccharide with anti-Xa activity	Renal; other	17 hr	NA	Not approved for HIT; not generally recommended for use in acute HIT
Warfarin	Vitamin K antagonist	Hepatic	35–45 hr	INR 2.0–3.0	Potential for microvascular thrombosis when given during acute HIT

Abbreviations: aa = amino acid; anti-Xa = anti-Factor Xa; aPTT = activated partial thromboplastin time; DTI = direct thrombin inhibitor; EU = European Union; FDA = US Food and Drug Administration; INR = international normalized ratio; IV = intravenous; SC = subcutaneous; NA = not applicable.

[a]Half-life determined in normal subjects and may be longer in many patients with HIT.

[b]Baseline is the patient's baseline aPTT off heparin or the laboratory mean if the patient's baseline value is notably elevated.

Table 15-12: Prospective Cohort Studies (with historical controls) of Lepirudin or Argatroban for Treatment of HIT Complicated by Thrombosis[12–16]

Trial (n = number of patients receiving DTI indicated)	% HIT Antibody Positive	Duration of DTI Therapy (days)	% Thrombosis (% of controls)	RRR[a]	% Major Bleeding (% of controls)
Lepirudin					
HAT-1,2 (n=113) (76)	100	13.3	10.1 (27.2)	0.63	18.8 (7.1)
HAT-3 (n=98) (77)	100	14.0	6.1	0.78	20.4
Postmarketing (n=496) (78)	77	12.1	5.2	0.81	5.4
Argatroban[b]					
Arg-911 (n=144) (87)	65	5.9	19.4 (34.8)	0.44	11.1 (2.2)
Arg-915 (n=229) (88)	N.A.	7.1	13.1	0.62	6.1

Abbreviations: Arg = Argatroban trial; DTI = direct thrombin inhibitor; HAT = heparin-associated thrombocytopenia trial; RRR = relative risk reduction.

[a]The RRR calculations shown for HAT-3/postmarketing studies and for Arg-915 were based on the historical control data reported for HAT-1,2 and Arg-911, respectively.

[b]Additional observations from the lepirudin trials[15]:

• Thrombosis occurred in 6.1% after enrollment but prior to starting the lepirudin. Thrombosis rates were 1.3% during therapy and 0.7% after.

• Thrombosis rates were higher if half the aPTT values were below 1.5 times control.

Table 15-13: Comparison Between Argatroban and Lepirudin Trials[17]

Argatroban	Lepirudin
Prospective	Prospective, intent to treat
Historical control	Historical control (27% receiving danaparoid)

(continued)

Table 15-13: (Continued)

Argatroban	Lepirudin
HIT diagnosis	HIT diagnosis
– Thrombocytopenia: 70% of patients had 50% drop or <100 K/mm³ – Prior history of HIT (acute HIT not required) – Lab confirmation not required (65% antibody positive)	– Thrombocytopenia (50%, 100 K/mm³) – With/without thromboembolic event during heparin therapy – Laboratory conformation required (treatment delayed 1.5–1.9 days)
Treatment initiated at diagnosis	Treatment initiated upon laboratory conformation of positive antibody
Duration of argatroban: 5.9 days	Duration of lepirudin: 13.3 days
Transitioned to warfarin: 62%	Transitioned to warfarin: 83%

American College of Chest Physicians' recommendation regarding patients with a confirmed history of HIT to avoid a recurrence[4]

- Patients with history of HIT or heparin allergy needing venous thromboembolism prophylaxis
    - If arterial disease present, consider warfarin, lepirudin, fondaparinux, or an antiplatelet agent.
    - Consider nonpharmacologic deep venous thromboembolism prophylaxis.
    - May consider cautiously using a heparin product if
        - Unable to avoid UFH or LMWH options
        - More than 100 days since HIT diagnosis
        - Duration of heparin therapy is limited

See Chapter 5 for insights/dosing of direct thrombin inhibitors in HIT. Information on danaparoid and fondaparinux is provided below.

Table 15-14: Danaparoid in HIT (currently not available in the US)[18]

Chemistry	Danaparoid is a mixture of depolymerized glycosaminoglycans: heparan sulfate (84%), dermatan sulfate (12%), and chondroitin sulfate (4%); a lower degree of sulfation and charge density compared to LMWH limits its binding to plasma proteins and platelets
Pharmacology	Indirect inhibition through antithrombin on factor Xa; Anti-Factor Xa: Anti-Factor IIa ratio >22:1; no effect unless at high doses on the aPTT, INR, or ACT
Cross reactivity with heparin antibodies	10% cross reactivity but not of any noted clinical significance in HIT
Observations in the management of HIT	In an assessment of 62 patients treated with danaparoid and transitioned to warfarin, compared to ancrod plus warfarin or warfarin alone; a new thrombosis, death or limb amputations and bleeding rates were significantly lower with danaparoid
	In a retrospective analysis of 1478 cases of HIT receiving danaparoid, a survival rate of 84% with new thrombosis during treatment of 9.7% and 16.4% having an inadequate treatment response (new/extended thrombosis, platelet count reduction, or unplanned amputation during treatment); major bleeding occurred in 8.1%
	Similar efficacy (80%) to lepirudin if at therapeutic doses with a lower bleeding rate (2.5% vs. 10.4%) in one analysis

Table 15-15: Danaparoid Dosing and Monitoring[3,4]

Indication	Danaparoid Dose	Anti-Factor Xa targets
Acute HIT management	2,250 units IV bolus followed by 400 units/hr x 4 hr then 300 units/hr x 4 hr then 200 units/hr subsequently adjusted by anti-Factor Xa activity levels	0.5–0.8 units/mL
VTE prophylaxis (history of HIT)	750 units SC q 8–12 hr	
VTE treatment	2,250 units IV bolus followed by 400 units/hr x 4 hr then 150–200 units/hr Option: 1,500–2,250 units SC q 12 hr	0.5–0.8 units/mL
Intermittent hemodialysis (for preventing thrombosis of the circuit)	3,750 IV prior to first two dialysis sessions, 3,000 units for third dialysis, then reduce to 2,250 units	Predialysis: <0.3 units/mL During dialysis: 0.5–0.8 units/mL
Continuous renal replacement therapy	2,250 units IV bolus followed by 400 units/hr x 4 hr then 300 units/hr x 4 hr, then 150–400 units/hr	During hemodialysis: 0.5–0.8 units/mL
Cardiac catheterization	≤75 kg: 2,250 units IV preprocedure 75–90 kg: 3,000 units >90 kg: 3,750 units	
PCI/balloon pump	Cardiac cath-preprocedure then 150–200 units for 1–2 days post-PCI until balloon pump removed	

(*continued*)

Table 15-15: (Continued)

Indication	Danaparoid Dose	Anti-Factor Xa targets
Cardiopulmonary bypass	125 units/kg IV bolus post-thoracotomy Prime circuit: 3 units/mL, 7 units/kg/hr IV infusion after bypass initiated, and stopping 45 min prior to going off circuit	
Embolectomy/vascular surgery	2,250 units IV preoperatively, 750 units in 250 mL 0.9% saline up to 50 mL uses as intraoperative flushes Postoperative: Low risk: 750 units SC q 8 hr High risk:150–200 units/hr starting 6 hr or more after procedure	

Table 15-16: Fondaparinux in HIT (see Chapter 4 for details on fondaparinux and use outside HIT)[19]

Evidence supporting fondaparinux	Several case reports, small series, or single center experiences have suggested that fondaparinux may be effective in the management of HIT In one small series, fondaparinux was effective in the management of acute HIT Clinical trials comparing fondaparinux to controls in HIT similar to those done with argatroban or lepirudin have not been published
Dosing	No dose in the management of HIT has been established; doses consistent with its use in other conditions may be one consideration (i.e., 5–10 mg SC daily initially, or in the presence of acute thrombosis; 2.5 mg SC daily for prolonged anticoagulation once platelet count has recovered)
Monitoring anti-Factor Xa activity	The use of anti-Factor Xa activity to monitor fondaparinux in HIT has not been established
Evidence suggesting caution	Several cases suggesting fondaparinux as the cause of HIT have been reported

Table 15-17: Use of Warfarin in HIT[3,4,10,20,21]

Initial recognition of HIT (Acute HIT)	Use of warfarin is not recommended, and if present at the time of HIT recognition, it should be reversed (ACCP grade 1C recommendation); monotherapy with warfarin as the initial means to manage HIT is not recommended; if possible, 5 days of overlapping therapy with a DTI until platelet count has recovered and the INR is above 2; evidence supporting this is weak
Place in therapy	A majority of patients in the lepirudin and argatroban trials were converted to warfarin for extended anticoagulation; duration for isolated HIT has been until stable recovery of platelets and reduced risk for thrombosis; in some settings, clinicians may complete 30 days of alternative anticoagulation; longer therapy may be considered in the presence of thrombosis or when other indications for continued anticoagulation are present; based on case reports, warfarin should be initiated during concurrent alternative anticoagulation therapy after complete or notable platelet count recovery has occurred; initial dosing should be conservative to decrease the risk for venous limb gangrene
Monitoring	INR, targeting a value of 2–3; in the setting of false INR elevations with concurrent DTI therapy; factor X levels of 11% to 42% (similar to an INR of 2.0–3.5) can be used (see Chapter 5)
Transitioning from a DTI to warfarin when a DTI is present	It is important to note that the assay for the INR and aPTT separately may be unique to each institution; further, other variables could be affecting the INR at a given DTI dose; these reasons can make the standard nomogram for argatroban provided in the prescribing information packet difficult to use One alternative approach is outlined below: 1. Draw a baseline INR with and an aPTT on DTI therapy alone 2. Initiate warfarin and identify a desired 1.5–2.0 point increase in the INR or a preselected INR, which considers the DTI-induced INR prolongation (with minimal change in the aPTT) 3. Once the desired number of overlap days and desired platelet recovery has occurred and the desired INR target is reached, hold the DTI for 4–8 hr and recheck the INR and aPTT; if the INR is between 2–3 with an aPTT value close to baseline (INR is being elevated by warfarin alone since aPTT close to baseline), then the DTI can be discontinued; it may take longer for the effects of a DTI to diminish if a very low infusion rate with aPTT values in the target range

See Figure 15-1 for recommendations on when to begin/stop therapy for HIT.

SPECIAL POPULATION CONSIDERATIONS

- Pediatrics
  - Pathophysiology and frequency similar to that of adult population
  - Most pediatric cases reported in critically ill or cardiac surgery patients
  - Use of LMWH may decrease likelihood of HIT.
  - Body weight may be correlated with DTI clearance.
- Pregnancy
  - HIT in this population is rare.
  - Special considerations: HIT antibodies cross the placenta.
  - Pregnancy-induced increases in cardiac output, renal clearance, blood volume, and weight may require doses different to that of the general population.
  - Alternative anticoagulants: danaparoid or a direct thrombin inhibitor
  - Danaparoid has the most supportive data for this population and condition.
  - Long-term anticoagulation: subcutaneous danaparoid, lepirudin, or fondaparinux
  - Target: not established, but consider monitoring aPTT (lepirudin); anti-Factor Xa (danaparoid)

Table 15-18: Suggested Alternative Anticoagulant Dosing in Pediatric Patients Under HIT Conditions[22]

Agent	Dose	
Argatroban	In normal hepatic function, doses similar to observations in adults may apply; younger patients <6 mo old may have lower clearance and require a lower dose	Higher doses may be necessary in the setting of ECLS

(*continued*)

Table 15-18: (Continued)

Agent	Dose	
Danaparoid	VTE prevention: 10 units/kg SC BID VTE treatment: Bolus: 30 units/kg IV Infusion: 1.2–2.0 units/kg/hr	Renal dialysis: <10 yr: 30 units/kg IV + 1,000 units before each of first two dialysis sessions ≥10–17 yr: 30 units/kg IV + 1,500 units before each of first two dialysis sessions Anti-Factor Xa target on day 3: 0.4–0.6 units/mL (0.5–0.8 units/mL for high dose)
Lepirudin	In normal renal function, initiate at 0.1 mg/kg/hr (no bolus)	Lower doses may be necessary in renal impairment; higher doses for selected procedures or ECLS (noting that ECLS can lead to impaired renal function and decreased lepirudin elimination)

Table 15-19: Considerations for Maintaining Lines in the Setting of HIT

Agent	Comments
0.9% saline	
Citrate	4% has been studied; volume depends on the line; flush drawn from the Abbott ACD-A solution has been used
Lepirudin	Double-lumen catheter: 1.3 mL of a 0.5-mg/mL dilution in each port Central venous device: 3 mL daily of 0.1-mg/mL dilution
Bivalirudin	Not recommended as a flush because of enzymatic degradation by thrombin

Acute coronary syndromes

- Identify cause of thrombocytopenia
  - Consider rapid onset HIT if recently exposed to heparin.
  - Other relevant causative drugs: glycoprotein IIb-IIIa inhibitor, IV contrast dyes, intraaortic balloon pump
- Alternative anticoagulant considerations
  - Antiplatelet inhibitor or direct thrombin inhibitor or combination
  - Fondaparinux
  - Ability of glycoprotein IIb-IIIa inhibitors to block platelet response in HIT during PCI or acute HIT is unknown.
- Percutaneous coronary intervention (PCI) dosing under HIT conditions
  - Bivalirudin often chosen due to the substantial data for use in PCI
  - Regimen may depend on whether the patient has unstable angina, NSTEMI, or STEMI (see Chapter 13 for bivalirudin dosing guidance).

Coronary bypass graft surgery[4,23,24]

- History of HIT
  - Antibody negative: UFH preferred during surgery (ACCP grade 1B)
  - Antibody positive; check washed platelets activation assay; if negative use UFH during surgery (ACCP grade 2C)
  - Consider using a nonheparin agent postoperatively if possible.
- Acute or subacute HIT
  - Delay surgery until HIT resolved and antibody negative or weak positive (ACCP grade 1C)
  - Bivalirudin intraoperative (ACCP grade 1B)
  - Lepirudin (if ECT available and renal function intact) (ACCP grade 2C)
  - UFH combined with antiplatelet agent (ACCP 2C) (Table 15-20)
  - Danaparoid (off-pump procedures) (ACCP grade 2C)

Table 15-20: Dosing of Alternative Agents in Bypass Graft
Surgery Procedures[23,24]

Agent	Dosing
DTI	See Chapter 5 for DTI dosing insights
Tirofiban	Of the parenteral GP IIb/IIIa inhibitors, tirofiban has a shorter duration of effect and complete binding to the PG IIB/IIIa receptor
	Regimen: stop DTI if being infused prior to cannulation; initiate tirofiban (bolus 10 mcg/kg followed by a continuous infusion of 0.15 mcg/kg/min) 10 min prior to cannulation for cardiopulmonary bypass and prior to starting heparin; initiate UFH at 400 units/kg targeting an ACT of 480 seconds; bolus UFH as necessary to maintain ACT of 480 nsec; stop tirofiban infusion 1 hr before conclusion of cardiopulmonary bypass; reverse UFH with protamine as necessary; begin thromboprophylaxis with DTI targeting a aPTT of 40–60 sec or 1.5–2.5 times control[24]
Epoprostenol	Prior to starting heparin, initiate infusion at 5 ng/kg/min, increasing as tolerated until target of 30 ng/kg/min is reached; standard heparin during surgery; norepinephrine may need to be used to manage hypotension; delay heparinization as long as possible (just prior to aortic canalization)

REFERENCES

*Key articles

1. Warkentin TE, Kelton JG. Temporal aspects of heparin-induced thrombocytopenia. *N Engl J Med.* 2001;344(17):1286–1292.

2. **Warkentin TE. Heparin-induced thrombocytopenia: pathogenesis and management.** *Br J Haematol.* **2003;121(4):535–555.**

3. **Warkentin TE, Greinacher A, eds.** *Heparin-Induced Thrombocytopenia.* **4th ed. New York, NY: Informa Healthcare USA Inc; 2008.**

4. **Warkentin TE, Greinacher A, Koster A, et al. Treatment and prevention of heparin-induced thrombocytopenia. American College of Chest Physicians Evidence-Based Clinical Practice Guidelines (8th ed.).** *Chest.* **2008;133:340S–380S.**

5. **Greinacher A, Warkentin TE. Recognition, treatment, and prevention of heparin-induced thrombocytopenia: review and update.** *Thromb Res.* **2006;118:165–176.**

6. Arepally GM, Ortel TL. Clinical practice. Heparin-induced thrombocytopenia. *N Engl J Med.* 2006;355:809–817.

7. Chong BH, Chong JH. Heparin-induced thrombocytopenia. *Expert Rev Cardiovasc Ther.* 2004;2:547–559.

8. Warkentin TE. Laboratory testing for heparin-induced thrombocytopenia. *J Thromb Thrombolysis.* 2001;10(Suppl 1):35–45.

* **9. Warkentin TE. New approaches to the diagnosis of heparin-induced thrombocytopenia. *Chest.* 2005;127(2 Suppl):35S–45S.**

* **10. Dager WE, Dougherty JA, Nguyen PH, et al. Heparin-induced thrombocytopenia: a review of treatment options and special considerations. *Pharmacotherapy.* 2007;27:564–587.**

11. Huhle G, Hoffmann U, Hoffmann I, et al. A new therapeutic option by subcutaneous recombinant hirudin in patients with heparin-induced thrombocytopenia type II: a pilot study. *Thromb Res.* 2000;99:325–334.

12. Greinacher A, Volpel H, Janssens U, et al. Recombinant hirudin (lepirudin) provides safe and effective anticoagulation in patients with heparin-induced thrombocytopenia: a prospective study. *Circulation.* 1999;99:73–80.

13. Greinacher A, Janssens U, Berg G, et al. Lepirudin (recombinant hirudin) for parenteral anticoagulation in patients with heparin-induced thrombocytopenia. Heparin-Associated Thrombocytopenia Study (HAT) investigators. *Circulation.* 1999;100:587–593.

14. Lubenow N, Eicher P, Lietz T, et al. HIT Investigators group. Lepirudin in patients with heparin-induced thrombocytopenia—results of the third prospective study (HAT-3) and a combined analysis of HAT-1, HAT-2, and HAT-3. *J Thromb Haemost.* 2005;3:2428–2436.

15. Lubenow N, Eichler P, Leitz T, et al. Lepirudin for prophylaxis of thrombosis in patients with acute isolated heparin-induced thrombocytopenia: an analysis of three prospective studies. *Blood.* 2004;104:3072–3077.

16. Lewis BE, Wallis DE, Berkowitz SD, et al. Argatroban anticoagulant therapy in patients with heparin-induced thrombocytopenia. *Circulation.* 2001;103:1838–1843.

17. Warkentin TE. Management of heparin-induced thrombocytopenia: a critical comparison of lepirudin and argatroban. *Thromb Res.* 2003;110:73–82.

18. Magnani HN, Gallus A. Heparin-induced thrombocytopenia (HIT). A report of 1478 clinical outcomes of patients treated with danaparoid (Orgaran) form 1982 to mid-2004. *Thromb Haemost.* 2006;95:967–981.

19. Grouzi E, Kyriakou E, Panagou I, et al. Fondaparinux for the treatment of acute heparin-induced thrombocytopenia: a single center experience. *Clin Appl Thromb Hemost.* 2009 Oct 13. [Epub ahead of print]

20. Arpino PA, Demirjian Z, Van Cott EM. Use of the chromogenic factor X assay to predict the international normalized ratio in patients transitioning from argatroban to warfarin. *Pharmacotherapy*. 2005;25:157–164.

21. Gosselin RC, Dager WE, King JH, et al. Effect of direct thrombin-inhibitors: bivalirudin, lepirudin and argatroban, on prothrombin time and INR measurements. *Am J Clin Path*. 2004;121:593–599.

22. Risch L, Fisher JE, Herklotz R, et al. Heparin-induced thrombocytopenia in paediatrics: clinical characteristics, therapy and outcomes. *Intensive Care Med*. 2004;30:1615–1624.

23. Greinacher A. The use of direct thrombin inhibitors in cardiovascular surgery in patients with heparin-induced thrombocytopenia. *Semin Thromb Hemost*. 2004;30:315–327.

24. Koster A, Meyer O, Fisher T, et al. One-year experience with the platelet glycoprotein IIb/IIIa antagonist tirofiban and heparin during cardiopulmonary bypass in patients with heparin-induced thrombocytopenia type II. *J Thorac Cardiovasc Surg*. 2001;122:1254–1255.

Pregnancy

16

Nancy L. Shapiro

INTRODUCTION[1-10]

Pregnancy is considered an acquired hypercoagulable state due to increased concentrations of several clotting factors, increased fibrinogen, and reductions in the natural anticoagulants free protein S and antithrombin. The increase in hypercoagulability during pregnancy predisposes the mother to deep vein thrombosis (DVT), pulmonary embolism (PE), and the fetus to gestational complications of recurrent pregnancy loss, intrauterine growth restriction, preeclampsia, and placental abruption. These complications affect up to 15% of pregnancies, and are a major cause of fetal morbidity and mortality. The risk of venous thromboembolism (VTE) composed of DVT and PE, is 2- to 5-fold higher in pregnancy compared to nonpregnant women of child-bearing age. The incidence of VTE ranges between 0.5 to 2 women per 1,000 pregnancies. Most symptomatic cases are DVT, with two thirds of cases occurring antepartum, and half of these events occurring before the third trimester. PE is the leading cause of mortality in pregnant women but occurs more often in the postpartum period than during pregnancy. In the postpartum period, the risk of VTE has been estimated to be increased 20-fold. VTE accounts for 1.1 deaths per 100,000 deliveries or 10% of all maternal deaths. Management of anticoagulation in pregnant patients with mechanical heart valves remains an area of controversy.

USE OF ANTICOAGULANTS DURING PREGNANCY

Table 16-1: Indications for Anticoagulation During Pregnancy

Prevention of thrombosis during pregnancy
Prophylaxis against VTE
Prophylaxis against arterial thrombosis
Stroke prevention in patients with mechanical heart valves
Stroke prevention in atrial fibrillation
Treatment of thrombosis during pregnancy
Treatment of VTE during pregnancy
Treatment of arterial events during pregnancy
Prevention of pregnancy loss

Safety of anticoagulants during pregnancy

Table 16-2: Safety to the Fetus[11–13]

Drug	Supporting Evidence
UFH	Does not cross placenta; FDA Category C
LMWH (dalteparin, enoxaparin, tinzaparin)	Do not cross placenta; FDA Category B
Aspirin	FDA category D; crosses placenta
	First trimester: safety remains uncertain, there is no clear evidence of harm to the fetus, and, if fetal anomalies are caused by early aspirin exposure, they are very rare; clinicians should offer first-trimester patients aspirin if the indication for aspirin is clear and there is no satisfactory alternative agent
	Second and third trimester: low-dose (50–150 mg/day) aspirin therapy given to women at risk for preeclampsia is safe for the mother and fetus

(continued)

Table 16-2: (Continued)

Drug	Supporting Evidence
Clopidogrel	FDA category B; unknown if crosses the placenta
Prasugrel	FDA category B; unknown if crosses the placenta
Warfarin	FDA category X; crosses placenta
	Any time: risk of fetal hemorrhage, particularly when given close to time of delivery
	Weeks 6–12 of pregnancy: nasal hypoplasia, stippled epiphyses, CNS abnormalities have been reported
	2nd and 3rd trimesters: CNS and neurodevelopmental abnormalities have been reported, including mental retardation and blindness
Danaparoid[a]	FDA category B
	No demonstrable fetal toxicity, low quality of evidence
DTIs (argatroban, bivalirudin, lepirudin)	FDA category B
	Insufficient data to evaluate its safety
	Limit to those with severe allergic reactions to heparin (including HIT) who cannot receive danaparoid
Fondaparinux	FDA category B
	Anti-Factor Xa activity (at approximately $\frac{1}{10}$ the concentration of maternal plasma) has been found in the umbilical cord plasma in newborns treated with fondaparinux
	Clinicians should avoid the use of fondaparinux during pregnancy whenever possible and reserve its use for those pregnant women with HIT or a history of HIT who cannot receive danaparoid

(continued)

Table 16-2: (Continued)

Drug	Supporting Evidence
Rivaroxaban[a]	Rivaroxaban crosses the placenta; in animal data it has shown increased risk of hemorrhagic complications, reproductive toxicity, including postimplantation loss, retarded/progressed ossification, hepatic changes, placental changes, and reduced viability of offspring. It is contraindicated during pregnancy
Dabigatran	FDA Category C
	In animal data, decreased implantations and an increase in preimplantation loss, decrease in fetal body weight and fetal malformations have been seen; women of child-bearing potential should avoid pregnancy during treatment with dabigatran etexilate, and should not use during pregnancy unless clearly necessary
Apixaban[a]	Limited data available; likely not safe in pregnancy

[a]Not available in the US market at this time.

Table 16-3: FDA Pregnancy Category Definitions

Category	Definition
Category A	Controlled studies in women fail to demonstrate a risk to the fetus in the first trimester and there is no evidence of a risk in later trimesters
Category B	Animal reproduction studies have failed to demonstrate a risk to the fetus and there are no adequate and well-controlled studies in pregnant women
	or
	Animal studies have shown an adverse effect, but adequate and well-controlled studies in pregnant women have failed to demonstrate a risk to the fetus in any trimester
Category C	Animal reproduction studies have shown an adverse effect on the fetus and there are no adequate and well-controlled studies in humans, but potential benefits may warrant use of the drug in pregnant women despite potential risks

(*continued*)

Table 16-3: (Continued)

Category	Definition
Category D	There is positive evidence of human fetal risk based on adverse reaction data from investigational or marketing experience or studies in humans, but potential benefits may warrant use of the drug in pregnant women despite potential risks
Category X	Studies in animals or humans have demonstrated fetal abnormalities and/or there is positive evidence of human fetal risk based on adverse reaction data from investigational or marketing experience, and the risks involved in use of the drug in pregnant women clearly outweigh potential benefits

Clinical Pearl

- Multidose vials of unfractionated heparin (UFH) and low molecular weight heparin (LMWH) contain benzyl alcohol, which has been reported to cause cases of fetal gasping syndrome in neonates. Use of preservative-free vials or single-dose syringes is advised.

Table 16-4: Maternal Safety[1–2,14]

Adverse Effect	Supporting Evidence
Bleeding	- Reported risk of major bleeding with therapeutic anticoagulants is comparable in pregnant and nonpregnant women
	- Primary postpartum hemorrhage (PPH) (blood loss greater than 500 mL within 24 hr of delivery) is seen in up to 5% of women receiving anticoagulant therapy; the frequency of this complication is dependant on a number of factors such as maternal age, parity, and mode of delivery; the rate of PPH does not appear to be appreciably higher in women receiving antepartum LMWH therapy than in other women when these are taken into account
	- Injection-site bruising is common throughout pregnancy and can vary by location and injection technique

(continued)

Table 16-4: (Continued)

Adverse Effect	Supporting Evidence

Bone	• Prolonged UFH use during pregnancy may reduce bone mineral density and lead to the development of symptomatic vertebral fractures in up to 2% of women
	
	   – Less bone loss seen with LMWH
	
	   – Supplemental calcium may be recommended for some

HIT	• Documented HIT in pregnancy is rare, at less than 1% of women – In the setting of serologically confirmed HIT in pregnancy, substitute UFH or LMWH for a DTI
Skin	• Skin rashes can be seen in up to 2% of pregnant women receiving LMWH and are usually managed with a change in brand; if there is skin necrosis around the injection sites, HIT-associated skin necrosis should be excluded

Table 16-5: Safety of Anticoagulants During Breast-feeding[11,15]

Anticoagulant	Potential Risks During Breast-feeding
Warfarin	Not secreted in breast milk and considered safe for nursing mothers Thomson Lactation Rating: infant risk is minimal AAP Rating: maternal medication usually compatible with breast-feeding ACCP Grade 1A for breast-feeding
UFH	Not secreted in breast milk and considered safe for nursing mothers Thomson Lactation Rating: infant risk is minimal AAP Rating: maternal medication usually compatible with breast-feeding ACCP Grade 1A for breast-feeding

(continued)

Table 16-5: (Continued)

Anticoagulant	Potential Risks During Breast-feeding
Danaparoid[a]	It is unknown if it passes into breast milk and the safety cannot be established
	Its high molecular weight make it unlikely to cause clinically significant effects on the nursing infant
	Thomson Lactation Rating: infant risk cannot be ruled out
	ACCP Grade 2C for breast-feeding
Dalteparin	Small amounts have been found in breast milk
	Thomson Lactation Rating: infant risk cannot be ruled out
	ACCP Grade 2C for breast-feeding
Enoxaparin	Unlikely that it passes into breast milk
	Thomson Lactation Rating: infant risk cannot be ruled out
	ACCP Grade 2C for breast-feeding
Tinzaparin	Very low levels have been detected in rat breast milk
	Thomson Lactation Rating: infant risk cannot be ruled out
	ACCP Grade 2C for breast-feeding
Fondaparinux	Animal data has detected it in milk of lactating rats
	Thomson Lactation Rating: infant risk cannot be ruled out
	ACCP Grade 2C that alternative anticoagulants are recommended other than pentasaccharides
	ACCP recommends limiting use to patients with HIT or those who cannot take danaparoid
DTIs argatroban, bivalirudin, and lepirudin	Available data is limited, weigh the potential risks and benefits before prescribing
	Thomson Lactation Rating: infant risk cannot be ruled out
	Argatroban: rat studies have shown the presence in breast milk
	Danaparoid and r-hirudin: ACCP Grade 2C for breast-feeding
	ACCP recommends limiting DTIs to patients with HIT or those who cannot take danaparoid

(continued)

Table 16-5: (Continued)

Anticoagulant	Potential Risks During Breast-feeding
Aspirin	Increased association between salicylates and Reye's syndrome
	Some available data have suggested that low intermittent doses can be used safely in breast-feeding
	Thomson Lactation Rating: infant risk cannot be ruled out
	AAP Rating: associated with significant effects on some nursing infants and should be given to nursing mothers with caution
	WHO Rating: avoid breast-feeding; enters breast milk; may pose risk to infant long term
Clopidogrel	Available data is limited, weigh the potential risks and benefits before prescribing
	Due to its molecular weight, it is theoretically possible that it is excreted in breast milk
	Animal data in rats showed that it enters breast milk
	Thomson Lactation Rating: infant risk cannot be ruled out
Prasugrel	Available data is limited; weigh the potential risks and benefits before prescribing
	Animal data in rats showed that its metabolites enter breast milk
	Thomson Lactation Rating: infant risk cannot be ruled out
Apixaban[a]	There are no clinical data of the effect on infants during breast-feeding
	Lactation should be discontinued during treatment
Dabigatran	There are no clinical data of the effect on infants during breast-feeding
	Lactation should be discontinued during treatment
Rivaroxaban[a]	Animal studies indicate it is secreted into milk; it is contraindicated during breast-feeding

[a]Not available in the US market at this time.

Preconception planning[1,2,16]

- Evaluation of a woman who may require anticoagulation during pregnancy should occur before conception, ideally, or at least early in pregnancy

- Patients with a high risk of maternal mortality due to thrombosis (mechanical heart valves, chronic thromboembolic pulmonary hypertension, history of recurrent thrombosis while fully anticoagulated, history of myocardial infarction) may be advised against pregnancy

- Patients already on anticoagulation prior to pregnancy will likely need to continue; counsel regarding the switch from a coumarin to a LMWH preconception

- Either LMWH (or UFH) can be substituted for warfarin before conception is attempted or frequent pregnancy tests undertaken and warfarin replaced once a positive test is achieved

Table 16-6: UFH and LMWH Regimens and Associated Doses as Defined by ACCP[15]

Regimen	Associated Doses
Prophylactic UFH	UFH 5,000 units SC q 12 hr
Intermediate-dose UFH	UFH SC q 12 hr in doses adjusted to target an anti-Factor Xa level of 0.1–0.3 units/mL
Adjusted-dose UFH	UFH SC q 12 hr in doses adjusted to target a midinterval aPTT into the therapeutic range
Prophylactic LMWH	Dalteparin 5,000 units SC q 24 hr
	Tinzaparin 4,500 units SC q 24 hr
	Enoxaparin 40 mg SC q 24 hr
	(At extremes of body weight modification of dose may be required)
Intermediate-dose LMWH	Dalteparin 5,000 Units SC q 12 hr
	Enoxaparin 40 mg SC q 12 hr

(*continued*)

Table 16-6: (Continued)

Regimen	Associated Doses
Adjusted-dose LMWH	Weight-adjusted, full treatment doses of LMWH, given once or twice daily
	Dalteparin 200 units/kg daily
	Tinzaparin 175 units/kg daily
	Dalteparin 100 units/kg q 12 hr
	Enoxaparin 1 mg/kg q 12 hr
Postpartum anticoagulants	Vitamin K antagonists for 4–6 weeks with a target INR of 2.0–3.0, with initial UFH
	Or
	LMWH overlap until the INR is ≥2.0, or prophylactic LMWH for 4–6 weeks

Source: reprinted with permission from reference 6.

PREVENTION OF THROMBOSIS DURING PREGNANCY

Pregnancy as a risk factor for VTE[1,2,17]

- Hypercoagulability
  - Coagulation is not fully corrected until 6 weeks postpartum.
  - True diagnosis of deficiencies (protein C, S, antithrombin) should wait until at least 6 weeks postpartum and off vitamin K antagonists (VKAs) for at least 2 weeks.
- Venous stasis
  - >30% reduction in flow by 15 week; >60% reduction by 36 weeks.
  - 90% of DVTs in left leg due to compression of left iliac vein by the right iliac artery where they cross.
- Vascular damage
  - Trauma to pelvic veins during delivery.
  - Pelvic vein thromboses, rare outside of pregnancy or pelvic surgery, account for approximately 10% of DVT during pregnancy and the postpartum period.

Table 16-7: Risk Factors for VTE in Pregnancy[1,2,18–20]

Age >35

Cesarean section

Weight >80 kg

Family history of thrombosis

Previous thrombosis

Thrombophilia

Smoking

Heart disease

Hypertension

Sickle cell disease

Anemia

Diabetes

Table 16-8: Complications of Pregnancy and Delivery Associated with Increased Risk of VTE

Multiple gestation

Immobility

In vitro fertilization

Cesarean section

Antepartum or postpartum hemorrhage

Infection

Preeclampsia

Fluid and electrolyte imbalance

Transfusion

Table 16-9: Risk of VTE in Pregnant Women with Thrombophilia[21]

Thrombophilia	OR (95% CI)
FVL homozygote	34.40 (9.86, 120.05)
Prothrombin G20210A homozygote	26.36 (1.24, 559.29)
FVL heterozygote	8.32 (5.44, 12.70)
Prothrombin G20210A heterozygote	6.80 (2.46, 18.77)
Protein C deficiency	4.76 (2.15, 10.57)
Antithrombin deficiency	4.69 (1.30, 16.96)
Protein S deficiency	3.19 (1.48, 6.88)
MTHFR homozygote	0.74 (0.22, 2.48)

Prevention of VTE during pregnancy

Table 16-10: When Prophylactic Therapy Should Be Utilized Thrombophilia[15,a]

No history of VTE	Recommendations
Thrombophilia with no prior VTE	Perform an individualized risk assessment rather than use routine pharmacologic antepartum prophylaxis (ACCP Grade 1C)
No history of VTE but have antithrombin deficiency	Antepartum and postpartum prophylaxis (ACCP Grade 2C)
All other pregnant women with thrombophilia and no prior VTE	Antepartum clinical surveillance or prophylactic LMWH or UFH, plus postpartum anticoagulants (ACCP Grade 2C)
Single episode of VTE	
Thrombophilia with single prior VTE, not receiving long-term anticoagulants	Antepartum prophylactic or intermediate dose LMWH or prophylactic or intermediate-dose UFH or clinical surveillance throughout pregnancy, plus postpartum anticoagulants, rather than routine care or adjusted-dose anticoagulation (ACCP Grade 1C)

(*continued*)

Table 16-10: (Continued)

No history of VTE	Recommendations
"Higher risk" thrombophilias (e.g., AT deficiency, APLAs, compound heterozygosity for prothrombin G20210A variant and factor V Leiden or homozygosity for these conditions) and a single prior episode of VTE, not receiving long-term anticoagulants	Antepartum prophylactic or intermediate-dose LMWH or prophylactic or intermediate-dose UFH, rather than clinical surveillance, plus postpartum prophylaxis (ACCP Grade 2C)

Source: reprinted with permission from reference 15.

Refer to Table 16-6 for corresponding dosing regimens.

Table 16-11: Previous VTE[15,a]

ACCP Recommendations	
Single episode of VTE	
Associated with a transient risk factor that is no longer present and no thrombophilia	Clinical surveillance antepartum and anticoagulant prophylaxis postpartum (ACCP Grade 1C)
If the transient risk factor associated with a previous VTE event is pregnancy- or estrogen-related	Antepartum clinical surveillance or prophylaxis (prophylactic LMWH/UFH or intermediate-dose LMWH/UFH) plus postpartum prophylaxis, rather than routine care (ACCP Grade 2C)
A single idiopathic episode of VTE but without thrombophilia and who are not receiving long-term anticoagulants	Prophylactic LMWH/UFH or intermediate-dose LMWH/UFH or clinical surveillance throughout pregnancy plus postpartum anticoagulants rather than routine care or adjusted dose anticoagulation (ACCP Grade 1C)
Multiple episodes of VTE	
Not receiving long-term anticoagulants	Antepartum prophylactic, intermediate-dose, or adjusted-dose LMWH or prophylactic, intermediate or adjusted-dose UFH followed by postpartum anticoagulants rather than clinical surveillance (ACCP Grade 2C)

(continued)

Table 16-11: (Continued)

ACCP Recommendations	
Multiple episodes of VTE	
Receiving long-term anticoagulants for prior VTE	Adjusted-dose LMWH or UFH, 75% of adjusted-dose LMWH, or intermediate-dose
	LMWH throughout pregnancy, followed by resumption of long-term anticoagulants postpartum (ACCP Grade 1C)
All pregnant women with previous DVT	Graduated elastic compression stockings both antepartum and postpartum (ACCP Grade 2C)

Source: reprinted with permission from reference 15.

aRefer to Table 16-6 for corresponding dosing regimens.

Clinical Pearl

- Multiple anticoagulants may be acceptable for use during pregnancy and the postpartum period. Drug decision depends on efficacy, safety to the mother and the fetus, including bleeding risk

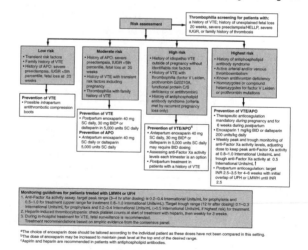

Figure 16-1: Risk Assessment and Prevention of VTE and Adverse Pregnancy Outcomes (APO) in Pregnant Patient[16]

and risk during lactation, but also includes patient preferences. Strategies may differ in the US and Europe.

Clinical Pearls

For dosing and monitoring of LMWH/UFH for VTE prophylaxis:

- LMWH recommended over UFH for the prevention and treatment of VTE (ACCP Grade 2C)

- Higher doses of LMWH may be needed to achieve target prophylactic anti-Factor Xa levels, especially in obese patients (i.e., enoxaparin 40 mg BID, dalteparin 5,000 units BID).

  - Monitoring of anti-Factor Xa levels in this setting is controversial; if performed, checking every 1–3 months is reasonable.

  - Target anti-Factor Xa levels of 0.1–0.3 International Units/mL have been recommended by some, while others recommend 0.2–0.6 International Units/mL. No comparative studies have been conducted.

- Monitoring aPTT levels is not generally recommended for prophylactic dosing of UFH.

Table 16-12: ACCP Considerations of Cesarean Section[15]

With at least one risk factor in addition to pregnancy	Consider prophylactic LMWH or UFH or GCS or IPC while in hospital following delivery (ACCP Grade 2C)
If multiple additional risk factors	Combine pharmacologic prophylaxis with GCS and/or IPC (ACCP Grade 2C)
If risk factors continue following delivery	Consider treatment for 4–6 weeks after delivery following hospital discharge (ACCP Grade 2C)

Source: reprinted with permission from reference 15.

Prevention of arterial events during pregnancy

Table 16-13: Mechanical Heart Valves During Pregnancy[15]

Anticoagulation Options for Mechanical Heart Valves	Recommendations
Adjusted dose BID LMWH throughout pregnancy (Grade 1C)	Adjust doses to achieve manufacturer's peak anti-Factor Xa LMWH 4 hr after SC injection (ACCP Grade 2C)
Adjusted-dose UFH throughout pregnancy (Grade 1C)	Subcutaneously q 12 hr in doses adjusted to keep the mid-interval aPTT at least twice control or attain an anti-Factor Xa heparin level of 0.35–0.70 units/mL
UFH or LMWH (as above) until the thirteenth week (Grade 1C)	After the 13th week, transition to warfarin until close to delivery when UFH or LMWH is resumed
Patients at very high risk of TE with concerns about the efficacy and safety of UFH or LMWH as dosed above (e.g., older-generation prosthesis in the mitral position, history of TE, or atrial fibrillation)	VKAs throughout pregnancy (target INR 3, range 2.5–3.5) with replacement by UFH or LMWH (as above) close to delivery, rather than one of the regimens above, after a thorough discussion of the potential risks and benefits of this approach (ACCP Grade 2C) A lower INR goal of 2.5 (range 2–3) can be used for patients with bileaflet aortic valves without AF or left ventricular dysfunction
For pregnant women with prosthetic valves at high risk of thromboembolism	Recommend the addition of low-dose aspirin, 75–100 mg/day (ACCP Grade 2C)

Source: reprinted with permission from reference 15.

Clinical Pearls

For dosing and monitoring of UFH and LMWH for mechanical heart valves:

- In pregnancy, particularly in the third trimester, an increase in heparin-binding proteins combined with elevated Factor VIII levels can attenuate the aPTT response leading to heparin resistance; consider plasma heparin levels if there is difficulty achieving a therapeutic aPTT response despite infusing 30,000–35,000 units IV per 24 hours.

- For SC UFH dosing to achieve therapeutic aPTT: initiate doses starting at 18 units X (wt in kg) x 24 hr x 1.2, divided q 12 hr (a correction factor of 1.2 can be applied to account for the 10% to 20% loss of bioavailability with SC absorption—see Chapter 3 for more information on dose adjustments).

    - For example, an 80-kg patient would start at 20,000 units SC q 12 hr.

    - Check aPTT levels 6 hours after dose is given.

    - Use 20,000 units/mL single dose, preservative-free heparin vials.

    - Increase or decrease dose by 2,000–5,000 units with followup aPTT levels every 3 days.

- The range for peak anti-Factor Xa levels in women with mechanical heart valves using LMWH is controversial. Current ACCP recommendations do not include a target anti-Factor Xa level. Some clinicians prefer to target higher peak anti-Factor Xa levels above 1.0 International Units/mL or 12-hour trough levels greater than 0.5 International Units/mL. Clinical judgment should include the type and location of the valve, previous history of TE, and other risk factors for TE and bleeding.

Atrial fibrillation during pregnancy[22]

- Current recommendations from the ACC/AHA/ESC 2006 Guidelines for atrial fibrillation:

    - Prevention against thromboembolism is recommended throughout pregnancy except for those patients with lone AF/low risk for embolism. Treatment (anticoagulant or aspirin) should be chosen based on the stage of pregnancy (Level of Evidence: C).

    - Adjusted dose UFH (Level B) or LMWH (Level C) are preferred for patients needing full anticoagulation, with warfarin considered an option during the second trimester (Level C).

- ACCP recommendations for atrial fibrillation are mentioned in the previous section.

TREATMENT OF THROMBOSIS DURING PREGNANCY

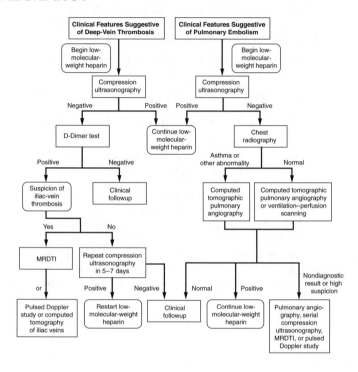

Figure 16-2: Diagnosis of VTE During Pregnancy[23]

Clinical Pearls

For VTE diagnosis:

- Compression ultrasound is the test of choice in women with suspected DVT but is less accurate for isolated calf and iliac vein thrombosis.

- Magnetic resonance direct thrombus imaging is useful for diagnosis of iliac vein thrombosis and causes no radiation exposure.

- Computed tomographic (CT scans) cause low radiation exposure to fetus but exposes maternal breast tissue to radiation.

- V/Q scans have a low amount of radiation exposure.

- Negative D-dimer is useful for ruling out DVT in combination with a negative compression ultrasound, but there may be false elevations during pregnancy.

Treatment of VTE during pregnancy[15]

- Initiate treatment prior to objective confirmation if no contraindication to anticoagulation.

- Initiate therapy with either adjusted dose SC LMWH or adjusted dose UFH (IV bolus, with continuous infusion to maintain aPTT within the therapeutic range or SC therapy adjusted to maintain the aPTT 6 hours after injection into the therapeutic aPTT range for at least 5 days [ACCP Grade 1A]).

Dosing and monitoring of UFH[15,24–27]

If the woman is potentially unstable (large PE with hypoxia), presents with extensive iliofemoral disease and extreme venous congestion, or has significant renal impairment (e.g., a creatinine clearance of less than 30 mL/min), initial inpatient intravenous adjusted-dose UFH should be considered.

Dosing and monitoring of LMWH[15,24–27]

- Based on the safety data for both mother and fetus, LMWH is the preferred drug for the treatment of VTE during pregnancy.
  - Better bioavailability, longer plasma-half-life, more predictable dose response, less monitoring, and improved safety profile with respect to osteoporosis and thrombocytopenia compared to UFH
- Alterations in volume of distribution
  - Elevated throughout pregnancy and declines postpartum
- Alterations in renal clearance
  - More rapid during early pregnancy, decreases as pregnancy progresses
- Some clinicians prefer to use twice daily LMWH during pregnancy because of alterations in renal clearance. No comparative studies have been conducted.

Monitoring strategies

- Controversy exists about the need for monitoring LMWH with anti-Factor Xa levels during pregnancy. Currently acceptable strategies include the following:
  - Initial dosing based on weight with no further dose adjustment
  - Dose adjustment guided by weight changes throughout pregnancy
  - Dose adjustment guided by manufacturer recommended peak anti-Factor Xa levels
    - Monthly monitoring throughout pregnancy is reasonable.
    - For therapeutic anticoagulation for VTE, peak anti-Factor Xa levels measured 4 hours postdose to reach 0.6–1.0 units/mL if a twice-daily regimen is used; slightly higher if a once-daily regimen is chosen.
    - Peak anti-Factor Xa levels greater than 1.0 units/mL or 12-hour trough levels greater than 0.5 units/mL may be targeted for patients with mechanical heart valves.

Duration of therapy[15]

- Treatment of VTE should be continued throughout pregnancy (ACCP Grade 1B) and continued until at least 6 weeks postpartum (ACCP Grade 2C).
- In general, at least 6 months of treatment in necessary for most patients.

PREVENTION OF PREGNANCY LOSS

Table 16-14: Risk Categories and Dosing Strategies[15,a]

Recurrent early pregnancy loss (three or more miscarriages) or unexplained late pregnancy loss	Recommend screening for APLAs (ACCP Grade 1A)
Women with severe or recurrent preeclampsia or IUGR	Suggest screening for APLAs (ACCP Grade 2C)
APLA and 3 or more pregnancy losses or late pregnancy loss and no history of venous or arterial thrombosis	Antepartum prophylactic or intermediate-dose UFH or prophylactic LMWH combined with aspirin (ACCP Grade 1B)

(continued)

Table 16-14: (Continued)

High risk for preeclampsia	Low-dose aspirin throughout pregnancy (ACCP Grade 1B)
History of preeclampsia	UFH and LMWH should not be used as prophylaxis in subsequent pregnancies (ACCP Grade 2C)

Source: reprinted with permission from reference 15.

ᵃRefer to Table 16-6 for corresponding dosing regimens.

USE OF ANTICOAGULANTS DURING LABOR AND DELIVERY[1,2,16,28]

Table 16-15: Anticoagulants During Labor and Delivery

Treatment doses of SC UFH	Prolonged aPTT can be seen more than 24 hr after the last q 12 hr dose; consider induction of labor with planned discontinuation of heparin prior to delivery; aPTT monitoring and/or administration of protamine sulfate around the time of delivery may be necessary
	• Protamine has been reported to cause neonatal respiratory depression
	• Neuraxial anesthesia should not be used in anticoagulated women
Treatment doses of LMWH	Consider induction of labor, with discontinuation of LMWH 24–36 hr prior to elective induction of labor or cesarean section
	• If induction of labor is not planned, caution patients to withhold further LMWH doses at the onset of regular contractions
	• Neuraxial anesthesia should not be used in anticoagulated women (i.e., within 24 hr of last dose of treatment-dose LMWH)

(*continued*)

Table 16-15: (Continued)

Prophylactic doses of UFH or LMWH	Stop treatment 12–24 hr before induction or cesarean delivery
	• Wait at least 10–12 hr after the last dose of prophylactic dose LMWH before placement of epidural catheter or spinal anesthesia
	• Prophylactic doses of UFH 5,000 units SC q 12 hr have no contraindications to neuraxial anesthesia; safety and recommendations with higher doses of UFH are uncertain; a delay of 12 hr may be warranted in this situation
Converting from LMWH to IV UFH prior to delivery	Wait 10–11 hr after the last dose of LMWH before initiating IV UFH
New VTE	In patients with new VTE within 4 weeks of delivery, consider hospital admission with planned induction of therapy with IV UFH, and/or placement of temporary IVC filter
Postpartum anticoagulants	May be started 12–24 hr after delivery as long as there are no bleeding concerns; consider IV UFH in women at high risk of bleeding, with LMWH reasonable for most women
	• Restart warfarin when hemostasis has occurred, bridging with UFH or LMWH until INR therapeutic
Postpartum anticoagulants in patients receiving epidural catheters	For patients receiving twice daily LMWH: administer the first dose no sooner than 24 hr postoperatively, and with adequate hemostasis in place; remove indwelling catheters prior to the initiation of LMWH; for patients with continuous technique, the epidural may be kept in place overnight but must be removed before the first dose of LMWH; delay the first dose of LMWH for at least 2 hr after catheter removal
	For patients receiving once daily LMWH: administer the first dose 6–8 hr postoperatively; the second dose should occur no sooner than 24 hr after the first; indwelling catheters may be maintained; the removal of the catheter should occur no sooner than 10–12 hr after the last LMWH dose; further dosing should occur at least 2 hr after catheter removal; no additional hemostasis-altering medications should be given due to additive effects

Clinical Pearl

- For patients that have undergone a miscarriage, withholding anticoagulation until 12–24 hours after a dilation and curettage has been performed may be necessary to help minimize risk of postpartum hemorrhage.

REFERENCES

*Key articles

1. Chunilal SD, Bates SM. Venous thromboembolism in pregnancy: diagnosis, management and prevention. *Thromb Haemost.* 2009;101:428–438.

2. James AH. Venous thromboembolism in pregnancy. *Arterioscler Thromb Vasc Biol.* 2009;29:326–331.

3. Heit JA, Kobbervig CE, James AH, et al. Trends in the incidence of venous thromboembolism during pregnancy or postpartum: a 30-year population-based study. *Ann Intern Med.* 2005;143:697–706.

4. James AH, Jamison MG, Brancazio LR, et al. Venous thromboembolism during pregnancy and the postpartum period: incidence, risk factors, and mortality. *Am J Obstet Gynecol.* 2006;194:1311–1315.

5. James AH, Tapson VF, Goldhaber SZ. Thrombosis during pregnancy and the postpartum period. *Am J Obstet Gynecol.* 2005;193:216–219.

6. Gherman RB, Goodwin TM, Leung B, et al. Incidence, clinical characteristics, and timing of objectively diagnosed venous thromboembolism during pregnancy. *Obstet Gynecol.* 1999;94(5 Pt 1):730–734.

7. Simpson EL, Lawrenson RA, Nightingale AL, et al. Venous thromboembolism in pregnancy and the puerperium: incidence and additional risk factors from a London perinatal database. *BJOG.* 2001;108:56–60.

8. De Stefano V, Martinelli I, Rossi E, et al. The risk of recurrent venous thromboembolism in pregnancy and puerperium without antithrombotic prophylaxis. *Br J Haematol.* 2006;135:386–391.

9. Dilley A, Austin H, El-Jamil M, et al. Genetic factors associated with thrombosis in pregnancy in a United States population. *Am J Obstet Gynecol.* 2000;183:1271–1277.

10. Gerhardt A, Scharf RE, Beckmann MW, et al. Prothrombin and factor V mutations in women with a history of thrombosis during pregnancy and the puerperium. *N Engl J Med.* 2000;342:374–380.

11. Micromedex® Healthcare Series [Internet database]. Greenwood Village, CO: Thomson Healthcare; updated periodically.

12. Pradaxa [summary of product characteristics—EU]. Rhein, Germany: Boerhinger Ingelheim GmbH; 2009.

13. Xarelto [summary of product characteristics—EU]. Berlin, Germany: Bayer Schering Pharma AG; 2009.

14. Kominiarek MA, Angelopoulos SM, Shapiro NL, et al. Low-molecular-weight heparin in pregnancy: peripartum bleeding complications. *J Perinatol.* 2007;27:329–334.

* **15. Bates SM, Greer IA, Pabinger I, et al. Venous thromboembolism, thrombophilia, antithrombotic therapy, and pregnancy: Evidence-Based Clinical Practice Guidelines American College of Chest Physicians.** *Chest.* **2008;133:844–886.**

* **16. Duhl AJ, Paidas MJ, Ural SH, et al. Antithrombotic therapy and pregnancy: consensus report and recommendations for prevention and treatment of venous thromboembolism and adverse pregnancy outcome.** *Am J Obstet Gynecol.* **2007;197:457.e1–457.e21.**

17. Bremme KA. Haemostatic changes in pregnancy. *Best Pract Res Clin Haematol.* 2003;16:153–168.

18. Lindqvist P, Dahlback B, Marsal K. Thrombotic risk during pregnancy: a population study. *Obstet Gynecol.* 1999;94:595–599.

19. Danilenko-Dixon DR, Heit JA, Silverstein MD, et al. Risk factors for deep vein thrombosis and pulmonary embolism during pregnancy or post partum: a population-based, case-control study. *Am J Obstet Gynecol.* 2001;184:104–110.

20. Anderson FA Jr, Spencer FA. Risk factors for venous thromboembolism. *Circulation.* 2003;107(23 Suppl 1):L9–16.

* **21. Robertson L, Wu O, Langhorne P, et al. Thrombophilia in pregnancy: a systematic review.** *Br J Haematol.* **2005;132:171–196.**

22. Fuster V, Rydén LE, Cannom DS, et al. ACC/AHA/ESC 2006 guidelines for the management of patients with atrial fibrillation: a report of the American College of Cardiology/American Heart Association Task Force on Practice Guidelines and the European Society of Cardiology Committee for Practice Guidelines (Writing Committee to Revise the 2001 Guidelines for the Management of Patients With Atrial Fibrillation). *Circulation.* 2006;114:e257–e354.

* **23. Marik PE and Plante LA. Venous thromboembolic disease and pregnancy.** *N Engl J Med.* **2008;359:2025–2033.**

24. Salas SP, Marshall G, Gutiérrez BL, et al. Time course of maternal plasma volume and hormonal changes in women with pre-eclampsia or fetal growth restriction. *Hypertension.* 2006;47:203–208.

25. Barbour L, Oja JL, Schultz LK. A prospective trial that demonstrates that dalteparin requirements increase in pregnancy to maintain therapeutic level of anticoagulation. *Am J Obstet Gynecol.* 2004;191:1024–1029.

26. Casele HL, Laifer SA, Woelker DA, et al. Changes in the pharmacokinetics of the low molecular weight heparin enoxaparin sodium during pregnancy. *Am J Obstet Gynecol.* 1999;181:1113–1117.

27. Chunilal SD, Young E, Johnston MA, et al. The aPTT response of pregnant plasma to unfractionated heparin. *Thromb Haemost.* 2002;87:92–97.

28. **Horlocker TT, Wedel DJ, Rowlingson JC, et al. Regional anesthesia in the patient receiving antithrombotic or thrombolytic therapy: American Society of Regional Anesthesia and Pain Medicine Evidence-Based Guidelines (3rd ed.). *Reg Anesth Pain Med.* 2010;35(1):64–101.**

SEVENTEEN

Chapter

Pediatrics

Kirsten H. Ohler

INTRODUCTION

Venous thromboembolism (VTE) is becoming an increasingly encountered disease state in pediatric patients in part due to advances in pediatric critical care medicine as well as improvements in diagnostic modalities. Although many recommendations regarding the management of this population are adapted from adult data, there are important differences between children with thromboembolic events and their adult counterparts that should be taken into consideration and warrant well-designed pediatric clinical trials.

INCIDENCE OF THROMBOSIS IN PEDIATRIC PATIENTS[1-5]

- Incidence of thromboembolic events is generally lower than in adults.
  - Overall incidence ranges from 0.07–0.14 per 10,000 children.
  - >90% of pediatric patients with VTE have at least one risk factor.
  - >60% of pediatric patients with VTE have two or more risk factors.
- Incidence related to risk factors
  - Age: highest incidence in infants <1 year old and adolescents >14 years old
  - Gender: teenage females have twice the rates of males.
  - Disease state
    - Central venous catheter—most common risk factor in pediatrics
      - Accounts for ~60% of VTE in children and 90% in neonates
      - Risk is higher with external catheters than indwelling ports.

- Cancer
  - Acute lymphoblastic leukemia (ALL) is the most common cancer type associated with TE in children.
  - Up to 93% of children with an underlying malignancy develop a VTE at the central venous catheter site.
- Trauma
  - 0.3% of children with severe trauma develop a VTE.
  - Severe spinal, thoracic, and abdominal injuries are associated with clinically significant VTE.
- Congenital heart disease
  - Risk of VTE is dependent on type of defect and surgical intervention performed.
- Incidence related to site of thrombosis
  - Thrombosis in an upper extremity is more common than in lower extremity.
  - Central nervous system—less common than upper and lower venous systems
    - Arterial ischemic events account for ~80% of pediatric strokes.
    - Cerebral sinovenous thrombosis, the second most common site, preferentially affects neonates; also children with ALL receiving asparaginase.
  - Renal vein thrombosis (RVT)—most commonly observed in neonates

DEVELOPMENTAL AND PHARMACOKINETIC DIFFERENCES AMONG PEDIATRIC POPULATIONS

Table 17-1: Definition of Age Groups

Pediatric	Birth–18 yr
Neonate	Birth–28 days
Infant	1–12 mo
Child	1–12 yr
Adolescent	12–18 yr

Table 17-2: Developmental Aspects of the Coagulation System[6]

	Pediatric Values Compared to Adults	**Age When Adult Values Are Achieved**
Liver function and development		
CYP2C9	Present within 1st week of life	3 mo
Vitamin K	Relative deficiency in newborns	
Coagulation factors		
• Maternal coagulation factors do not cross the placental barrier		
Vitamin K dependent clotting factors (II, VII, IX, X)	Decreased by ~50% in neonates	Increase during first 6 mo but remain 20% below adult values through childhood
Thrombin production	Delayed and decreased	Increase during first 6 mo but remain 20% below adult values through childhood
Antithrombin	Decreased by ~50% in neonates	6 mo
Protein C	Decreased by ~65% to 70% in neonates	Adolescence
Protein S	Decreased by ~65% to 70% in neonates	3 mo

Table 17-3: Recommendations for VTE Prophylaxis and Treatment in Pediatrics[5,a]

VTE Prophylaxis		
Indication	**Agent**	**Duration**
CVL for long-term home TPN	Warfarin (target INR 2–3)	Until catheter removal
AIS secondary to dissection or cardioembolism	LMWH or warfarin	6 weeks

(continued)

Table 17-3: (Continued)

VTE Prophylaxis		
Indication	**Agent**	**Duration**
AIS excluding SCD, dissection or cardioembolism related	Aspirin	At least 2 yr
Modified Blalock-Taussig shunt	Aspirin (1–5 mg/kg/day) or no post-op anticoagulation	Optimal duration unknown
Stage I Norwood procedure	Aspirin (1–5 mg/kg/day) or no post-op anticoagulation	Optimal duration unknown
Glenn shunt	Aspirin (1–5 mg/kg/day) or warfarin (target INR 2–3) or no post-op anticoagulation	Optimal duration unknown
Fontan procedure	Aspirin (1–5 mg/kg/day) or warfarin (target INR 2–3)	Optimal duration unknown
Cardiomyopathy	Warfarin (target INR 2–3)	Until resolved
PPH requiring medical therapy	Warfarin (target INR varies by center, 1.7–2.5 or 2–3)	Until resolved
Biological and mechanical prosthetic heart valves	Follow adult recommendations	Follow adult recommendations

[a]VTE prophylaxis is *not* routinely recommended in the following circumstances: (1) cancer and CVAD; (2) CVL; (3) hemodialysis catheter; and (4) neonates with an initial AIS.

Table 17-4: VTE Treatment[a]

Indication	**Agent**	**Duration**
Idiopathic VTE	Warfarin or LMWH	At least 6 mo[b]
VTE secondary to resolved risk factor	Warfarin or LMWH	At least 3 mo
VTE secondary to ongoing risk factor	Therapeutic or prophylactic anticoagulation	Until risk factor resolved
Recurrent idiopathic VTE	Warfarin	Indefinitely

(continued)

Table 17-4: (Continued)

Indication	Agent	Duration
CVL-related VTE with ongoing need for access	Therapeutic anticoagulation followed by prophylaxis with warfarin or LMWH	Therapeutic for 3 mo Prophylactic until CVL removed
Cancer and VTE	LMWH	At least 3 mo and until risk factors[c] resolved
Unilateral RVT without renal impairment or extension into the IVC	Observation for thrombus extension or LMWH	3 mo
Unilateral RVT extending into IVC without renal impairment	LMWH	3 mo
Bilateral RVT with any degree renal impairment	UFH and tPA thrombolysis[d] followed by UFH or LMWH	Until resolved

[a]Clinicians are referred to the American College of Chest Physicians practice guidelines for recommendations in other less common clinical scenarios.[5]

[b]Lifelong anticoagulation is not generally recommended as the known bleeding risk of long-term anticoagulation outweighs the unknown incidence of thrombosis recurrence in children without an identifiable risk factor.

[c]Risk factors include asparaginase, mediastinal mass, and CVL.

[d]Limited data exist for the use of tPA for this indication. Doses of 0.04–0.5 mg/kg/hr have been used with variable success. Monitor closely for adverse events such as intracranial hemorrhage.[7–9]

INITIATING AND MONITORING ANTICOAGULATION THERAPY

Unfractionated heparin[5]

Neonatal heparin considerations

- More rapid clearance and larger volume of distribution than older children and adults generally results in higher dose requirements.

- Reduced plasma concentrations of antithrombin may lead to a reduced response to heparin therapy.

Dosing recommendations

- Loading dose: 75 units/kg
- Initial maintenance dose:

  Infants <1 year: 28 units/kg/hr

  Children >1 year: 20 units/kg/hr

Table 17-5: Sample Nomogram for Heparin Dosage Adjustments in Pediatrics[a]

aPTT (seconds)	Bolus(units/kg)	Stop infusion (minutes)	Rate change (% of current rate)	Repeat aPTT
<50	50	0	Increase by 10%	4 hr
50–59	0	0	Increase by 10%	4 hr
60–85	0	0	0	Next day
86–95	0	0	Decrease by 10%	4 hr
96–120	0	30	Decrease by 10%	4 hr
>120	0	60	Decrease by 15%	4 hr

Source: adapted from reference 10.

[a]Target aPTT range will be institution specific (refer to Chapter 18 for more details).

Clinical Pearl

- Due to the low infusion rates often utilized in neonatal and pediatric patients, clinicians should insure that the concentration of heparin infusions is sufficiently diluted to allow for the above suggested rate changes. Many syringe pumps will allow for rate measurements to the hundredth decimal place (e.g., 0.25 mL/hr). However, the actual dosage change in terms of units/kg/hr should be considered because a percentage change in the infusion rate, as suggested above, may or may not result in a clinically signifi-cant change in the amount of heparin delivered depending on the concentration of the infusion and the current dose.

Considerations when monitoring heparin therapy

- "Normal" aPTT is significantly prolonged in infants compared to older children; adult values are not achieved until late adolescence.
- Use of pedi-tubes for lab draws should be considered to reduce blood loss. Blood should not be transferred from a citrated tube to a pedi-tube.
- Variability in aPTT by age has lead to a suggestion that heparin therapy be monitored by correlating aPTT values with therapeutic anti-Factor Xa levels (0.35–0.70 units/mL) normalized for UFH activity. Some institutions directly monitor heparin therapy using anti-Factor Xa levels.

Table 17-6: Sample Nomogram for Heparin Dosage Adjustments Using Anti-Factor Xa Levels

Anti-Factor Xa Level (units/mL)	Bolus Dose (units/kg)	Stop Heparin Infusion (min)	Rate change (round to nearest whole number)	Repeat Anti-Factor Xa Level
Less than or equal to 0.1[a]	50	0	Increase rate by 20%	4 hr
0.1–0.34	0	0	Increase rate by 10%	4 hr
0.35–0.7	0	0	No change	4 hr after first anti-Factor Xa level between 0.35–0.7, then every AM
0.71–0.89	0	0	Decrease rate by 10%	4 hr
0.9–1.2	0	30 min	Decrease rate by 10%	4 hr
≥1.2[a]	0	60 min	Decrease rate by 15%	4 hr

Source: used with permission from Sanford Children's Hospital, Sioux Falls, SD.

[a]Goal anti-Factor Xa level = 0.35–0.70 units/mL.

Low Molecular Weight Heparins (LMWH)

- Potential advantages of LMWH in pediatrics: reduced monitoring requirements, which minimizes the need for needlesticks and venous access, lack of drug-drug and drug-food interactions, reduced risk of HIT

Enoxaparin[5,11-13]

- Neonates require higher per kg doses than older children to achieve therapeutic anti-Factor Xa levels likely due to decreased antithrombin concentrations in neonates and larger volume of distribution.

- Premature neonates have been shown to require higher enoxaparin doses than term neonates.

- Effective dose to attain a therapeutic anti-Factor Xa level has been shown to be inversely related to age.

- Enoxaparin dosing (Table 17-7)

Table 17-7: Enoxaparin Dosing

	Age	Dose
Standard treatment dose		
	Neonates	1.5 mg/kg SC q 12 hr
	Children	1 mg/kg SC q 12 hr
Suggested modified dose		
	Preterm neonates	2 mg/kg SC q 12 hr
	Term neonates	1.7 mg/kg SC q 12 hr
	3–12 mo	1.5 mg/kg SC q 12 hr
	1–5 yr	1.2 mg/kg SC q 12 hr
	6–18 yr	1.1 mg/kg SC q 12 hr
Prophylactic dose		
	<2 mo	0.75 mg/kg SC q 12 hr
	≥2 mo	0.5 mg/kg SC q 12 hr

Clinical Pearls

Utilizing higher initial SC doses of enoxaparin than usually recommended may reduce the number of venopunctures required for monitoring therapy and shorten the time to therapeutic anti-Factor Xa levels.

- SC administration may be problematic in critically ill children with significant edema or peripheral vasoconstriction due to vasopressor support or in preterm neonates with very little subcutaneous fat.

- IV administration has been shown to result in an earlier peak anti-Factor Xa level (1–2 hours after administration) with subtherapeutic levels by 6–8 hours suggesting the need for dose modification if this route of administration is used.

Dalteparin[14]

- Dalteparin dosing recommendations are based on a small study of 48 children (ages 31 weeks preterm neonate to 18 years old).
  - Treatment dose: 129 ± 43 units/kg q 24 hr
  - Prophylaxis dose: 95 ± 52 units/kg q 24 hr
  - Required dose per kg of body weight was found to be inversely related to age.

Table 17-8: Sample Nomogram for LMWH Therapeutic Dosage Adjustment

Anti-Factor Xa Level (units/mL)	Hold Next Dose?	Dose Change	Repeat Anti-Factor Xa Level
<0.35	No	↑ by 25%	4 hr after next dose
0.35–0.49	No	↑ by 10%	4 hr after next dose
0.5–1.0	No	No change	Next day

(continued)

Table 17-8: (Continued)

Anti-Factor Xa Level (units/mL)	Hold Next Dose?	Dose Change	Repeat Anti-Factor Xa Level
1.1–1.5	No	No change if once daily dosing (1.5–2.0 mg/kg enoxaparin; 150–200 units/kg dalteparin) ↓ by 20% if twice daily dosing (1 mg/kg enoxaparin; 100 units/kg dalteparin)	Before next dose
1.6–2.0	3 hr	↓ by 30%	Before next dose, then 4 hr after next dose
>2	Until anti-Factor Xa level <0.5	↓ by 40%	Before next dose, if not <0.5 units/mL repeat q 12 hr

Source: adapted from reference 10.

Dilution Data for Enoxaparin and Dalteparin[15–17]

- Enoxaparin diluted with sterile water to a final concentration of 20 mg/mL has been shown to be stable in tuberculin syringes for at least 2 weeks under refrigeration or at room temperature without a significant loss of anti-Factor Xa activity. A slight, but statistically nonsignificant, loss of anti-Factor Xa activity occurred at 4 weeks of storage.

- Due to potential errors associated with the dilution of any medication, some practitioners recommend combining rounded, whole milligram dosing with the use of undiluted enoxaparin 100 mg/mL measured in an insulin syringe such that 1 unit on the syringe measures 1 mg of enoxaparin.

  - This approach was shown to achieve therapeutic anti-Factor Xa levels in 514 of 514 children with no associated hemorrhagic side effects despite five of the children having an initial supratherapeutic anti-Factor Xa level (1.04–1.36 units/mL). Additionally there were no reported medication errors.

- Dalteparin diluted with preservative-free normal saline to a final concentration of 2,500 units/mL has been shown to be stable in tuberculin syringes for 4 weeks under refrigeration without a significant loss of anti-Factor Xa activity.

Monitoring LMWH with anti-Factor Xa levels

- Therapeutic anti-Factor Xa level of 0.5–1.0 units/mL (obtained 4–6 hours after the dose) has been extrapolated from adult data; safety and efficacy of this range has not been validated in children.
- Prophylactic anti-Factor Xa level = 0.1–0.3 units/mL
- Target levels are based on twice daily dosing of LMWH.

Fondaparinux[18–20]

- In vitro study suggests no age-related differences in anticoagulation effect.
- Case reports suggest an initial dose of 0.15 mg/kg q 24 hr.

Direct thrombin inhibitors

Heparin-induced thrombocytopenia in the pediatric population[21–23]

- Reported incidence ranges from 0% to 2.3%, which is similar to adult rates
- Highest risk in intensive care unit patients and those undergoing cardiac surgery
- Highest incidences in those 0–2 years and 11–17 years
  - This effect may be influenced by the higher likelihood of heparin exposure in these age groups rather than an age-related phenomenon.

Controversy exists over the occurrence of HIT in neonates[24,25]

- Detection assays have not been well-studied and validated in this population.
- The immature immune system of neonates especially those born prematurely may be unable to mount an adequate antibody response to heparin exposure and therefore would not be detected by available assays.
- In a small prospective study, 24 of 42 premature neonates receiving heparin developed thrombocytopenia without clinical thrombosis; no patient had antiheparin/platelet factor 4 antibodies detected by ELISA or serotonin release assay (SRA).

Argatroban use in pediatrics[26–30]

- Case reports and uncontrolled studies have reported doses ranging from 0.1–15 mcg/kg/min; some have reported the use of a bolus dose ranging from 50–250 mcg/kg, typically targeting an aPTT 1.5–2.0 times baseline.

- Argatroban prescribing information suggests initiating therapy at 0.75 mcg/kg/min in children with normal hepatic function with dose adjustments of 0.1–0.25 mcg/kg/min based on aPTT levels drawn 2 hours after dose adjustment.

- Hepatically metabolized, therefore, dosage adjustment is required in hepatic dysfunction.

  - Dosing in children with hepatic dysfunction or the effect of various stages of liver maturation has not been specifically evaluated; however, argatroban prescribing information suggests an initial dose of 0.2 mcg/kg/min with dosage adjustments made in increments of 0.05 mcg/kg/min.

Warfarin

Dosing considerations[5,31]

- Warfarin is generally avoided in neonates due to relative vitamin K deficiency and reduced concentrations of vitamin K dependent clotting factors (II, VII, IX, X).

- Infants (≤1 year old) have been shown to require a larger dose per kg of body weight (0.33 mg/kg) than adolescents (0.09 mg/kg) and adolescents require a larger per kg dose than adults to maintain a therapeutic INR.

Table 17-9: Sample Nomogram for Warfarin Dosing Administration and Dosage Adjustment

Day of therapy	INR	Adjustment
Day 1	Baseline = 1–1.3	Loading dose = 0.2 mg/kg
Days 2–4	1.1–1.3	Repeat initial loading dose
	1.4–1.9	50% of initial loading dose
	2–3	50% of initial loading dose
	3.1–3.5	25% of initial loading dose
	>3.5	Hold until INR <3.5, then restart at 50% less than previous dose

(*continued*)

Table 17-9: (Continued)

Day of therapy	INR	Adjustment
Maintenance	1.1–1.3	Increase current dose by 20%
	1.4–1.9	Increase current dose by 10%
	2–3	No change
	3.1–3.5	Decrease current dose by 10%
	>3.5	Hold until INR <3.5, then restart at 25% less than previous dose

Source: adapted from reference 10.

Dosage formulation and dispensing considerations

- No commercially available liquid preparation
- Relatively poor solubility of warfarin creates difficulty in compounding liquid formulations; no stability data.
- Children are often prescribed antibiotics that may interact with warfarin.
- Commercially available enteral infant formulas are high in vitamin K while breast milk contains low amounts.

INR monitoring[32–35]

- No clinical trials have assessed the optimal INR range for children.
- Target INR range is based on recommendations for adult patients despite differences in the coagulation system, which may suggest the need for age-related INR ranges.
- Prophylactic target INR = 1.5–1.9
- Therapeutic target INR = 2–3
  - 2.5–3.5 if indication is mitral valve replacement

Frequency of monitoring

- Frequent INR monitoring is required in neonates due to rapid physiologic changes in vitamin K dependent factors.

- It has been estimated that monthly monitoring is safe in only about 10% to 20% of children with most requiring more frequent INR monitoring and dose adjustments.
- Whole blood point-of-care monitors including CoaguChek S (Roche Diagnostics), CoaguChek XS (Roche Diagnostics), and ProTime (International Technidyne Corp.) have been validated in pediatric patients

Potential factors affecting anticoagulation in children

- CYP2C9*2 and CYP2C9*3 polymorphisms have been identified in children and may be a risk factor for overanticoagulation.[36]
- Children with disease states associated with fat malabsorption (e.g., cystic fibrosis) may be at risk for vitamin K deficiency and, therefore, overanticoagulation.

Monitoring considerations specific to pediatric patients

- Whenever possible, arrange blood collection for INR with other necessary labs to avoid excessive blood loss.
- Additionally, venipuncture may be more difficult in children due to poor peripheral vascularity and fear of needlesticks.
- Frequent laboratory blood draws result in missed school days and parental work absences, which may contribute to noncompliance.

Adverse effects[31,37]

- Minor bleeding—approximately 20% of children
- Serious bleeding—less than 3.2% in children with mechanical prosthetic heart valves and approximately 1.7% with other indications for anticoagulation
- Reduced bone density—case controlled study suggested risk in children with congenital heart disease receiving warfarin for longer than 12 months

Patient and family education[38,39]

- A standardized, comprehensive, developmentally appropriate educational program has been shown to improve patient and family understanding of warfarin therapy and improve time within a target INR range.
- Education should also include practical issues related to anticoagulation therapy (e.g., no contact sports, no aspirin, or NSAIDs, etc.).

Special considerations

Injections in pediatric patients

- Injectable therapies may pose several difficulties in this population. For example, neonates especially those born prematurely have very little subcutaneous fat making this route of administration less than ideal. Poor venous access and reduced peripheral perfusion in critically ill children create additional challenges. Finally, a child's fear of "shots" can make the outpatient use of agents such as LMWH problematic.

Insurance coverage

- Because most anticoagulant therapies and outpatient monitoring devices are not FDA-approved for children, obtaining coverage/reimbursement from insurance companies may require special measures such as a letter of medical necessity with supporting literature to justify their use in the outpatient setting. Verification of insurance coverage for both the anticoagulant agent and the monitoring tests is important.

ECMO considerations[40–41]

- UFH is typically used for anticoagulation of the ECMO circuit.
- Higher doses (e.g., 20.0–69.5 units/kg/hr) are needed due to binding to the ECMO circuit and a large volume of distribution.
    - A retrospective review of 604 pediatric ECMO patients demonstrated a correlation between higher heparin doses and improved survival; for heparin doses of 30, 40, 50, 60, and 70 units/kg/hr, the corresponding probability of survival was 50%, 58%, 64%, 70%, and 75%. Survival benefit declined at doses above 70 units/kg/hr.
- Low response ACT testing is often used for bedside monitoring of anticoagulation but has been shown to correlate poorly with heparin effect and have significant variability among available monitoring devices; anti-Factor Xa levels have been suggested as a better monitoring method.
- Please refer to Chapter 5 for a discussion on the use of direct thrombin inhibitors in ECMO.

Interpretation of laboratory tests

- Whenever possible, age-specific "normal" ranges should be used.
- Practitioners should be mindful that all therapeutic ranges for anticoagulant therapy in children have been extrapolated from adult data.

Intravenous catheter occlusions

- Because sites for venous access are limited in children, especially neonates, preventing catheter occlusion and ultimately the loss of the catheter are of utmost importance.

Considerations for maintaining IV catheter patency[21,42–44]

- Saline flushes and locks have been shown to be as effective as heparin in maintaining the patency of peripheral intravenous catheters while avoiding the potential complications of heparin therapy (e.g., HIT, accidental overdose).

- Heparin is commonly added to fluids infusing through peripheral catheters and PICC to prolong catheter patency; however, this practice has not been shown to provide a clinically significant benefit.

- Heparin at a concentration of 5 units/mL (vs. 1 units/mL) in normal saline has been shown to prolong the patency of peripheral arterial catheters when continuously infused at 1 mL/hr.

- Heparin low dose (0.25–1 units/mL) continuous infusion has been shown to reduce umbilical artery catheter (UAC) occlusions.

- A positive pressure device can be attached to the catheter hub of PICC to prevent backflow of blood, which has been shown to reduce catheter occlusion.

Considerations for restoring IV catheter patency[45–49]

Developmental aspects of the fibrinolytic system

- Plasminogen concentrations are decreased by 50% in full-term and 75% in premature neonates compared to adults.

- Adult values are reached by 6 months of age.

- Decreased plasminogen concentrations in neonates may result in a limited response to thrombolytic agents. Increasing doses of thrombolytic agents do not seem to result in an improved response in this patient population. However, no study has specifically evaluated the clinical implications of this developmental difference on catheter clearance.

Recombinant tissue plasminogen activator (tPA) for catheter clearance

- If a thrombotic (vs. nonthrombotic) occlusion is deemed to be the cause of intravenous catheter dysfunction, tPA has been shown to be effective in restoring catheter patency.

- tPA should be diluted to a final concentration of 1 mg/mL and dosed as follows:
  - Patients <30 kg: dose equal to 110% of internal catheter volume, maximum dose 2 mg (2 mL of the 1-mg/mL concentration).
    - This dose has been shown to be safe and effective in neonates; however, some investigators suggest a lower dose of 0.5 mg diluted in a sufficient volume of normal saline to fill the catheter for infants weighing less than 10 kg.
  - Patients ≥30 kg: 2 mg (2 mL of the 1-mg/mL concentration)
- tPA should be allowed to dwell within the catheter for at least 30 minutes (up to 120 minutes) prior to attempting aspiration.
- If the initial dose fails to restore patency after 120 minutes of dwell time, the benefit of a second dose has been shown.

REFERENCES

*Key articles

1. Stein PD, Kayali FK, Olson RE. Incidence of venous thromboembolism in infants and children: data from the national hospital discharge survey. *J Pediatr.* 2004;145:563–565.

2. Newall F, Wallace T, Crock C, et al. Venous thromboembolic disease: a single-centre case series study. *J Paediatr Child Health.* 2006;42:803–807.

3. Cyr C, Michon B, Pettersen G, et al. Venous thromboembolism after severe injury in children. *Acta Haematol.* 2006;115:198–200.

4. Wiernikowski JT, Athale UH. Thromboembolic complications in children with cancer. *Thromb Res.* 2006;118:137–152.

5. **Monagle P, Chalmers E, Chan A, et al. Antithrombotic therapy in neonates and children: American college of chest physicians evidence-based clinical practice guidelines (8th ed.). *Chest.* 2008;133:887S–968S.**

6. **Kuhle S, Male C, Mitchell L. Developmental hemostasis: pro- and anticoagulant systems during childhood. *Semin Thromb Hemost.* 2003;29:329–337.**

7. Dillon PW, Fox PS, Berg CJ, et al. Recombinant tissue plasminogen activator for neonatal and pediatric vascular thrombolytic therapy. *J Pediatr Surg.* 1993;28:1264–1269.

8. Farnoux C, Camard O, Pinquier D, et al. Recombinant tissue-type plasminogen activator therapy of thrombosis in 16 neonates. *J Pediatr.* 1998;133:137–140.

9. Weinschenk N, Pelidis M, Fiascone J. Combination thrombolytic and anticoagulant therapy for bilateral renal vein thrombosis in a premature infant. *Am J Perinatol.* 2001;18:293–297.

10. Michelson AD, Bovill E, Monagle P, et al. Antithrombotic therapy in children. *Chest.* 1998;114(suppl):748S–769S.

* **11. Malowany JI, Monagle P, Knoppert DC, et al. Enoxaparin for neonatal thrombosis: a call for a higher dose in neonates. *Thromb Res.* 2008;122:826–830.**

12. Bauman ME, Belletrutti MJ, Bajzar L, et al. Evaluation of enoxaparin dosing requirements in infants and children. *Thromb Haemost.* 2009;101:86–92.

13. Crary SE, Van Orden H, Journeycake J. Experience with intravenous enoxaparin in critically ill infants and children. *Pediatr Crit Care Med.* 2008;9:647–649.

14. Nohe N, Flemmer A, Rumler R, et al. The low molecular weight heparin dalteparin for prophylaxis and therapy of thrombosis in childhood: a report on 48 cases. *Eur J Pediatr.* 1999;158(suppl 3):S134–S139.

15. Dager WE, Gosselin RC, King JH, et al. Anti-Xa stability of diluted enoxaparin for use in pediatrics. *Ann Pharmacother.* 2004;38:569–573.

16. Bauman ME, Black KL, Bauman ML, et al. Novel uses of insulin syringes to reduce dosing errors: a retrospective chart review of enoxaparin whole milligram dosing. *Thromb Res.* 2009;123:845–847.

17. Goldenberg NA, Jacobson L, Hathaway H, et al. Anti-Xa stability of diluted dalteparin for pediatric use. *Ann Pharmacother.* 2008:42:511–515.

18. Ignjatovic V, Summerhayes R, Yip YY, et al. The in vitro anticoagulant effects of danaparoid, fondaparinux, and lepirudin in children compared to adults. *Thromb Res.* 2008;122:709–714.

19. Mason AR, McBurney PG, Fuller MP, et al. Successful use of fondaparinux as an alternative anticoagulant in a 2-month-old infant. *Pediatr Blood Cancer.* 2008;50:1084–1085.

20. Sharathkumar AA, Crandall C, Lin JJ, et al. Treatment of thrombosis with fondaparinux (Arixtra) in a patient with end-stage renal disease receiving hemodialysis therapy. *J Pediatr Hematol Oncol.* 2007;29:581–584.

21. Klenner AF, Fusch C, Rakow A, et al. Benefit and risk of heparin for maintaining peripheral venous catheters in neonates: a placebo-controlled trial. *J Pediatr.* 2003;143:741–745.

22. Schmugge M, Risch L, Huber AR, et al. Heparin-induced thrombocytopenia-associated thrombosis in pediatric intensive care patients. *Pediatrics.* 2002;109:e10.

23. Warkentin TE. Heparin-induced thrombocytopenia: pathogenesis and management. *Br J Haematol.* 2003;121:535–555.

24. Spadone D, Clark F, James E, et al. Heparin-induced thrombocytopenia in the newborn. *J Vasc Surg.* 1002;15:306–311.

25. Kumar P, Hoppensteadt P, Pretchel M, et al. Prevalance of heparin-dependent platelet-activating antibodies in preterm newborns after exposure to unfractionated heparin. *Clin Appl Thromb Hemost.* 2004;10:335–339.

26. John TE, Hallisey RK. Argatroban and lepirudin requirements in a 6-year-old patient with heparin-induced thrombocytopenia. *Pharmacotherapy.* 2005;25:1383–1388.

27. Potter KE, Raj A, Sullivan JE. Argatroban for anticoagulation in pediatric patients with heparin-induced thrombocytopenia requiring extracorporeal life support. *J Pediatr Hematol Oncol.* 2007;29:265–268.

28. Schmitz ML, Massicotte P, Faulkner SC. Management of a pediatric patient on the Berlin heart excor ventricular assist device with argatroban after heparin-induced thrombocytopenia. *ASAIO Journal.* 2008;54:546–547.

29. Hursting MJ, Dubb J, Verme-Gibboney CN. Argatroban anticoagulation in pediatric patients. *J Pediatr Hematol Oncol.* 2006;28:4–10.

30. Argatroban [package insert]. Research Triangle Park, NC: GlaxoSmithKline; 2009.

31. **Streif W, Andrew M, Marzinotto V, et al. Analysis of warfarin therapy in pediatric patients: a prospective cohort study of 319 patients. *Blood.* 1999;94: 3007–3014.**

32. Marzinotto V, Monagle P, Chan A, et al. Capillary whole blood monitoring of oral anticoagulants in children in outpatient clinics and the home setting. *Pediatr Cardiol.* 200;21;347–352.

33. Nowatzke WL, Landt M, Smith C, et al. Whole blood international normalization ratio measurements in children using near-patient monitors. *J Pediatr Hematol Oncol.* 2003;25:33–37.

34. Bradbury MJE, Taylor G, Short P, et al. A comparative study of anticoagulant control in patients on long-term warfarin using home and hospital monitoring of the international normalised ratio. *Arch Dis Child.* 2008;93:303–306.

35. Bauman ME, Black KL, Massicotte MP, et al. Accuracy of the CoaguChek XS for point-of-care international normalized ratio (INR) measurement in children requiring warfarin. *Thromb Haemost.* 2008;99:1097–1103.

36. Ruud E, Holmstrom H, Bergan S, et al. Oral anticoagulation with warfarin is significantly influenced by steroids and CYP2C9 polymorphisms in children with cancer. *Pediatr Blood Cancer.* 2008;50:710–713.

37. Barnes C, Newall F, Ignjatovic V, et al. Reduced bone density in children on long-term warfarin. *Pediatr Res.* 2005;57:578–581.

38. Bauman ME, Black K, Kuhle S, et al. KIDCLOT©: the importance of validated educational intervention for optimal long term warfarin management in children. *Thromb Res.* 2009;123:707–709.

39. Ronghe MD, Halsey C, Goulden NJ. Anticoagulation therapy in children. *Pediatr Drugs.* 2003;5:803–820.

40. Nankervis CA, Preston TJ, Dysart KC, et al. Assessing heparin dosing in neonates on venoarterial extracorporeal membrane oxygenation. *ASAIO*. 2007;53: 111–114.

41. Baird CW, Zurakowski D, Robinson B, et al. Anticoagulation and pediatric extracorporeal membrane oxygenation: impact of activated clotting time and heparin dose on survival. *Ann Thorac Surg*. 2007;83:912–920.

42. Kleiber C, Hanrahan K, Fagan, CL, et al. Heparin vs. saline for peripheral i.v. locks in children. *Pediatr Nurs*. 1993;19:405–409.

43. Paisley MK, Stamper, M, Brown J, et al. The use of heparin and normal saline flushes in neonatal intravenous catheters. *Pediatr Nurs*. 1997;23:521–524.

44. Kamala F, Boo NY, Cheah FC, et al. Randomized controlled trial of heparin for prevention of blockage of peripherally inserted central catheters in neonates. *Acta Paediatr*. 2002;91:1350–1356.

45. Albisetti M. The fibrinolytic system in children. *Semin Thromb Hemost*. 2003;29:339–347.

46. Deitcher SR, Fesen MR, Kiproff PM, et al. Alteplase treatment of occluded venous catheters: results of the cardiovascular thrombolytic to open occluded lines (COOL-2) trial. *J Clin Oncol*. 2002;20:317–324.

47. Jacobs BR, Haygood M, Hingl J. Recombinant tissue plasminogen activator in the treatment of central venous catheter occlusion in children. *J Pediatr*. 2001;139:593–596.

48. Choi M, Massicotte P, Marzinotto V, et al. The use of alteplase to restore patency of central venous lines in pediatric patients: a cohort study. *J Pediatr*. 2001;139:152–156.

49. Blaney M, Shen V, Kerner JA, et al. Alteplase for the treatment of central venous catheter occlusion in children: results of a prospective, open-label, single-arm study (The Cathflo Activase Pediatric Study). *J Vasc Interv Radiol*. 2006;17:1745–1751.

Note: the following key articles are not cited in the text.

* **Goldenberg NA, Bernard TJ. Venous thromboembolism in children. *Pediatr Clin N Am*. 2008;55:305–322.**

* **Risch L, Huber AR, Schmugge M. Diagnosis and treatment of heparin-induced thrombocytopenia in neonates and children. *Thromb Res*. 2006;118:123–135.**

PART III: Practical Monitoring and Coagulation Laboratory Insights

EIGHTEEN

Chapter

18

Coagulation Laboratory Considerations

Robert C. Gosselin, Maureen A. Smythe

INTRODUCTION

Coagulation testing is used in a variety of settings: screen for factor deficiencies (PT/aPTT), monitoring drug efficacy (PT/aPTT), and exclude disease states (D-dimer). Variables affecting coagulation testing include preanalytical (e.g., timing of blood collection, processing, timing, and suitability) and analytical (e.g., instrument and reagent systems), which may impact the accuracy of the reported result. These variables can lead to notable differences in reported results between laboratories and should be taken into consideration when using observations in the literature or from an outside hospital, and in developing or adjusting the anticoagulant management plan. Lastly, the laboratory evaluation/testing should be interpreted as a surrogate marker of the hemostasis process, as these data may not be an absolute reflection of in vivo coagulation or hard outcomes.

COAGULATION TESTING: METHODS

Coagulation testing typically measures either the functional or amount (antigen) of coagulation protein(s) using four basic testing principles:

- Clotting endpoint (functional test)—addition of patient plasma to reagent(s), then determining the time to clot formation

- Chromogenic testing (functional test)—addition of patient plasma to reagent(s) then determining the amount of color formation

- Immunologic (mostly antigenic, occasionally functional)—addition of patient plasma or serum to beads or microwells containing target antigen or antibody then assess color changes, changes in agglutination, hemagglutination, etc.

- Aggregation (other functional)—addition of patient plasma (platelet poor or containing platelets) to platelets and/or agonist(s) and measuring light scattering (agglutination) or platelet clumping (aggregation)

Most clotting, chromogenic, and aggregation studies use 3.2% sodium citrate anticoagulant. Immunologic testing can be done using either citrate anticoagulated blood or serum. Consult testing laboratory for specific sample requirements.

Table 18-1: Available Tests and Methods for Coagulation-Related Assays

	PT	aPTT	ACT	Fbg	Fx	TT	Heparin Level	XDP	HIT	AT	PLT Function
Clotting	•	•	•	•	•	•					
Chromogenic					•		•			•	
Immunologic				•	•			•	•	•	
Aggregation									•		•
Point-of-care	•	•	•				•	•	•		•

Abbreviations: PT = prothrombin time; aPTT = activated partial thromboplastin time; Fbg = fibrinogen; Fx = factor activity; TT = thrombin time; XDP = D-dimer, HIT = heparin induced thrombocytopenia test; AT = antithrombin; PLT = platelet.

Clinical Pearl

- Different testing approaches can occur between laboratories leading to different reported values or target ranges. Clinicians should be aware of the method used and the potential differences in reported values between methods when interpreting results or comparing target values to the literature.

Table 18-2: Principles of Coagulation Testing Using Clot-Based Assays

Citrated platelet poor plasma ($<$10,000 platelets/mL) used for analysis[1,2]

Sample, reagents, and testing performed at 37°C; aPTT testing requires a short incubation period (3–5 min) to allow activators and phospholipids to interact with plasma factors; this incubation phase is not feasible for point-of-care aPTT testing thus accounting for difference between laboratory methods

Clotting endpoint: changes in light scattering due to increased turbidity secondary to fibrin formation over time; waveform analysis can assist laboratory professionals in evaluating abnormal clotting results

Mechanical endpoint: decreased movement of a rotating ball within the cuvette secondary to fibrin formation; no waveform analysis possible

Point-of-care instruments are designed for whole blood testing and have no incubation period

Principles of coagulation testing: antibody-based assays

Antibody-related assays incorporate an antibody:antigen target pair to measure a specific *measurand* (something of which there is a desire to measure). For testing antibodies present in a patient (as seen in patients with heparin-induced thrombocytopenia), the antibody in the patient attaches to the target antigen affixed to a solid phase well (see Figure 18-1, ELISA testing below). For testing a specific measurand in a patient sample (e.g., von Willebrand's antigen), an antibody directed to that specific target protein is affixed to a solid phase well or bead (Figure 18-1).

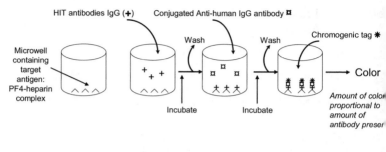

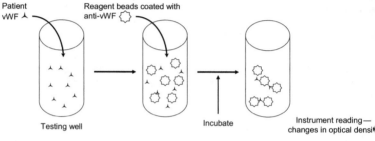

Figure 18-1: Antibody-Based Coagulation Assays

Table 18-3: Antibody-Based Coagulation Assays

ELISA Testing

- Microwells can be coated with target antigen or antibody directed to target protein (e.g., von Willebrand's factor)

- Specialized equipment required (microplate reader)

- Conjugated antihuman antibody can be monoclonal (e.g., antihuman IgG only), or polyclonal (e.g., antihuman IgG, IgM, and IgA); using monoclonal antibodies that are more specific to a given substance will typically improve test specificity

- Incubation periods vary (15–60 min per incubation period)

(continued)

Table 18-3: (Continued)

- Wash cycles are to eliminate unbound plasma/reagent
- Typically sensitive to low levels of measurand
- Some kit manufacturers may employ a secondary confirmation phase for positive screen assays (e.g., HIT testing)

Immunolatex Testing

- Fast tests; test usually completed within 3–5 min
- Fairly routine method on most larger coagulation instruments
- May not be as accurate at lower measurand levels

Table 18-4: Calibration of Assays

Coagulation Assays	Method
Routine screening tests: PT, aPTT, thrombin time, and platelet function testing have no calibration	• Abnormal results based on normal population • Normal ranges influenced by reagent, instrument, and population tested (age), and therefore no universal normal PT or aPTT range • INR calibration is recommended[3] but limited commercial material is available
Fibrinogen, factor assays, anti-Factor Xa activity	• Standardized commercially-prepared assay calibration (reference) material most often used • Calibration performed with each new reagent lot or at least every 6 mo[4,5]

Clinical Pearl

- Note that screening tests for coagulation are typically not calibrated, and new lots are needed relatively frequently. Changes in these reagent lots should be assessed appropriately (see below) prior to clinical use.

IMPLEMENTING A LABORATORY TEST FOR CLINICAL USE

Regulatory requirements

Implementing a new laboratory test: although most laboratories use commercially available kits and/or reagents, the following evaluations are required by the performing laboratory (CLIA regulation, Subpart K, §493.1253) prior to clinical use[4]:

Table 18-5: Approaches to Determining the Accuracy, Imprecision, and Reportable Range for a Test[a]

Test Evaluation Parameter	Definition/Requirements
Accuracy	Comparison of a new method to an existing method or reference method; the "closer" the new method is to the reference standard, the better the accuracy
Imprecision	Determining the imprecision of running a single sample multiple times concurrently (within-run imprecision) as well as the same sample (usually control material) over a period of days (day-to-day imprecision) to determine the coefficient of variation (CV); the lower the CV, the more likely the same value will occur for a sample on repeat testing
Reportable range (linearity)	Assesses the reportable range (high and low), as well as reproducibility of diluted samples; values that exceed the reportable range may undergo further testing in the lab (dilute out the sample), or may be reported as "<" or ">" the lower or upper limit of the range respectively as determined by the lab
Verify manufacturer's reference interval (normal range)	Appropriate for laboratory's patient population; many tests may not have age-related reference ranges, and therefore in patients <18 yr old, reference ranges may be cited from acceptable references

[a]If modifications to an FDA-approved test is used, or if in-house test is used, then additional performance characteristics must be evaluated and documented to include aforementioned accuracy, imprecision, reportable range, reference intervals, but also the following:
- Analytical sensitivity (see next below for description of sensitivity)
- Analytical specificity, including interfering substances (see below for description of specificity)
- Other performance characteristics required for testing (e.g., reagent stability)

Table 18-6: Sensitivity

Ability for test to detect abnormality (diagnostic or monitoring) formula:

$$\frac{\text{True Positive}}{\text{True Positives} + \text{False Negatives}}$$

Ideal coagulation reagent: 100% sensitive to all clinical and therapeutic needs

Realistic coagulation reagent

- Variable sensitivity for unfractionated heparin or DTI

- Variable sensitivity for lupus anticoagulant

- Variable sensitivity for factor deficiencies (e.g., factor VIII or XI)

- Variability between reagent manufacturers for same test (e.g., aPTT)

- Preanalytical and analytical variables can influence test results causing false negative results

Sensitivity is also used to describe the relative response of a test to drug or disease

- INR is more sensitive to vitamin K antagonists than the aPTT

- aPTT is more sensitive for measuring UFH treatment for DVT than the activated clotting time (ACT)

- Low response ACT is more sensitive to low dose UFH anticoagulation than to the high response ACT cartridges

Clinical Pearl

- Regarding sensitivity of laboratory testing, if a highly sensitive test is negative, then the presence of the substance or diagnosis is unlikely.

Table 18-7: Specificity

Ability for test to detect a specific pathologic condition (clinical sensitivity) or abnormality formula:

$$\frac{\text{True Negative}}{\text{True Negatives} + \text{False Positives}}$$

Ideal coagulation reagent: 100% specific to all clinical and therapeutic needs

Realistic coagulation reagent and anticoagulant monitoring or diagnostic testing

- Screening tests (e.g., PT and aPTT) measure multiple proteins
    - PT and aPTT testing can be influenced by increased factor levels (shortened clotting times) or decreased factor levels (increased clotting times)
- Preanalytical and analytical variables can influence test results causing falsely increased or decreased results:
    - Improperly derived reference range
    - Improperly assigned ISI and normal mean for INR calculation
    - Sample age >4 hr for aPTT
    - Sample age >24 hr for PT
    - Expired reagent(s)
- Monoclonal antibody testing (e.g., IgG isotype for HIT testing) may be more specific for diagnosing HIT than using a polyclonal test (measures IgG, IgM, and IgA antibodies)
- Abnormal result does not necessarily imply pathology
    - D-dimer can be elevated as normal physiological response to surgery, trauma, etc., and elevated result does not imply DIC or venous thromboembolism
    - Elevated PT/aPTT from diluted sample drawn above an IV line
    - Positive presence of HIT antibodies does not mean they are pathogenic causing clinical disease

Clinical Pearl

- Regarding specificity of laboratory testing, if a highly specific test is positive, then diagnosis or presence of a specific substance is more likely.

VARIABLES THAT AFFECT COAGULATION TESTING

Coagulation study sample in many situations must be placed in a tube containing citrate, which binds calcium and inhibits the coagulation process from occurring in vitro. Delays in transferring sample to a citrate environment may affect results.

Table 18-8: Potential Flaws with Collecting Samples[1]

Problem	Test Outcome
Samples submitted on ice	• Decrease PT due to cold activation of factor VII
	• Decreased platelet function
Samples acquired from syringes	• Delay in anticoagulating blood (>60 sec from syringe to citrate tube)
	• Increased PT/aPTT—clotted sample
	• Decreased PT/aPTT—activated sample
	• Increased platelet function—activated platelets more responsive to agonist
	• Decreased platelet function—platelet clumping, spent platelet function
Samples acquired from in-dwelling lines	• Increase PT/aPTT due to hemodilution (e.g., above IV site)
	• Increased PT/aPTT due to poor clearance of line prior to adding blood to citrate tube
	• Increased PT/aPTT due to heparin contamination from line

Clinical Pearl

• Regarding collecting blood samples for coagulation testing, the longer the sample remains in the syringe, the greater the error (can be either shortened or prolonged clotting times).

Table 18-9: Variables That Impact PT/INR and aPTT Testing

Possible Causes of ↑ INR and/or aPTT	Possible causes of ↓ INR and/or aPTT
Preanalytical	**Preanalytical**
Short draw—excess sodium citrate in plasma	Low HCT (<25%)
Elevated HCT (>55%)—common in neonates; excess citrate in plasma	Elevated calcium levels
	Poorly collected sample ↓ INR and/or aPTT due to activated sample
Clotted sample	Samples placed on ice ↓ INR
Sample >4 hr old: ↑ aPTT	Samples >2 hr for patients on UFH: ↓ aPTT due to platelet degranulation and PF4 release, which neutralizes heparin
Sample >24 hr old: ↑ INR	
Hemodilution drawn above IV site; drawn via arterial line without proper clearance	
Surgical hypothermia	
Factor deficiencies	
PT factors VII, X, V, II and to a lesser degree, fibrinogen	**Elevated factor levels**
aPTT factors XII, XI, IX, VIII, X, V, II, and to a lesser degree, fibrinogen	Inflammatory response ↓ aPTT due to elevated factor VIII and/or fibrinogen
Physiological decrease	Cryoprecipitate—contains high levels of factor VIII and fibrinogen
Hereditary deficiencies: Factor VIII and IX most common with higher incidence of factor XI deficiencies in Azhkenazi Jewish population	Drugs
	INR
	Activated factor VII
Immature liver: premature infants and neonates	Prothrombin complexes
	aPTT
Liver disease ↑ INR with normal or slight ↑ aPTT	Prothrombin complexes
	Direct factor therapy

(continued)

Table 18-9: (Continued)

Possible Causes of ↑ INR and/or aPTT	Possible causes of ↓ INR and/or aPTT
Consumptive coagulopathy	
Hemodilution	
RBC transfusion without FFP	
Blood volume expanders	
Deficiencies can also be associated with antibody directed against factors	
Drugs	
PT: oral vitamin K antagonists	
Daptomycin	
Direct thrombin inhibitors	
Argatroban > bivalirudin > lepirudin/ desirudin/dabigatran	
Activated protein C	
Rivaroxaban	
Systemic fibrinolytic activators (e.g., urokinase)	
aPTT: unfractionated heparin	
Direct thrombin inhibitors	
Activated protein C	
Systemic fibrinolytic activators (e.g., urokinase)	
Hydroxy-ethyl starch, hematin, Suramin, Taularidine	
Antiphospholipid antibodies—varies with reagent, may ↑ INR in addition to aPTT	

EVALUATING LABORATORY DATA

Table 18-10: Evaluation Methods Used for Comparison Studies

Evaluation Method	Comments
Regression analysis (or equivalent)	• Will assist in assessing relative accuracy to comparison method • When R value is one, there is perfect agreement between methods • When R value is low, there is poor correlation between methods Does not identify areas of biases
Bland-Altman plots (see Figure 18-2)	• Graphically depicts area(s) of bias Difference: new method $- \left[\dfrac{\text{currrent method} + \text{new method}}{2} \right]$ Modified bias plot: difference = new lot − current lot
Students paired t-test (or equivalent)	• Will determine if statistical differences exist between methods • Statistical software should be used to determine whether sample size and distribution are acceptable for valid analysis <0.05 considered not significantly different between methods

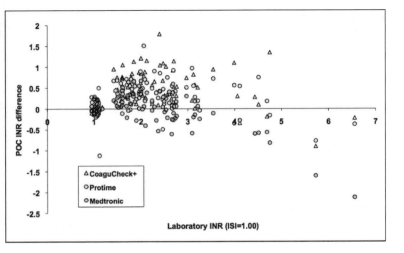

Figure 18-2: Bland Altman Bias Plot Demonstrating the Differences Between Methods

In this example, a modified Bland Altman bias plot was used to delineate the areas of bias between three different POC INRs and laboratory INRs. Note in this study, the POC INRs tend to be higher (positive bias) than laboratory INRs.

Table 18-11: Comparison of INR Measurements Between POC and Central Laboratory

- INR biases are mostly polar: POC provides values higher than laboratory methods on low end of therapeutic range (1.5–2.0), and provide values lower than laboratory methods at high INR levels (>4.0)[6]

- Laboratory should establish areas of bias between POC and lab INR methods[6] using Bland-Altman plots (see Figure 18-2)

- Newer methods with lower ISI (<1.5) may demonstrate better correlation with lab

- POC methods do not match each other

- Avoid interchanging monitoring methods during course of therapy

- Consider laboratory INR for POC values >5.0

Clinical Pearl

- Using different laboratories or methods may increase the variability in reported PT/INR results between samples and dose response assessment, leading to more instability in a regimen.

Table 18-12: Comparison of aPTT Measurements Between POC and Central Laboratory

- There is typically a bias between lab and POC aPTTs
- POC instrument manufacturers may use a mathematical correction factor to partially offset the bias to more closely correlate with laboratory aPTT results
- Since no incubation period for POC aPTT, results tend to be *lower* than laboratory aPTT, despite internal correction factor[7,8]
- Avoid interchanging monitoring methods (lab vs POC) during course of monitoring
- Consider laboratory aPTT if POC aPTT does not correlate with clinical picture

Prothrombin time [PT] and International Normalized Ratio [INR]

Table 18-13: Overview of PT and INR

- The PT is a measure of the extrinsic and final common pathway (II, V, VII, X)
- Vitamin K antagonists decrease the functional activity of factors II, VII, IX, X, protein C and protein S; the INR only describes the activity of factors II, VII, and X, and *not* factor IX
- The PT measures the time it takes for plasma to clot after the addition of calcium and an activator; the result is expressed in seconds
- Significant variation in PTs can occur due to differences in the source of thromboplastin (tissue factor, phospholipids, calcium) and the type of instrument used for clot detection
- Thromboplastin reagent sensitivity is expressed using the term ISI (International Sensitivity Index)

  - History: established to mitigate observed differences between US and European reported PT results; ultimately the INR replaced PT ratio for determining oral vitamin K antagonist effects

  - ISI provides an indicator of the thromboplastin responsiveness to the reduction in vitamin K dependent factors as compared with the WHO reference preparation

  - Thromboplastin with low ISI values correlate well with reference standard

  - Highly sensitive thromboplastins have an ISI of ~1.0 and are comprised of human or recombinant tissue factor

(*continued*)

Table 18-13: (Continued)

- Less sensitive thromboplastins have higher ISI values and are comprised of rabbit brain tissue factor

- Reagents with ISI values <1.4 are recommended for warfarin monitoring

- The INR was created as a mechanism to adjust for variation in PTs due to thromboplastin reagent sensitivity

$$INR = \left[\frac{patient\ PT(s)}{normal\ reference\ mean} \right]^{ISI}$$

Note: mean is geometric mean

- CLSI INR calibration guidelines, but limited commercial products and/or availability[3]

- Although the INR is an improvement, variations still occur due to the following:

  - Inaccurate reporting of the ISI by the manufacturer

  - Pretest variables

  - Differences resulting from lab instrumentation

- In hospitalized patients, the PT/INR is typically performed from a venipuncture acquired sample and analyzed using a laboratory-based coagulation analyzer

- Once collected in sodium citrate tube, the PT and INR is stable for 24 hours, when maintained at room temperature

- The PT/INR is also available as a POC test using a portable coagulation device, which is available from several different manufacturers

  - Capillary blood is used

  - The device converts the result to a plasma equivalent PT or INR

  - Results vary across manufacturers

  - Variations from lab assays are not typically considered clinically significant, except for elevated INRs

- Alternative strategies for monitoring oral vitamin K antagonist anticoagulation

  - Monitoring using factor levels

  - Most common is factor X levels (not anti-Factor Xa activity levels)

  - Differences exist between chromogenic and clot-based factor X results (see Figure 18-3)

  - Target factor level results of INRs between 2–3[9,10]:

    Factor II: ~20% to 35% for INR 2–3

    Factor X: 11% to 42% for INR 2.0–3.5 (chromogenic method); small variations in the % factor range for a given INR value can exist between assays (see Chapter 5)

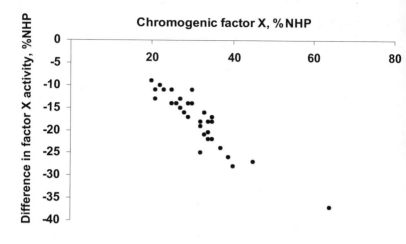

Figure 18-3: Difference in Factor X Activity, %NHP

Bias plot depicting the difference in reportable results between chromogenic determined factor X activity and clot-based determined factor X activity. Literature targeting therapeutic factor X activity levels using chromogenic assays should be used with caution if the more standard clot-based factor X activity assay is available. Note: clot-based factor X activity results are lower than chromogenic-based factor X activity results in normal human plasma (NHP).

Clinical Pearl

- When an INR is needed and only the aPTT was recently collected, the laboratory can be requested to run an INR off the aPTT sample to expedite the reporting of the result and avoid additional needle sticks or blood draws.

Table 18-14: Clinical Applications of PT and INR

Less accurate during initiation of warfarin therapy as the INR is most responsive initially to reductions of Factor VII, which has the shortest half-life

Can be prolonged by lupus anticoagulant, liver disease

Heparin can prolong the PT/INR

- Therapeutic dose heparin may increase the PT by 1.2 to 1.8 sec if no heparin neutralizing agent (e.g., polybrene) contained in reagent

- High dose heparin may have a more pronounced effect

- Can obtain an accurate PT in patients on heparin by using a heparin neutralizer like polybrene to neutralize heparin effect up to 2.0 units/mL of anti-Factor Xa activity, but can vary between reagents

Direct thrombin inhibitors exert a drug laboratory interaction and prolong the INR; this INR prolongation is not representative of a hemostatic effect

- The elevation is greatest with argatroban followed by bivalirudin and then lepirudin or desirudin

Clinical Pearls

- The INR target range (2 to 3) assumes steady state anticoagulation.

- Considering that the half-life of factor II is longer than VII or X, a INR value that is rising rapidly during the initiation of VKA therapy may not fully represent the measured degree of anticoagulation occurring at steady state dosing because the decline in factors VII and X are faster than II.

  - Early increases in INR values after initiating warfarin therapy may represent the early loss of predominantly factor VII.

  - In contrast, recovery of factor II may lag behind VII and X after holding the VKA, suggesting a greater degree of anticoagulation for a given INR value. Thus, declining INR values may represent a higher level of anticoagulation compared to the same INR value rising.

- If a PT reagent has heparin neutralization capabilities, there will be minimal effect on the INR for patients receiving heparin. If heparin neutralization is not part of the PT reagent system, then the baseline INR may be elevated in the presence of heparin.

ACTIVATED PARTIAL THROMBOPLASTIN TIME [APTT]

Table 18-15: Overview of the aPTT Test

- A global assay of coagulation

- The aPTT is referred to as partial thromboplastin due the absence of tissue factor in the thromboplastin

- Can be used to screen for inhibitors and deficiencies of the intrinsic pathway (factors XII, XI, IX, and VIII) and common pathway (factors X, V, prothrombin), and to a lesser degree, fibrinogen (of note is that some DTIs can decrease measured fibrinogen values)

- Many preanalytic variables that may affect aPTT results include sample timing, site of sample, concentration of citrate, and sample handling including centrifugation and processing time

- Instruments to detect the presence of clot may be dependent on plasma turbidity; lipemic or icteric specimens can affect plasma turbidity; in vitro hemolyzed samples should not be used for coagulation testing

- aPTT reagents vary in the type of contact activator, phospholipid composition, and concentration

- The relationship between factor activity in the blood and the aPTT result is logarithmic; therefore, for longer baseline aPTTs, a lower level of change is needed for additional prolongation

- aPTT has circadian variation (higher during sleep), which can result in difficulty in maintaining a therapeutic aPTT once achieved (see Chapter 3)

- Point-of-care (POC) testing for aPTT adds to the test variability

- Once appropriately collected into sodium citrate tubes, the aPTT is stable for the following:

  - Monitoring unfractionated heparin: 2 hr at room temperature

  - All other indications: 4 hr at room temperature

Table 18-16: Considerations of Heparin Monitoring Using the aPTT

- The most common test to monitor unfractionated heparin

- The heparin therapeutic aPTT range will vary depending on the aPTT reagent and instrument employed

- aPTT reagents vary in their responsiveness by manufacturer and lot number (see Figure 18-4)

- aPTT reagents vary in their responsiveness to heparin; therefore, an empiric aPTT ratio (i.e., 1.5–2.5 x control) is not appropriate for heparin monitoring

Clinical Pearls

- The correlation between anti-Factor Xa activity and aPTT is stronger with a laboratory-based aPTT than with a POC aPTT.

- The heparin therapeutic range *may* need to be reestablished with each new lot number of reagent or change in reagent manufacturer.[11]

  - Compare new lot aPTT vs. old lot aPTT reagents in at least 30 patients on UFH treatment (no concomitant warfarin). No more than ≤2 samples per single patient is acceptable.

  - Determine the differences of the means between each lot (current and new).

    - If the difference is <5 seconds, no change in therapeutic range is necessary.

    - If the difference is between 5–7 seconds, change may be necessary.

    - If the difference is >7 seconds, a new therapeutic range may be necessary.

- The approach recommended by ACCP and CAP to establish the aPTT therapeutic range uses regression analysis between aPTT and heparin levels (anti-Factor Xa activity) on samples from patients receiving therapeutic UFH only (no warfarin). The aPTT therapeutic range corresponds to 0.3–0.7 units/mL anti-Factor Xa activity, by chromogenic methods (see Figure 18-5).[11]

- The aPTT response when heparin is added to plasma is different than the response to ex vivo samples from patients on therapeutic heparin treatment (see Figure 18-6).

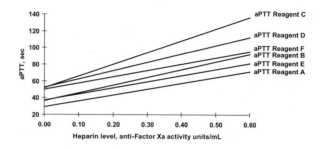

Figure 18-4: Heparin Response Curve

aPTT results tested concurrently using six different reagent/instrument combinations on UFH-treated patients. Note that aPTT reagents that are more sensitive to UFH (steeper slope and higher aPTT clotting times) may yield different aPTT ratios (patient's aPTT/baseline aPTT). Note that literature-based therapeutic ranges (e.g., 60–80 seconds) will also not be equivalent between reagent systems.

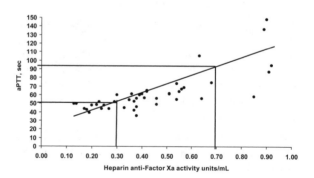

Figure 18-5: Heparin Response Curve

The recommended method for laboratory determination of unfractionated heparin therapeutic range by comparing anti-Factor Xa activity levels to aPTTs results in patients receiving therapeutic doses and no concomitant anticoagulant therapy (warfarin). In this example, the laboratory determined unfractionated heparin therapeutic range would be 50–95 seconds.

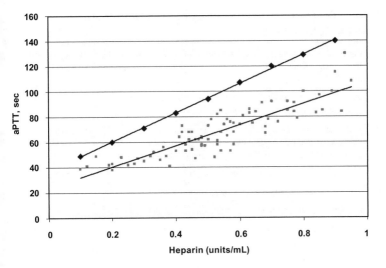

Figure 18-6: Heparin Response Curve

Comparison of regression data from recommended method of determining the unfractionated heparin therapeutic range using anti-Factor Xa activities compared to patient aPTTs (small squares) and using in vitro unfractionated heparin spiking of plasma (larger triangles in bold). The therapeutic range for the recommended method is 45–85 seconds, and the therapeutic range from in vitro spiking would be 70–120 seconds.

Clinical Pearl

UFH therapeutic range:

- Using UFH-spiked plasma to determine therapeutic range may overestimate drug requirement and lead to excessive anticoagulation. This method should not be used even though often attractive to facilities that rarely utilize heparin.

Table 18-17: aPTT Testing of UFH Anticoagulation: Clinical Applications

- Decisions to adjust heparin infusion therapy based on the aPTT will not always agree with those based on other tests such as heparin concentration (anti-Factor Xa activity level) or the ACT

- It is reasonable to validate by repeating the aPTT when results are unexpectedly prolonged during monitoring for VTE treatment with IV UFH

- Data supporting a relationship between an elevated aPTT to major bleeding in patients for VTE is weak; some correlation between bleeding and the frequency of aPTT values above the target range beyond 48 hr of therapy has been observed

- Data from ACS trials supports a relationship between increased aPTT and major bleeding

- Heparin resistance/altered heparin responsiveness

    - Consider when heparin infusion rate exceeds 25 units/kg/hr

    - Suspect when patients fail to obtain a therapeutic aPTT despite progressive heparin infusion rate increases

    - Possible causes:

        - Antithrombin deficiency

        - Increase in heparin binding proteins

        - Increase in Factor VIII levels or fibrogen; these are acute phase reactants, patients with increased levels of FVIII and fibrinogen (i.e., pregnancy) will have a downward shift in their heparin dose response curve and demonstrate less aPTT prolongation at a given heparin concentration; if failure to prolong the aPTT with increased heparin dose, monitor heparin using the heparin anti-Factor Xa activity level

            - If aPTT is subtherapeutic on heparin infusion and the patient is receiving >40,000 units of heparin/day and the heparin anti-Factor Xa activity level is at least 0.35 units/mL, further dose increases may not be necessary

- LMWH heparin and aPTT

    - Therapeutic doses have minimal impact on aPTT—cannot be used to monitor therapy

Clinical Pearl

- One way to assess for potential resistance is to measure an aPTT shortly after a heparin bolus to see if a response is observed.

Table 18-18: Considerations with Monitoring the aPTT During Direct Thrombin Inhibitor Therapy

- The DTI aPTT therapeutic range is not the heparin aPTT therapeutic range

- Varying aPTT reagents will produce different aPTT ratios for a clinically relevant concentration of DTI[12]

- The aPTT therapeutic range for DTIs was established in multicenter trials, which used multiple aPTT reagents

- With increasing concentrations of DTI, the aPTT dose response curve flattens and significant changes in plasma level result in only minor change in aPTT (see Figure 18-7)

- Per CAP requirements, each laboratory should determine a therapeutic range for a test used to monitor an anticoagulant; for the use of the aPTT during DTI therapy, the following is one approach to consider (see Figure 18-8)

  – Spiked normal plasma with DTI corresponding to drug concentrations of 0.1–1.2 mcg/mL

  – Run aPTT and PT/INR

  – Repeat with each new lot of reagents (PT and aPTT)

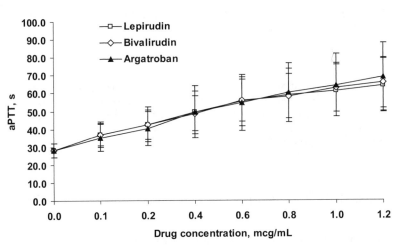

Figure 18-7: Graphic Representation of the Mean Seconds and Errors Bars for aPTT Results from 14 Different aPTT Reagents

Note plateau effect with increasing drug concentration, with slope changes beginning at 0.6 mcg/mL of drug.

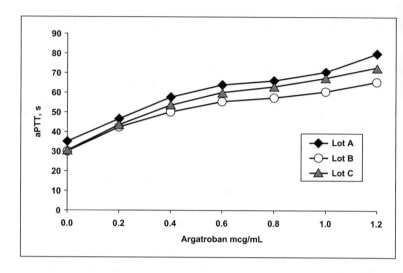

Figure 18-8: Comparison of Different aPTT Reagent Lots for Response to Argatroban Concentrations In Vitro

Lot A represents increased sensitivity and the possibility of higher reported aPTT values. However, the base line value may be elevated as well, reducing the impact on the ratio. A flattening of the curve (or change in the slope) may be observed at higher DTI concentrations. Note: the target serum DTI level related to clinical outcomes has not been established. The curve above describes how the aPTT range observed may vary between reagents and could lead to different results if a set range in seconds is established instead of a ratio.

Table 18-19: Clinical Application of the aPTT Test for Parenteral DTI Monitoring

Note: refer to Chapter 5 for further information about parenteral DTIs

- Warfarin can increase the aPTT, which can result in underdosing of DTI if not reversed at time of HIT diagnosis

- Elevated aPTTs are associated with increased bleeding

(continued)

Table 18-19: (Continued)

- Consider aPTT ratio 1.5–2.0 x baseline or low end of the therapeutic range if high bleeding risk is present

- If no elevation in aPTT with increasing dose, verify the amount of drug or switch to another DTI; an elevation in the ACT may suggest an anticoagulation effect is present and a problem exists with the aPTT assay in use; consider sending sample to an outside laboratory for verification using either alternative aPTT method or chromogenic thrombin inhibitor assay

- Check aPTT any time thrombosis or major bleeding is suspected

- With excessive aPTT prolongation verify aPTT has returned to therapeutic range before restarting therapy

- Degree of INR prolongation varies with DTI and PT reagent[13]; the amount of DTI will also impact the elevation in the INR; higher rates can result in higher INR values

- **Bivalirudin**

  – Monitor aPTT 2–4 hr after initiation and any dose change, then at least daily

  – Consider extending the interval for aPTT monitoring in patients with significant renal impairment to assess steady state effect; earlier values may be requested to determine the rate of rise for a given infusion dose (see Chapter 5)

- **Argatroban**

  – Monitor aPTT 4 hr after initiation of therapy and any dose change

- **Lepirudin**

  – Not recommended for use if (lab normal PT/patient PT) baseline aPTT ratio of ≥2.5

  – aPTT monitoring at baseline, every 4 hr until therapeutic then daily

  – Monitor 4 hr after dose change

  – Prolonged lepirudin therapy can result in the formation of anti hirudin antibodies, which can enhance the anticoagulation effect as evidenced by an increased aPTT on the same dose

  – Clinical trial data supports relationship between low aPTT and thrombosis and high aPTT and bleeding

  – Extend interval for aPTT monitoring in critically ill patients and those with renal insufficiency when assessing a steady state response; earlier values may be considered prior to steady state to minimize excessive anticoagulation (see Chapter 5)

Heparin Level Monitoring

Table 18-20: Overview of Heparin Level Monitoring

- Heparin levels can be determined from two different types of assay methods; anti-Factor Xa activity assay and protamine sulfate titration; of these the anti-Factor Xa activity assay is more routinely available

Anti-Xa Level Monitoring

- Anti-Factor Xa activity assays can be clot-based or chromogenic; clot-based assays may underestimate anti-Factor Xa activity relative to chromogenic assays; chromogenic assays are most often used (see Figure 18-9 for chromogenic method description)

- UFH anti-Factor Xa activity must be determined from a UFH derived calibration curve

- Assay variability comes from different instrumentation and manufacturers, the addition of exogenous AT in some assay systems, different lots of heparin, and differences in process for creating the standard curve

- The heparin anti-Factor Xa activity level therapeutic range was initially established by identifying the anti-Factor Xa activity level, which corresponds to a known therapeutic heparin level by the protamine sulfate titration assay (0.2–0.4 International Units/mL); the limitation of this approach is that there is significant assay variability in the anti-Factor Xa activity assay

- Anti-Factor Xa activity assays have an advantage over aPTT for heparin monitoring in that results are less affected by preanalytic and biologic variables

- Some institutions monitor heparin infusion therapy using the heparin anti-Factor Xa activity levels directly instead of aPTT

Heparin anti-Xa level considerations

- Considerable variability in LMWH anti-Factor Xa activity assays exist, which can result in significant variation in the anti-Factor Xa activity results reported; characteristics shown to contribute to variability include the following:

    - Addition of exogenous AT

    - Anti-Factor Xa activity of the LMWH

    - Method manufacturer of kit

    - Instrument that level is performed on

    - Appropriate calibration is required

    - Using the UFH curve for measuring LMWH can underestimate LMWH effect

    - Using the LMWH curve for measuring UFH anticoagulation can overestimate UFH effect

    - Heparin levels determined by chromogenic heparin anti-Factor Xa activity are numerically higher than levels determined by protamine titration; avoid interchange of heparin level/activity results

(*continued*)

Table 18-20: (Continued)

- Pentasaccharide anti-Factor Xa activity monitoring also requires a different calibration curve than UFH or LMWH as the drug concentration is measured in different units (mg vs. anti-Factor Xa activity respectively)

  Note: although pentasaccharide anti-Factor Xa activity correlates with dose, a relationship between fondaparinux dose and clinical outcomes is lacking

Protamine Titration Method

- A heparin neutralization assay, not a routinely performed assay

- Estimates the heparin activity by identifying the lowest titer of protamine, which neutralizes the heparin induced clotting test prolongation; this amount is then compared to the amount needed to neutralize a known correlation of heparin

- The therapeutic range of 0.2–0.4 International Units/mL is based on a thrombogenic model in rabbits

- The CAP and ACCP indicate that heparin levels by protamine sulfate titration of 0.2–0.4 International Units/mL are equivalent to chromogenic heparin anti-Factor Xa activity levels of ~0.3–0.7 International Units/mL; not all data supports these equivalencies

- In patients undergoing cardiopulmonary bypass the Hepcon device can measure heparin levels using protamine sulfate titration; this method can be used for monitoring heparin anticoagulation during cardiopulmonary bypass, dosing protamine sulfate reversal after bypass, and residual heparin anticoagulation after protamine administration

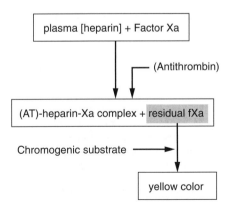

plasma [heparin] + Factor Xa

Optional supplementing of antithrombin

— (Antithrombin)

(AT)-heparin-Xa complex + residual fXa

Chromogenic substrate ⟶

yellow color

Amount of yellow color produced is inversely proportional to amount of anti-Factor Xa activity

Figure 18-9: Schematic of the Chromogenic Process for Determining Anti-Factor Xa Activity

Table 18-21: Clinical Applications of UFH Anti-Factor Xa Activity Testing (See Chapter 3)

- Anti-Factor Xa activity should be drawn at the time interval as recommended for aPTT monitoring of UFH anticoagulation

- Consider anti-Factor Xa activity monitoring over aPTT monitoring in

  - situations of suspected heparin resistance such as increased levels of factor VIII, heparin binding proteins, or fibrinogen

  - failure to increase aPTT despite heparin dose increases

  - lupus anticoagulant

  - pregnancy

  - situations where a lab cannot adequately perform regression analysis due to a lack of samples (small facilities, etc.)

- Warfarin does not affect the heparin anti-Factor Xa activity levels

- Heparin monitoring with anti-Factor Xa activity levels instead of the aPTT has been shown to result in fewer monitoring tests, fewer dose changes, and a higher percentage of therapeutic test results; earlier values within the anti-Factor Xa activity target range may result in fewer upward dosing titrations and a lower level of anticoagulation compared to the use of the aPTT, especially if aPTT targets are set at the upper end of the range (i.e., equivalent of 0.5–0.7 anti-Factor Xa activity units for VTE treatment)

- The relationship between anti-Factor Xa activity levels and clinical outcomes (thrombosis or major bleeding) is poorly defined; limited data suggests increased risk of bleeding when heparin concentration exceeds 0.7–0.8 units/mL by anti-Factor Xa activity analysis; patient-related factors are the most important determinants for bleeding complications

Clinical Pearl

Anti-Factor Xa activity testing:

- AT supplemented as part of the test may demonstrate a greater anti-Factor Xa activity effect (higher value) in patients with depressed AT activity or levels (<70%) compared to testing methods that do not include this step. Infusion of a source of AT such as FFP can increase reported anti-Factor Xa activity in tests that do not include AT.

  - Chromogenic anti-Factor Xa activity testing is most commonly used.

  - It is important to verify that the correct, calibrated curve is being used for the agent being tested.

- Anti-Factor Xa activity targets are different depending on method used.

- UFH anti-Xa activity cannot be differentiated from LMWH anti-Factor Xa activity in patients converting from one to the other.

Table 18-22: Clinical Applications of LMWH Anti-Factor Activity Xa Testing[a]

- The relationship between anti-Factor Xa activity levels and clinical outcomes (thrombosis or major bleeding) is not well defined in VTE and ACS

- The level of anti-Factor Xa activity accumulation in renal impairment varies by LMWH

   - Enoxaparin demonstrates an inverse linear relationship between CrCl and anti-Factor Xa activity level

   - With enoxaparin, anti-Factor Xa activity levels accumulate significantly with CrCl <40 mL/min

   - Dalteparin and tinzaparin do not appear to demonstrate significant anti-Factor Xa activity accumulation with renal impairment (CrCl >20 mL/min) when used for a short duration of therapy

- If anti-Factor Xa activity monitoring is desired, monitoring the trough level will allow for detection of accumulation

Potential candidates for LMWH anti-Factor Xa activity monitoring

- Renal insufficiency

- Newborn

- Low body weight

- Pediatrics

- Unexpected thrombosis on therapy

- Pregnant women

- Morbid obesity—BMI >40 kg/m^2 or actual body weight >190 kg

- Long-term therapy with therapeutic anticoagulation in patients with moderate renal impairment

- Data supporting beneficial outcomes of LMWH dose adjustment based on anti-Factor Xa activity levels do not yet exist

[a]Other substances influencing the effects of these agents that may have a larger role in renal failure (i.e., plasminogen activating inhibitor) on thrombosis and bleeding may not be reflected with singular measurement such as the anti-Factor Xa activity. Reported results should be used with caution in this setting until outcomes data is available. Poor correlation between anti-Factor Xa activity and estimated renal function or weight has been observed.[14]

Activated Clotting Time (ACT)
Table 18-23: Overview of the ACT Test

- A POC method, with normal range typically 80–130 sec (can vary)
- Used to monitor moderate to high dose heparin and DTI monitoring during cardiopulmonary bypass and other invasive intravascular procedures including cardiac angiography and intervention, intra-aortic balloon pumps, extracorporeal membrane oxygenation (ECMO), vascular surgery and carotid endarterectomy
- Results are affected by numerous factors including platelet count, platelet function, lupus anticoagulants, factor deficiency, test method, blood volume, technique employed, ambient temperature, and hemodilution
- Warfarin and glycoprotein IIb/IIIa inhibitors can increase the ACT; aprotinin effect is dependent on the contact activator used (celite >kaolin)
- Devices have a low range and a high range card, which will differ in heparin anticoagulation response (see Figure 18-10)
- Devices vary in contact activator used (celite and/or kaolin), method of clot detection and results therefore ACT values between devices are not comparable[15]
- There are differences between ACT devices, with Medtronic ACT device having positive bias as compared to Hemochron results

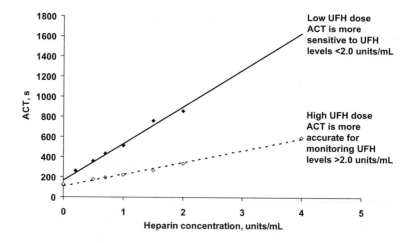

Figure 18-10: Heparin Response in Two Different ACT Cartridges: Low-Dose UFH and High-Dose UFH Anticoagulation

Clinical Pearls

ACT testing:

- If ACT is not responding to UFH anticoagulation, be sure that appropriate cartridge is being used prior to increasing drug. An aPTT or a heparin anti-Factor Xa activity level can also be checked to affirm drug effect.

- In the rare circumstance that a laboratory value such as the ACT is not responding despite sufficient administration of an anticoagulant (verification of the correct concentration and dose used), alternative testing such as a different ACT, aPTT, anti-Factor Xa activity should be considered. Selected patients transiently or long term may be uniquely nonresponsive to a selected test.

Table 18-24: Clinical Applications of the ACT

UFH Anticoagulation

- Relationship between ACT and ischemic complications during PCI is controversial; therefore, the optimal ACT range for heparin in PCI is not well established
- LMWH does not significantly prolong the ACT
- Options for patients with lupus anticoagulant undergoing cardiovascular surgery:
  - Double the baseline ACT
  - Use spiked samples to create a patient specific ACT heparin level titration curve to identify the ACT, which corresponds to the desired heparin level in the operating room, typically a whole blood concentration of >3 units/mL
  - Hepcon point-of-care device can be used to measure the ACT, which corresponds to a therapeutic heparin level (heparin levels measured with this device use protamine titration)

THROMBOELASTOGRAPHY [THEG] (SEE FIGURE 18-11)

Thromboelastography measures the viscoelastic properties of whole blood or recalcified citrated blood after inducing clot formation under low shear conditions.[16] The results of a TEG provides insights on all stages of thrombin formation in addition to clot stability. There are two primary instruments used: TEG analyzer (Haemoscope Corporation, Niles, IL) primarily used in the US, and ROTEM (Tem International GmbH, Munich, GE) is also FDA approved and available. THEG testing has been used in a variety of clinical settings to monitor hemostasis, including cardiopulmonary bypass surgery, hepatic surgeries, such as transplantation, monitoring efficacy of drug therapy, transfusion replacement requirements, and screening for hypercoagulable conditions.[16]

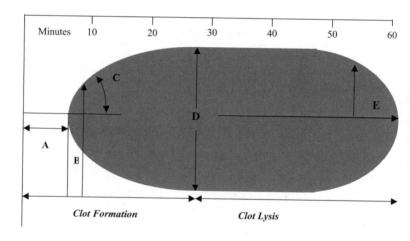

Figure 18-11: Thromboelastography Recording

Table 18-25: Interpretation of TEG and ROTEM
Thromboelastogram

Area	TEG	ROTEM	Process
A	r: clotting time	CT: clotting time	Initiation of thrombin formation, start of clot polymerization
B	k: amplitude to 20 mm	CFT: clot formation time, amplitude to 20 mm	Rate of clot formation, fibrin polymerization/crosslinking and platelet interaction
C	α°: slope between r and k	α° : angle of tangent a 2 mm amplitude	
D	MA: maximum amplitude	MCF: maximum clot firmness	Increased stabilization of clot by platelets and factor XIII
E	CL45; CL60: lysis after 45 and 60 min	LY30; LY 45 or ML: lysis at 30 or 45 min; maximum lysis	Degree of fibrinolysis after defined time/hr

Clinical Pearls

- Bleeding can sometimes be the result of a coagulopathy or low platelet function. The TEG can identify which system is impaired and guide management.

- Thrombosis driven by thrombin formation can be platelet or thrombin mediated, or a combination of both.

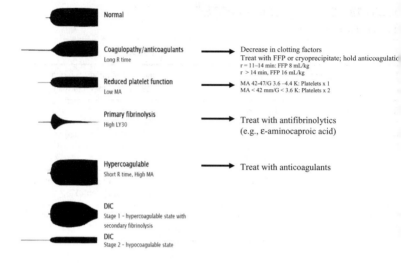

Figure 18-12: Thromboelastography: Interpretations and Treatments[17,18]

Note: treatment is only suggested if the patient is bleeding or if thrombosis risk is high enough to warrant the intervention.

REFERENCES

*Key articles

1. Clinical and Laboratory Standards Institute Document H21-A5. Collection, transport, and processing of blood specimens for testing plasma-based coagulation assays and molecular hemostasis assay: approved guideline (5th ed.). Available at: http://www.clsi.org www.clsi.org.

2. Clinical and Laboratory Standards Institute Document H47-A2. One-stage prothrombin time (PT) test and activated partial thromboplastin time (APTT) test: approved guideline (2nd ed.). Available at: http://www.clsi.org.

3. Clinical and Laboratory Standards Institute Document H54-A. Procedures for validation of INR and local calibration of PT/INR Systems: approved guideline (1st ed.). Available at: http://www.clsi.org.

4. US Department of Health and Human Services. Title 42 Public Health, Chapter IV Centers for Medicare & Medicaid Services, part 493: laboratory requirements. Available at: http://www.cms.gov.

5. **College of American Pathologists 2009 Hematology and Coagulation Checklist. Available at: http://www.cap.org www.cap.org.**

6. Gosselin R, Owings JT, White RH, et al. A comparison of point-of-care instruments designed for monitoring oral anticoagulation with standard laboratory methods. *Thromb Haemost.* 2000;83:698–703.

7. **Kemme MJ, Faaij RA, Schoemaker RC, et al. Disagreement between bedside and laboratory activated partial thromboplastin time and international normalized ratio for various novel anticoagulants. *Blood Coagul Fibrinolysis.* 2001;12:583–591.**

8. **Reiss RA, Haas CE, Griffis DL, et al. Point-of-care versus laboratory monitoring of patients receiving different anticoagulant therapies. *Pharmacotherapy.* 2002;22:677–685.**

9. Le DT, Weibert RT, Sevilla BK, et al. The international normalized ratio (INR) for monitoring warfarin therapy: reliability and relation to other monitoring methods. *Ann Intern Med.* 1994;120:552–558.

10. McGlasson DL, Romick BG, Rubal BJ. Comparison of a chromogenic factor X assay with international normalized ratio for monitoring oral anticoagulation therapy. *Blood Coagul Fibrinolysis.* 2008;19:513–517.

11. **Olson JD, Arkin CF, Brandt JT, et al. College of American Pathologists Conference XXXI on laboratory monitoring of anticoagulant therapy: laboratory monitoring of unfractionated heparin therapy. *Arch Pathol Lab Med.* 1998;122:782–798.**

12. Gosselin RC, King JH, Janatpour K, et al. Comparing direct thrombin inhibitors using aPTT, ecarin clotting time and thrombin inhibitor management testing. *Ann Pharmacother.* 2004;38:1383–1388.

13. Gosselin RC, Dager WE, King JH, et al. Effect of direct thrombin inhibitors, bivalirudin, lepirudin, and argatroban, on prothrombin time and INR values. *Am J Clin Pathol.* 2004;121:593–599.

14. Bazinet A, Almanric K, Brunet C, et al. Dosage of enoxaparin among obese and renal impairment patients. *Thromb Res.* 2005;116:41–50.

15. Despotis GJ, Filos KS, Levine V, et al. Aprotinin prolongs activated and nonactivated whole blood clotting time and potentiates the effect of heparin in vitro. *Anesth Analg.* 1996;82:1126–1131.

16. Luddington RJ. Thromboelastography/thromboelastometry. *Clin Lab Haem.* 2005;27:81–90.

17. Shore-Lesserson L, Manspeizer HE, DePerio M, et al. Thromboelastography-guided transfusion algorithm reduces transfusions in complex cardiac surgery. *Anesth Analg.* 1999;88:312–319.

18. Mallett SV, Cox DJ. Thrombelastography. *Br J Anaesth.* 1992;69:307–313.

Hypercoagulability Testing

Jessica B. Michaud

INTRODUCTION

Testing for hypercoagulable states, also called *thrombophilias*, is used to determine patients' risk of thrombosis. Hypercoagulable states can be inherited or acquired, and not all hypercoagulable states have been identified. Most hypercoagulable states have been associated with venous thromboembolism; there is limited information about any hypercoagulable state causing arterial thrombosis, except for hyperhomocysteinemia and antiphospholipid antibody (APLA) syndrome.[1] Hypercoagulability testing is controversial with regard to when, who, and what to test, and how positive hypercoagulability tests influence treatment decisions. Since several methods can be used for a given test for hypercoagulability, it is important to know which is used and any potential downfalls of the test. Testing should be considered if the results alter the management approach.

HYPERCOAGULABILITY TESTING

Basics of the hypercoagulable states

Table 19-1: Basic Information About Hypercoagulable States

Hypercoagulable State Category	Basic Information About Hypercoagulable States
Increased levels or function of natural procoagulants	Activated protein C resistance occurs when factor Va is resistant to inactivation by activated protein C • More factor Va results in higher factor IIa (thrombin) production

(continued)

Table 19-1: (Continued)

Hypercoagulable State Category	Basic Information About Hypercoagulable States
	• 90% to 95% of activated protein C resistance is caused by the factor V Leiden mutation[1-3]
	• Factor V Leiden mutation is a point mutation on the factor V gene that codes for the cleavage site of factor V by activated protein C[2,3]
	• Factor V Leiden mutation is one of the most common hypercoagulable states
	Prothrombin G20210A mutation on the prothrombin gene causes elevated circulating levels of otherwise normal prothrombin[2,4,5]
	Elevated levels of otherwise normal factors, especially of factors VIII, IX, and XI, can also result in a hypercoagulable state[2,6]; the cause is unknown but could be genetic[2]
Deficiencies of the natural anticoagulants	Deficiencies of antithrombin (formerly termed *antithrombin III*), protein C, and protein S are caused by >100 mutations each, making genetic testing impractical[4]
	Antithrombin inhibits factor IIa (thrombin), factor Xa, and other factors[2]
	Activated protein C, with its cofactor protein S, inhibits factors Va and VIIIa[2,4]
APLA syndrome	APLA syndrome is an acquired hypercoagulable state where auto-antibodies bind to phospholipids (e.g., cardiolipin), phospholipid-binding proteins (e.g., β_2-glycoprotein I), or both, causing arterial or venous thrombosis[7]
	APLA syndrome may be classified into patients with positive lupus anticoagulant tests, elevated anticardiolipin antibody levels, and/or elevated anti-β_2-glycoprotein I levels; the association between thrombosis and lupus anticoagulant (OR 11.0) is stronger than that for anticardiolipin antibody (OR 1.6)[8]
	APLA syndrome is its own distinct disorder but may coexist with rheumatologic diseases such as systemic lupus erythematosus

(*continued*)

Table 19-1: (Continued)

Hypercoagulable State Category	Basic Information About Hypercoagulable States
	The presence of APLAs is associated with anticoagulant (hence the term *lupus anticoagulant*) and procoagulant effects on the clotting system, but the usual eventual net result is a procoagulant effect[7]
	APLA syndrome may involve recurrent pregnancy loss, chronic thrombotic microangiopathy (causing organ dysfunction), thrombocytopenia, hemolytic anemia, and livedo reticularis, in addition to venous and arterial thromboembolism[7]
Hyperhomocysteinemia	Hyperhomocysteinemia, the elevation of the amino acid homocysteine in the plasma, signifies increased risk of arterial or venous thrombosis; mutations in several genes that code enzymes involved in homocysteine metabolism can lead to hyperhomocysteinemia[9]; it is not clear whether hyperhomocysteinemia causes thrombosis or whether venous thrombosis and ischemic cardiovascular disease elevate homocysteine[1,10]; lowering homocysteine levels with B vitamins does not lower thrombotic risk[11-17]

PREVALENCE AND RISK FOR THROMBOSIS OF HYPERCOAGULABLE STATES

Table 19-2: Prevalence and Thrombosis Risk for Selected Hypercoagulable States

Hypercoagulable State	Prevalence	Risk for Thrombosis
Activated protein C resistance (factor V Leiden mutation)	5% to 15%	3.8-fold increase[a] for heterozygotes
Prothrombin G20210A mutation	2% to 6%	2- to 3-fold increase
Elevated factor VIII levels	10%	>150 International Units/dL increases risk by 4.8-fold compared to <100 International Units/dL

(*continued*)

Table 19-2: (Continued)

Hypercoagulable State	Prevalence	Risk for Thrombosis
Antithrombin deficiency	<1%	8.1-fold increase 1% annual risk
Protein C deficiency[b]	0.2%	25- to 50-fold increase 1% annual risk
Protein S deficiency[b]	<1%	10- to 15-fold increase 1% annual risk
Antiphospholipid antibody syndrome	2% to 4%	5.5% annual risk
Hyperhomocysteinemia	5% to 10%	2.6-fold increase

[a]Factor V Leiden homozygotes carry a higher risk for VTE (about 18-fold increase).

[b]True combined protein C and protein S deficiency is rare. The more likely explanation for low levels of both proteins is poor timing of testing (e.g., during vitamin K antagonist therapy or acute thrombosis).

DIAGNOSTIC CONSIDERATIONS FOR HYPERCOAGULABLE STATES/TESTS

Types of hypercoagulable lab tests

Table 19-3: Types of Hypercoagulable Lab Tests

Type of Hypercoagulable Lab Test	Definition and Examples
Functional (activity)	Measures function of coagulation factors, sometimes based on a clotting test (e.g., antithrombin functional level, lupus anticoagulant)[18-20]
Quantitative (antigenic)	Measures quantitative levels of coagulation factors or antibodies using immunoassays such as ELISA (e.g., free protein S level, anticardiolipin antibody)[18-21]
Genetic	Genetic test (e.g., factor V Leiden mutation, prothrombin G20210A mutation); genetic tests can be done at any time

Available laboratory tests

Table 19-4: Available Laboratory Tests for Hypercoagulable States

Hypercoagulable State	Available Laboratory Tests	Comments
		Increased Levels or Function of Natural Procoagulants
Activated protein C resistance (factor V Leiden mutation)	Activated protein C resistance assay	The second-generation assay that uses factor V-deficient plasma is more accurate than the first-generation assay that does not use factor V-deficient plasma[3,22]; the APC resistance assay is easier to perform and less expensive than the factor V Leiden mutation genetic test[1]
	Factor V Leiden mutation genetic test (by polymerase chain reaction)	The genetic test by itself could miss the small percentage of patients that have activated protein C resistance not caused by factor V Leiden mutation; consider as a first test in patients with lupus anticoagulant or family history of factor V Leiden mutation; the genetic test is the only way to determine whether the patient is homozygous or heterozygous for factor V Leiden mutation
Prothrombin G20210A mutation	Prothrombin G20210A mutation genetic test (by polymerase chain reaction)	Because the range of factor II (prothrombin) values overlap considerably in patients with and without prothrombin G20210A mutation, testing for factor II functional or antigenic is not useful[1]
Elevated factor levels	Factors VIII, IX, or XI functional or antigenic[2,4]	A value of 100% is equivalent to 100 International Units/dL; inconsistent interlaboratory test results, unknown interactions, and unclear reference ranges makes testing challenging[9]
		Deficiencies of Natural Anticoagulants
Antithrombin deficiency	Antithrombin functional	A positive test should be rechecked to confirm the diagnosis[18,23]

(*continued*)

Table 19-4: (Continued)

Hypercoagulable State	Available Laboratory Tests	Comments
	Antithrombin antigenic	Testing just antithrombin antigenic can miss functionally abnormal antithrombin; although this test does not improve upon antithrombin functional to diagnose antithrombin deficiency, it has been suggested that antigenic testing can differentiate the subtype of deficiency, which could be important since certain subtypes confer greater thrombotic risk[1,18,23]; most tests ordered as "antithrombin test" are antigenic[1,4]
Protein C deficiency	Protein C functional	A positive test should be rechecked to confirm the diagnosis[19,24]
	Protein C antigenic	Testing just protein C antigenic can miss functionally abnormal protein C[4]
Protein S deficiency	Protein S functional	A positive functional or antigenic test should be rechecked to confirm the diagnosis[4,25,26]; this test may occasionally produce falsely normal results, so also testing total and free protein S antigenic is prudent[4,25]
	Total protein S antigenic	60% to 70% of total protein S is bound to the transport protein C4b-binding protein and is not available as a cofactor for activated protein C[9]
	Free protein S antigenic	The levels of C4b-binding protein, an acute-phase reactant, can fluctuate, influencing the proportion of free protein S[9]; free protein S antigenic is the preferred test for patients with lupus anticoagulant[25]

Antiphospholipid Antibody Syndrome
(see Table 19-7 for the APLA syndrome diagnostic criteria)

Lupus anticoagulant	Various clotting times (functional)	One positive lupus anticoagulant test is sufficient for diagnosis; two different negative tests are required to rule out lupus anticoagulant[27]; various lupus

(continued)

Table 19-4: (Continued)

Hypercoagulable State	Available Laboratory Tests	Comments
		anticoagulant tests exist, including those that measure the intrinsic pathway (aPTT, CSCT, KCT), the extrinsic pathway (dPT), and the final common pathway (dRVVT, taipan venom time, textarin time, ecarin time)[7]; INRs, especially point-of-care INRs, can be inaccurate (typically falsely elevated) in patients with positive lupus anticoagulant—correlation with chromogenic factor X or clot-based factor II or X activity should be done at least once during stable anticoagulation (see Chapter 18)[1]
Anticardiolipin antibody	Anticardiolipin antibodies (IgG, IgM, IgA) (antigenic)	Only anticardiolipin IgG and IgM are included in the APLA syndrome diagnostic criteria
Anti-β_2-glycoprotein I antibody	Anti-β_2-glycoprotein I antibodies (IgG, IgM, IgA) (antigenic)	Only anti-β_2-glycoprotein I IgG and IgM are included in the APLA syndrome diagnostic criteria
	Hyperhomocysteinemia	
Hyperhomocysteinemia	Homocysteine plasma level	There are many acquired causes of hyperhomocysteinemia (see Table 19-5); although fasting levels are often recommended, it is probably not clinically relevant whether a patient is fasting or not[1,10]
	Genetic tests	Genetic tests for mutations causing hyperhomocysteinemia are not directly associated with thrombosis; examples of these genes are MTHFR (most commonly C677T and A1298C mutations), cystathione β synthase, or methionine synthase[9]

Clinical Pearl

- Some laboratories may batch routine hypercoagulable tests into a panel that includes multiple tests. In some situations (i.e., suspicion for antithrombin deficiency), a selected hypercoagulable test may be requested on a more emergent basis. Check with the laboratory on the assay turnaround time and to see if ordering differently will expedite the process.

HYPERCOAGULABLE LABORATORY INTERACTIONS WITH MEDICAL CONDITIONS AND NONANTITHROMBOTIC MEDICATIONS

As detailed in Table 19-5, many hypercoagulable tests can be inaccurate in the setting of acute thrombosis. Other medical conditions can also influence hypercoagulability tests; therefore, how long an interacting factor takes to resolve should be considered when determining appropriate timing of testing. Genetic tests can be checked at anytime, without regard to medications or medical conditions. Nongenetic tests must be ordered before anticoagulation therapy is started or when therapy is discontinued/on hold (see Table 19-6). Suspicious diagnoses (e.g., positive protein C and positive protein S deficiency in a single patient) should be rechecked.

Table 19-5: Hypercoagulable Laboratory Interactions with Medical Conditions and Nonantithrombotic Medications

Hypercoagulable Laboratory Test	Factors That May Decrease Value of Laboratory Test[a]	Factors That May Increase Value of Laboratory Test
Increased Levels or Function of Natural Procoagulants		
Activated protein C resistance assay with factor V-deficient plasma	Lupus anticoagulant (false positive)[3,22,28]	None
Factor V Leiden mutation genetic test	None	None
Prothrombin G20210A mutation genetic test	None	None
Factors VIII, IX, and XI tests	<ul><li>Conditions associated with vitamin K deficiency, such as malnutrition and hepatic or biliary disease (for factor IX)[29]</li><li>Acute, large trauma</li><li>Nephrotic syndrome (for factor IX)[29]</li><li>O blood type compared to A or B blood types (for factor VIII)[29]</li></ul>	<ul><li>Acute illness</li><li>Chronic inflammation</li><li>Estrogen, pregnancy, oral contraceptives</li><li>Recent aerobic exercise</li><li>Aging[9,29,30]</li></ul>

(continued)

Table 19-5: (Continued)

Hypercoagulable Laboratory Test	Factors That May Decrease Value of Laboratory Test[a]	Factors That May Increase Value of Laboratory Test
	Deficiencies of Natural Anticoagulants	
Antithrombin tests	• Acute thrombotic event • Acquired conditions that impair antithrombin synthesis (e.g., liver disease, malnutrition, premature infancy, IBD, extensive burns) • Conditions that result in loss of protein (e.g., DIC, acute hemolytic transfusion reaction, thrombotic microangiopathy, malignancy, L-asparaginase therapy, nephrotic syndrome) • After major vascular surgery with lowest levels noted the 3rd post-op day[9]	• Postmenopausal period[9]
Protein C tests	• Acute thrombotic event • Vitamin K deficiency • Liver disease • DIC • Sepsis • Renal insufficiency • Nephrotic syndrome (functional level can be low or high)	• Diabetes • Ischemic heart disease • Pregnancy • Postmenopausal period • Hormone replacement therapy • Oral contraceptive therapy

(continued)

Table 19-5: (Continued)

Hypercoagulable Laboratory Test	Factors That May Decrease Value of Laboratory Test[a]	Factors That May Increase Value of Laboratory Test
	• Postoperative state	• Nephrotic syndrome (functional level can be low or high)[19]
	• Adult respiratory distress syndrome	• Lupus anticoagulant[19]
	• After plasma exchange	
	• In breast cancer patients with some types of chemotherapy	
	• After massive hemorrhage and dilution with crystalloid solutions	
	• Elevated factor VIII (falsely low protein C functional)	
	• Newborns have naturally lower protein C[9]	
Protein S tests	• Acute thrombotic event	• Adults compared to newborns
	• Female gender compared to male gender	• Postmenopausal state
	• Oral contraceptive use (depends on product and type of progestin used)	• Increasing age in women (although hormonal status may account for this difference)[9]
	• Pregnancy	
	• Liver disease	
	• Nephrotic syndrome	
	• DIC	
	• High factor VIII levels and lupus anticoagulant (falsely low protein S functional)[9]	

(continued)

Table 19-5: (Continued)

Hypercoagulable Laboratory Test	Factors That May Decrease Value of Laboratory Test[a]	Factors That May Increase Value of Laboratory Test
Antiphospholipid Antibody Syndrome		
Lupus anticoagulant tests	None	None
Anticardiolipin antibodies (IgG, IgM, IgA)	None	None
Anti-β_2-glycoprotein I antibodies (IgG, IgM, IgA)	None	None
Hyperhomocysteinemia		
Homocysteine	None	• Acute thrombosis (for up to several months) • Vitamin B6, B12, or folate deficiency • Renal insufficiency • Hypothyroidism • Psoriasis • IBD • Rheumatoid arthritis • Organ transplantation • Drugs (anticonvulsants, L-dopa, niacin, methotrexate, thiazides, cyclosporine)

Table 19-5: (Continued)

Hypercoagulable Laboratory Test	Factors That May Decrease Value of Laboratory Test[a]	Factors That May Increase Value of Laboratory Test
		• Lifestyle factors (physical inactivity, smoking, coffee consumption) • Increasing age • Postmenopausal state • Male gender[10]
Mutations associated with hyperhomocysteinemia	None	None

[a]See Clinical Pearl below.

Clinical Pearl

- If a hypercoagulable laboratory test is normal during a medical condition that could potentially reduce the test value, the laboratory test can be considered normal (e.g., a normal antithrombin test during an acute thrombotic event rules out antithrombin deficiency).

HYPERCOAGULABLE LABORATORY INTERACTIONS WITH ANTITHROMBOTIC MEDICATIONS

Table 19-6: Hypercoagulable Laboratory Interactions with Concurrent Antithrombotic Medications

Hypercoagulable Laboratory Test	Warfarin[a]	Heparin or Low Molecular Weight Heparins (LMWHs)[a]
Increased Levels or Function of Natural Procoagulants		
Activated protein C resistance assay with factor V-deficient plasma	Reliable[9]	Reliable if factor-V deficient plasma used[9]
Factor V Leiden mutation genetic test	Reliable[9]	Reliable[9]
Prothrombin G20210A mutation genetic test	Reliable[9]	Reliable[9]
Factor VIII tests	Reliable[4]	Reliable[4]
Factor IX tests	Likely to be decreased[4,29]	Reliable[4]
Factor XI tests	Reliable[4]	Reliable[4]
Deficiencies of Natural Anticoagulants		
Antithrombin tests	May be increased[9]	May be decreased, although the amidolytic assays should not be affected (waiting at least 5 days after cessation of heparin to test is safe)[4,9,18,23]

(*continued*)

Table 19-6: (Continued)

Hypercoagulable Laboratory Test	Warfarin[a]	Heparin or Low Molecular Weight Heparins (LMWHs)[a]
Protein C tests	Likely to be decreased (wait until 2–4 weeks after warfarin is discontinued before testing; the functional amidolytic assays may also be overestimated)[9,19]	May be increased (clot-based functional tests are most likely to be affected; may also be increased by direct thrombin inhibitors)[19]
Protein S tests	Likely to be decreased (wait until 2–4 weeks after warfarin is discontinued before testing)[9,26]	Reliable[9]
Antiphospholipid Antibody Syndrome		
Lupus anticoagulant tests	May be increased (resulting in a false positive)[31]	May be increased (resulting in a false positive) depending on heparin level[31]
Anticardiolipin antibodies (IgG, IgM, IgA)	Reliable	Reliable
Anti-β_2-glycoprotein I antibodies (IgG, IgM, IgA)	Reliable	Reliable
Hyperhomocysteinemia		
Plasma homocysteine level	Reliable[9]	Reliable[9]
Mutations associated with hyperhomocysteinemia	Reliable[9]	Reliable[9]

[a]See Clinical Pearl below.

Clinical Pearl

- If a hypercoagulable laboratory test is normal during use of a medication that could potentially reduce the test value, the laboratory test can be considered normal (e.g., a normal protein C test during warfarin therapy rules out protein C deficiency).

ANTIPHOSPHOLIPID ANTIBODY SYNDROME DIAGNOSTIC CRITERIA

Table 19-7: APLA Syndrome Diagnostic Criteria

Criteria for Definite APLA Syndrome (revised Sapporo criteria; one clinical and one laboratory criteria must be met)

Clinical criteria	Vascular thrombosis: ≥1 clinical episode of arterial, venous, or small vessel thrombosis (excluding superficial venous thrombosis) in any tissue or organ, OR
	Pregnancy morbidity: 1. ≥1 unexplained death of a morphologically normal fetus at or beyond the 10th week of gestation, OR
	2. ≥1 premature birth of a morphologically normal neonate before the 34th week of gestation because of (1) eclampsia or severe preeclampsia or (2) recognized features of placental insufficiency, OR
	3. ≥3 unexplained consecutive spontaneous abortions before the 10th week of gestation, with maternal anatomic or hormonal abnormalities and paternal and maternal chromosomal causes excluded
Laboratory criteria (must be present on ≥2 occasions at least 12 weeks apart)	Lupus anticoagulant present in plasma, OR
	Anticardiolipin antibody of IgG and/or IgM isotype in serum or plasma, present in medium or high titer (i.e., >40 GPL or MPL, or >the 99th percentile), OR
	Anti-β_2-glycoprotein I antibody of IgG and/or IgM isotype in serum or plasma (in titer >the 99th percentile)

Source: adapted from reference 27.

SUMMARY OF RECOMMENDED HYPERCOAGULABLE LAB TESTS

Table 19-8: Summary of Recommended Hypercoagulable Lab Tests[a]

Hypercoagulable State	Recommended Laboratory Tests
Increased Levels or Function of Natural Procoagulants	
Activated protein C resistance (factor V Leiden mutation)	APC resistance assay with factor V-deficient plasma or FVL genetic test (or use FVL genetic test as a confirmatory test for a positive APC resistance assay)[1,3,4,32,33]
Prothrombin G20210A mutation	Prothrombin G20210A mutation genetic test
Elevated factor levels	Factor VIII antigenic or functional[1,29,34,35]
Deficiencies of Natural Anticoagulants	
Antithrombin deficiency	Antithrombin functional (amidolytic assay)[18]
Protein C deficiency	Protein C functional[4,19,24]
Protein S deficiency	Protein S functional and/or free protein S antigenic +/− total protein S antigenic[4,25]
Antiphospholipid Antibody Syndrome	
Lupus anticoagulant	Various (see Table 19-4)
Anticardiolipin antibody	Anticardiolipin antibodies (IgG, IgM, IgA)
Anti-β_2-glycoprotein I antibody	Anti-β_2-glycoprotein I antibodies (IgG, IgM, IgA)
Hyperhomocysteinemia	
Hyperhomocysteinemia and associated mutations	Possibly plasma homocysteine level[1,34,36]

[a]Testing for hypercoagulable states should include all recommended tests, since the presence of more than one hypercoagulable state (e.g., factor V Leiden mutation + prothrombin G20210A mutation) increases the risk beyond that of one hypercoagulable state.[37]

TREATMENT CONSIDERATIONS

Table 19-9: General Treatment Considerations

Topic	Treatment Considerations
General treatment considerations	• Except for APLA syndrome and hyperhomocysteinemia, the drug choice for thrombosis associated with a hypercoagulable state is the same as treatment of the thrombosis without a hypercoagulable state
	• The presence of the hypercoagulable state may influence decisions about duration of therapy or what to do during high-risk situations (surgical procedures, hospitalizations, pregnancy, subtherapeutic INRs, etc.)
	• Although the 2008 ACCP guidelines do not cite the presence of a hypercoagulable state as a major factor to guide duration of therapy for VTE, the authors go on to detail hereditary thrombophilia as one of the most clinically useful risk factors in patients with unprovoked VTE[38]
	• According to the ACCP guidelines, when designing periprocedure anticoagulation, the presence of "severe thrombophilic conditions (deficiency of protein C, protein S, or antithrombin, antiphospholipid antibodies, or multiple thrombophilic abnormalities)" is one of the factors that signifies patients as "high risk", the presence of "nonsevere thrombophilic conditions (heterozygous carrier of factor V Leiden mutation or factor II mutation)" implies "moderate risk"[39]
General treatment considerations for VTE	• For duration of therapy for patients with unprovoked VTE, the ACCP guidelines currently state, " ...we recommend treatment with a VKA for at least 3 months (Grade 1A). We recommend that after 3 months of anticoagulant therapy, all patients with unprovoked DVT should be evaluated for the risk-to-benefit ratio of long-term therapy (Grade 1C). For patients with a first unprovoked VTE that is a proximal DVT, and in whom risk factors

(continued)

Table 19-9: (Continued)

Topic	Treatment Considerations
	for bleeding are absent and for whom good anticoagulant monitoring is achievable, we recommend long-term treatment (Grade 1A). For patients with a second episode of unprovoked VTE, we recommend long-term treatment (Grade 1A). For patients with a first isolated distal DVT that is unprovoked, we suggest that 3 months of anticoagulant therapy is sufficient rather than indefinite therapy (Grade 2B)."[38]
	• In making decisions about duration of therapy for unprovoked VTE, it may be reasonable to consider hypercoagulable states, especially higher-risk hypercoagulable states—deficiency of antithrombin, protein C, or protein S; APLA syndrome (see below); or multiple hypercoagulable states—in determining thrombotic risk
	• It is important to use the presence of hypercoagulable states as only one factor in evaluating thrombotic risk
	• Many prospective studies have shown no increased risk of *recurrent thromboembolism* in patients with hypercoagulable states, but there are no studies designed to evaluate recurrence in patients with hypercoagulable states randomized to intermediate-term vs. indefinite durations of therapy[38]
	• When determining patients' thrombotic risk, acquired hypercoagulable states such as cancer, pregnancy, estrogen-containing oral contraceptives, and hormone replacement therapy should be considered, in addition to hereditary hypercoagulable states and other clinical factors[9]
General treatment considerations for ischemic CVA or TIA	• Because activated protein C resistance/factor V Leiden mutation, prothrombin G20210A mutation, and MTHFR C677T mutation have been linked (although weakly) to ischemic CVA, it may be reasonable to evaluate patients with a CVA or TIA for hypercoagulable states; DVT, and an atrial or ventricular septal defect (such as patent foramen ovale) in order to determine whether an undiagnosed DVT caused the CVA via a septal defect[40]; if a DVT is found, it may be reasonable to use an oral vitamin K antagonist to prevent future ischemic events

(continued)

Table 19-9: (Continued)

Topic	Treatment Considerations
General treatment considerations for ischemic CVA or TIA	• The AHA/ASA stroke guidelines recommend evaluating for a DVT in patients with an established hypercoagulable state who have a CVA or TIA (Class IIa [there is conflicting evidence and/or divergence of opinion but weight of evidence is in favor of the treatment], Level of Evidence B [data derived from single randomized trial or nonrandomized studies])[40] • Based on the WARSS/APASS study, the AHA/ASA guidelines state that antiplatelet therapies are reasonable for patients with an ischemic CVA or TIA and positive APLAs (Class IIa, Level of Evidence B, see above for definitions of Class and Level)[40,41]; however, the guidelines state that oral anticoagulation with goal INR of 2–3 is reasonable for patients with ischemic CVA or TIA who have APLA syndrome including venous and arterial occlusive disease in multiple organs, miscarriages, and livedo reticularis (Class IIa, Level of Evidence B, see above for definitions of Class and Level)[40]; the WARSS/APASS study showed that APLAs did not have a significant effect on the risk of CVA recurrence and found that aspirin 325 mg daily was equivalent to warfarin titrated to an INR goal of 1.4–2.8 in preventing a composite endpoint of death from any cause, ischemic CVA, TIA, myocardial infarction, DVT, PE, and other systemic thrombo-occlusive events[41]

Table 19-10: Treatment Considerations for Increased Levels or Function of Natural Procoagulants

Hypercoagulable State	Treatment Considerations
	Increased levels or function of natural procoagulants
Activated protein C resistance (factor V Leiden mutation) and prothrombin G20210A mutation	• Although some studies have shown a significant effect on *recurrence* of VTE (4- to 5-fold higher), most studies have shown little effect[34,42]; for this reason, these mutations are less likely to result in a decision to anticoagulate indefinitely
Elevated factor levels	• Elevation of factor VIII has shown some utility in predicting VTE recurrence[35,43] although not in all studies[34]

Table 19-11: Treatment Considerations for Deficiencies of Natural Anticoagulants

Hypercoagulable State	Treatment Considerations
	Deficiencies of Natural Anticoagulants
Antithrombin deficiency	• Patients with antithrombin deficiency may have difficulty reaching therapeutic anticoagulation with UFH, LMWH, or fondaparinux despite high doses, since they rely on antithrombin for their mechanism of action; in this case, it may be advisable to use a direct thrombin inhibitor (e.g., argatroban, lepirudin) instead[9]

(continued)

Table 19-11: (Continued)

Hypercoagulable State	Treatment Considerations
	Deficiencies of Natural Anticoagulants
Antithrombin, protein C, and protein S deficiencies	• Replacement of antithrombin, protein C, or protein S in patients with a deficiency could be considered in certain situations (e.g., difficulty achieving adequate anticoagulation, very severe thrombosis, neonatal purpura fulminans, recurrent thrombosis despite adequate anticoagulation, or need for prophylaxis perioperatively or peripartum) • Replacement products are antithrombin concentrate for antithrombin, fresh frozen plasma or prothrombin complex concentrate for protein C or S, and protein C concentrate for protein C[9,44]
Protein C and S deficiency	• Patients with protein C or S deficiency starting or restarting warfarin should be given UFH, LMWH, or fondaparinux at the same time until the INR is therapeutic and stable • Warfarin initiation rapidly lowers protein C and S levels before factors II, VII, IX, and X are sufficiently suppressed, which can precipitate warfarin skin necrosis or other thrombotic event, especially in patients with underlying deficiency of protein C or S; "loading" doses of warfarin should also be avoided in these patients[9]

Table 19-12: Treatment Considerations for APLA Syndrome and Hyperhomocysteinemia

Hypercoagulable State	Treatment Considerations
	Antiphospholipid Antibody Syndrome
Antiphospholipid antibody syndrome	• Treatment of pregnant patients with APLA syndrome is covered in Chapter 16
	• Generally, patients with APLA syndrome and VTE are treated indefinitely due to the high risk of recurrence
	• In patients with arterial thromboembolism and APLA syndrome, it is not clear whether long-term warfarin should be used or whether antiplatelet therapy is sufficient[45,46]
	• There are no data to support pharmacologic therapy in patients with APLA syndrome and no arterial thrombosis, but low-dose aspirin could be considered, especially in patients with other cardiovascular risk factors[46]
	• There has been some controversy about the appropriate goal INR for patients with APLA syndrome
	• Two randomized trials have shown that INRs of >3.0 or 3.1 do not reduce thrombotic events compared to INRs of 2–3, although there was considerable overlap in the INR ranges[47,48]
	• These trials did not include many patients with arterial thrombosis, so conclusions cannot be made on the appropriate goal INR for these patients
	• The ACCP guidelines recommend a goal INR of 2.5 (range 2–3), except for patients who have had a recurrent thromboembolic event at a therapeutic INR or who have other additional risk factors for a thromboembolic event, in which case the recommended goal is 3 (range 2.5–3.5)[49]
	• Lupus anticoagulant can falsely elevate the aPTT and INR, at baseline and in patients treated with antithrombotics, potentially causing patients to be undertreated

(*continued*)

Table 19-12: (Continued)

Hypercoagulable State	Treatment Considerations
	• In patients treated with UFH, an antifactor Xa assay can be used in place of the aPTT for monitoring, and in patients treated with warfarin, a chromogenic factor X assay can be used in place of or in conjunction with the INR[9,50]
	• It may be reasonable to target a higher INR range for warfarin therapy in patients with elevated baseline INR
	• False INR elevation occurs in a small subset (~19%) of patients with lupus anticoagulant taking warfarin and depends on the thromboplastin used[50]
	• Point-of-care testing was shown to be comparable to plasma-based testing, except when the point-of-care INR was >4 and in 5 of 59 patients whose INR was unreadable on one of the point-of-care meters tested[50]
	• However, in 88% of patients with INRs >3 on the point-of-care meter, the chromogenic factor X assay was therapeutic[50]
	• A reasonable approach would be to check a chromogenic factor X assay at least once during a stable interval in a patient's course of therapy to verify that the point-of-care or plasma-based INR is accurate in that patient, and to recheck point-of-care INRs >4 with a plasma-based INR or chromogenic factor X assay[4]
Hyperhomocysteinemia	
Hyperhomocysteinemia and associated mutations	• For patients with ischemic CVA or TIA and hyperhomocysteinemia, a daily multivitamin containing adequate vitamin B6 (1.7 mg), vitamin B12 (2.4 mcg), and folate (400 mcg) is recommended in the AHA/ASA guidelines due to its safety and low cost, even though it is recognized that reducing homocysteine does not lead to reduced CVA (Class IIa, Level of Evidence B, see Table 19-9 for definitions of Class and Level)[40]

PROS AND CONS OF HYPERCOAGULABILITY TESTING

Table 19-13: Pros and Cons of Hypercoagulability Testing

Pros	Cons
• Identification of patients who may benefit from indefinite anticoagulation	• High cost of testing
• Identification of patients who may benefit from anticoagulation during high-risk periods	• Low likelihood of detecting hereditary hypercoagulable states
	• Inconclusive and conflicting data for indefinite anticoagulation in hereditary hypercoagulable states
• Prevention of pregnancy complications	
• Detection of potential increased thrombotic risk for family members	• Lack of universal physician awareness of how to interpret test results
• Explanation of possible cause of thrombosis	• Risk of being denied health insurance coverage or of higher premium payments
	• Potential for laboratory error
	• False reassurance to patients with negative results

SUMMARY

Testing for hypercoagulable states is controversial because there are conflicting data about the risk of initial and recurrent thrombosis for many of the thrombophilias. However, testing may help determine thrombotic risk, which may ultimately help guide clinical decisions regarding duration of anticoagulation or therapy during high-risk periods. Recommendations for specific laboratory tests are made, should a hypercoagulability workup be performed. There are numerous lab–disease and lab–drug interactions; therefore, laboratory tests must be carefully timed, and unclear diagnoses should be confirmed by repeat testing. Understanding hypercoagulable laboratory tests is essential to appropriate diagnosis and treatment of these disorders.

REFERENCES

*Key articles

1.   Moll S. Blood coagulation, thrombosis, antithrombotics, and hypercoagulable states. In: Ansell JE, Oertel LB, Wittkowski AK, eds. *Managing Oral Anticoagulation Therapy Clinical and Operational Guidelines.* 3rd ed. St. Louis, MO: Wolters Kluwer Health; 2009:85–104.

* 2. Crowther MA, Kelton JG. Congenital thrombophilic states associated with venous thrombosis: a qualitative overview and proposed classification system. *Ann Intern Med.* 2003;138:128–134.

3. Press RD, Bauer KA, Kujovich JL, et al. Clinical utility of factor V Leiden (R506Q) testing for the diagnosis and management of thromboembolic disorders. *Arch Pathol Lab Med.* 2002;126:1304–1318.

* 4. Moll S. Thrombophilias—practical implications and testing caveats. *J Thromb Thrombolysis.* 2006;21:7–15.

5. McGlennen RC, Key NS. Clinical and laboratory management of the prothrombin G20210A mutation. *Arch Pathol Lab Med.* 2002;126:1319–1325.

6. Chandler WL, Rodgers GM, Sprouse JT, et al. Elevated hemostatic factor levels as potential risk factors for thrombosis. *Arch Pathol Lab Med.* 2002;126:1405–1414.

* 7. Levine JS, Branch DW, Rauch J. The antiphospholipid antibody syndrome. *N Engl J Med.* 2002;346:752–763.

8. Lim W, Crowther MA, Eikelboom JW. Management of antiphospholipid antibody syndrome: a systematic review. *JAMA.* 2006;295:1050–1057.

* 9. Nutescu EA, Michaud JB, Caprini JA. Evaluation of hypercoagulable states and molecular markers of acute venous thrombosis. In: Gloviczki P, ed. *Handbook of Venous Disorders.* 3rd ed. London, UK: Hodder Arnold; 2009 113–128.

10. Key NS, McGlennen RC. Hyperhomocyst(e)inemia and thrombophilia. *Arch Pathol Lab Med.* 2002:126:1367–1375.

11. Ray JG, Kearon C, Yi Q, et al. Homocysteine-lowering therapy and risk for venous thromboembolism. *Ann Intern Med.* 2007;146:761–767.

12. Ebbing M, Bleie Ø, Ueland PM, et al. Mortality and cardiovascular events in patients treated with homocysteine-lowering B vitamins after coronary angiography. *JAMA* 2008;300:795–804.

13. Bazzano LA, Reynolds K, Holder KN, et al. Effect of folic acid supplementation on risk of cardiovascular diseases. *JAMA.* 2006;296:2720–2726.

14. Lonn E, Yusuf S, Arnold MJ, et al. Homocysteine lowering with folic acid and B vitamins in vascular disease. *N Engl J Med.* 2006;354:1567–1577.

15. den Heijer M, Willems HPJ, Blom HJ, et al. Homocysteine lowering by B vitamins and the secondary prevention of deep-vein thrombosis and pulmonary embolism: a randomized, placebo-controlled, double blind trial. *Blood.* 2007;109:139–144.

16. Toole JF, Malinow MR, Chambless LE, et al. Lowering homocysteine in patients with ischemic stroke to prevent recurrent stroke, myocardial infarction, and death: the vitamin intervention for stroke prevention (VISP) randomized controlled trial. *JAMA* 2004;291:565–575.

17. Bønaa KH, Njølstad I, Ueland PM, et al. Homocysteine lowering and cardiovascular events after acute myocardial infarction. *N Engl J Med.* 2006;354:1578–1588.

18. Kottke-Marchant K, Duncan A. Antithrombin deficiency: issues in laboratory diagnosis. *Arch Pathol Lab Med.* 2002;126:1326–1336.

19. Kottke-Marchant K, Comp P. Laboratory issues in diagnosing abnormalities of protein C, thrombomodulin, and endothelial cell protein C receptor. *Arch Pathol Lab Med.* 2002;126:1337–1348.

20. Goodwin AJ, Rosendaal FR, Kottke-Marchant K, et al. A review of the technical, diagnostic, and epidemiologic considerations for protein S assays. *Arch Pathol Lab Med.* 2002;126:1349–1366.

21. Ortel TL. The antiphospholipid syndrome: What are we really measuring? How do we measure it? And how do we treat it? *J Thromb Thrombolysis.* 2006;21:79–83.

22. Rosendorff A, Dorfman DM. Activated protein C resistance and factor V Leiden: a review. *Arch Pathol Lab Med.* 2007;131:866–871.

23. Patnaik MM, Moll S. Inherited antithrombin deficiency: a review. *Haemophilia.* 2008;14:1229–1239.

24. Goldenberg NA, Manco-Johnson MJ. Protein C deficiency. *Haemophilia.* 2008;14:1214–1221.

25. Goodwin AJ, Rosendaal FR, Kottke-Marchant K, et al. A review of the technical, diagnostic, and epidemiologic considerations for protein S assays. *Arch Pathol Lab Med.* 2002;26:1349–1366.

26. Ten Kate MK, Van der Meer J. Protein S deficiency: a clinical perspective. *Haemophilia.* 2008;14:1222–1228.

27. Miyakis S, Lockshin MD, Atsumi T, et al. International consensus statement on an update of the classification criteria for definite antiphospholipid syndrome (APS). *J Thromb Haemost.* 2006;4:295–306.

28. Le DT, Griffin JH, Greengard JS, et al. Use of a generally applicable tissue factor-dependent factor V assay to detect activated protein C-resistant factor Va in patients receiving warfarin and in patients with a lupus anticoagulant. *Blood.* 1995;85:1704–1711.

29. Chandler WL, Rodgers GM, Sprouse JT, et al. Elevated hemostatic factor levels as potential risk factors for thrombosis. *Arch Pathol Lab Med.* 2002;126:1405–1414.

30. Lippi G, Maffulli N. Biological influence of physical exercise on hemostasis. *Semin Thromb Hemost.* 2009;35:269–276.

31. Teruya J, West AG, Suell MN. Lupus anticoagulant assays. *Arch Pathol Lab Med.* 2007;131:885–889.

32. Van Cott EM, Laposata M, Prins MH. Laboratory evaluation of hypercoagulability with venous or arterial thrombosis. *Arch Pathol Lab Med.* 2002;126:1281–1295.

33. Van Cott EM, Soderberg BL, Laposata M. Activated protein C resistance, the factor V Leiden mutation, and a laboratory testing algorithm. *Arch Pathol Lab Med.* 2002;126:57–582.

* 34. **Christiansen SC, Cannegieter SC, Koster T, et al. Thrombophilia, clinical factors, and recurrent venous thrombotic events. *JAMA*. 2005;293:2352–2361.**

35. Pabinger I, Ay C. Biomarkers and venous thromboembolism. *Arterioscler Thromb Vasc Biol*. 2009;29:332–336.

36. Eldibany MM, Caprini JA. Hyperhomocysteinemia and thrombosis. *Arch Pathol Lab Med*. 2007;131:872–884.

* 37. **Dalen J. Should patients with venous thromboembolism be screened for thrombophilia? *Am J Med*. 2008;121:458–463.**

38. Kearon C, Kahn SR, Agnelli G, et al. Antithrombotic therapy for venous thromboembolic disease. *Chest*. 2008;133:454S–545S.

39. Douketis JD, Berger PB, Dunn AS, et al. The perioperative management of antithrombotic therapy. *Chest*. 2008;133:299S–339S.

40. Sacco RL, Adams R, Albers G, et al. Guidelines for prevention of stroke in patients with ischemic stroke or transient ischemic attack: a statement for healthcare professionals from the American Heart Association/American Stroke Association Council on Stroke co-sponsored by the Council on Cardiovascular Radiology and Intervention. *Stroke* 2006;37:577–617.

41. Levine SR, Brey RL, Tilley BC, et al. Antiphospholipid antibodies and subsequent thrombo-occlusive events in patients with ischemic stroke. *JAMA* 2004;291:576–584.

42. Ho WK, Hankey GJ, Quinlan DJ, et al. Risk of recurrent venous thromboembolism in patients with common thrombophilia: a systematic review. *Arch Intern Med*. 2006;166:729–736.

43. Cosmi B, Legnani C, Cini M, et al. D-dimer and factor VIII are independent risk factors for recurrence after anticoagulation withdrawal for a first idiopathic deep vein thrombosis. *Thromb Res*. 2008;122:610–617.

44. Bauer KA. Management of inherited thrombophilia. In: Basow DS, ed. *UpToDate*. Waltham, MA: UpToDate; 2009.

45. Albers GW, Amarenco P, Easton JD, et al. Antithrombotic and thrombolytic therapy for ischemic stroke. *Chest*. 2008;133:630S–669S.

46. Brey RL. Management of the neurological manifestations of APS—what do the trials tell us? *Thromb Res*. 2004;114:489–499.

47. Crowther MA, Ginsberg JS, Julian J, et al. A comparison of two intensities of warfarin for the prevention of recurrent thrombosis in patients with the antiphospholipid antibody syndrome. *N Engl J Med*. 2003;349:1133–1138.

48. Finazzi G, Marchioli R, Brancaccio V, et al. A randomized clinical trial of high-intensity warfarin vs. conventional antithrombotic therapy for the prevention of recurrent thrombosis in patients with the antiphospholipid syndrome (WAPS). *J Thromb Haemost*. 2005;3:848–853.

49. Ansell J, Hirsh J, Hylek E, et al. Pharmacology and management of the vitamin K antagonists. *Chest*. 2008;133:160S–198S.

50. Perry SL, Samsa GP, Ortel TL. Point-of-care testing of the international normalized ratio in patients with antiphospholipid antibodies. *Thromb Haemost*. 2005;94: 1196–1202.

Appendix

Coagulation Cascade

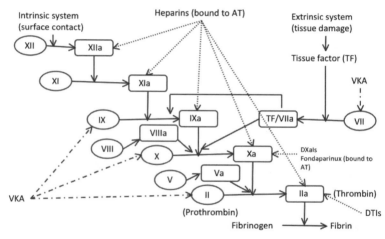

Key

VKA= vitamin K antagonist (example warfarin)
AT= antithrombin
DTIs= direct thrombin inhibitors (example argatroban)
DXaIs= direct Xa inhibitors (example rivaroxaban)

⬭ = inactive clotting factor

▭ = active clotting factor

– · – · – > = inhibits production

———> = enhances/promotes production

···········> = inactivates factor

Child-Pugh Score for Liver Impairment

Child-Pugh Score			
Score	**1**	**2**	**3**
Bilirubin (mg/dL)	1–2	2–3	Greater than 3
Albumin (mg/dL)	Greater than 3.5	2.8–3.5	Less than 2.8
Ascites	None	Mild	Moderate
Encephalopathy (grade)[a]	None	1 and 2	3 and 4
Prothrombin time (seconds prolonged)	1–4	4–6	Greater than 6

[a]Encephalopathy grades: Grade 1: disordered sleep, mild confusion; Grade 2: lethargic, moderate confusion; Grade 3: somnolent but rousable, confused, disoriented; Grade 4: coma, unrousable. Total up score from five rows. Score interpretation: Grade A (mild disease) less than 7; Grade B (moderate disease) 7–9; Grade C (severe disease) 10–15.

Appendix

Anticoagulants in Management of Ischemic Stroke or Transient Ischemic Attacks

---

Cardioembolic Stroke or TIA

Atrial fibrillation	See Chapter 12
	(Noncardiogenic: antiplatelet therapy preferred over warfarin)
Acute MI with LV thrombus	Warfarin (INR 2–3) for 3 mo minimum
Cardiomyopathy	The benefits of warfarin with a cardiomyopathy and history of a stroke of TIA has not been determined; considerations to prevent recurrent ischemic events include
	• Warfarin (INR 2–3)
	• ASA 81 mg daily
	• Clopidogrel 75 mg daily
	• ASA 25 mg/dipyridamole 200 mg twice daily
Native valvular disease	Warfarin (INR 2–3) is reasonable; avoid combination with antiplatelet agent if possible
	Antiplatelet therapy can be considered:
	• Mitral annular calcification
	• Native aortic/nonrheumatic mitral valve and no AF
	• Mitral valve prolapsed (long-term antiplatelet therapy)

(*continued*)

(continued)

| Prosthetic heart valve | Mechanical valves—warfarin (INR 2.5–3.5), avoid addition of antiplatelet agents; add ASA 75–100 mg/day if stroke or TIA occurs with therapeutic anticoagulation and bleeding risk is not high |
| | Bioprosthetic—warfarin (INR 2–3) if no other source identified[a] |

Anticoagulation Postintracranial Hemorrhage

ICH, SAH, and SDH	Consider stopping all anticoagulants and antiplatelet agents and reversing their effects; hold anticoagulation for 1–2 weeks
	Restarting therapy after an ICH will depend on the risk of recurrent thrombosis or ICH; in patients with a high risk of thromboembolism, warfarin may be restarted 7–10 days after the onset of the original ICH
Hemorrhagic cerebral infarction	Depending on the situation and risk of thromboembolism, it may be reasonable to continue anticoagulation

[a]ACCP 2008: "In patients with mechanical heart valves who have additional risk factors for thromboembolism, such as AF, hypercoagulable state, or low ejection fraction, or who have a history of atherosclerotic vascular disease, we recommend the addition of low-dose ASA (50 to 100 mg/day) to long-term VKA therapy (Grade 1B). We suggest ASA not be added to VKA therapy in patients with mechanical heart valves who are at particularly high risk of bleeding, such as in patients with history of GI bleed or in patients >80 years of age (Grade 2C)."

Sources: Furie KL, Kasner SE, Adams RJ, et al. on behalf of the American Heart Association Stroke Council, Council on Cardiovascular Nursing, Council on Clinical Cardiology, and Interdisciplinary Council on Quality of Care and Outcomes Research. Guidelines for the prevention of stroke in patients with stroke or transient ischemic attack. A guideline for healthcare professionals from the American Heart Association/American Stroke Association. *Stroke.* 2010, Published online October 21, 2010, http://stroke.ahajournals.org/cgi/content/full/42/1/227; Salem DN, O'Gara PT, Madias C, et al. American College of Chest Physicians. Valvular and structural heart disease: American College of Chest Physicians Evidence-Based Clinical Practice Guidelines (8th ed.). *Chest.* 2008;133(6 Suppl):593S–629S.

Appendix

 # Citrate Anticoagulation

Mechanism	Regional citrate anticoagulation chelates calcium required for the coagulation cascade to create clotting factors involved in thrombus formation
Cautions	Hypocalcemia will occur, requiring supplemental calcium during use; metabolic complications including hyponatremia, metabolic acidosis and citrate toxicity can occur Note: blood products are preserved in citrate to prevent clotting; transfusion of a large amount of blood products or use of systemic citrate infusions can lead to hypocalcemia and reduced blood pressure unless concurrent calcium supplementation is provided
ACD-A Solution (224 mmo/L sodium, 112.8 mmol/L citrate)	• Dextrose 2.45 g/100 mL • Sodium citrate 2.2 g/100 mL • Citric acid 730 mg/100 mL
Catheter Flush	4% citrate solutions have been assessed in maintaining catheter patency, but are not commercially available in large quantities; ACD-A solution has been used as an alternative; more concentrated citrate solutions have been explored for additional antimicrobial properties but can lead to metabolic effects if instilled into the systemic circulation
Renal Replacement Therapy	Regional citrate is one option to heparin to prevent thrombosis of the hemodialysis circuit; protocols for its use should be developed in advance and personal responsible for managing trained; protocols will vary between dialysis circuits; in general, citrate anticoagulation can maintain circuits and preserve filters longer than heparin related anticoagulants

(continued)

(continued)

Example Citrate and Calcium Protocol (using ACD-A solution in CRRT)	Citrate infusion:
	• Rate = circuit blood flow x 0.03
	• Check ionized calcium q 6 hr
	• Adjust rate according to circuit ionized calcium level (1.0–1.4 mg/dL (e.g., if rate 200 mL/hr, increase rate 30 mL/hr if <1 mg/dL, decrease by 30 mL/hr if >1.4 mg/dL)
	Calcium infusion:
	• Make a calcium gluconate IV solution of 12 g in 0.9% NaCl total volume of 250 cc (or 24 g in 500 cc 0.9% NaCl)
	• Infuse 30 mL/hr via the central line
	• Calcium level every 6 hr (target ionized calcium of 3.7–4.4 mg/dL)
	• <3 mg/dL: stop citrate for 30 min; give 4 g calcium gluconate IV over 2 hr via central line; increase calcium infusion by 20 mL/hr and decrease citrate infusion by 30 mL/hr
	• 3.0–3.19 mg/dL: give 2 g calcium gluconate IV over 1 hr via central line; increase calcium infusion by 15 mL/hr
	• 3.2–3.6 mg/dL: increase calcium gluconate infusion by 10 mL/hr
	• 4.5–4.8 mg/dL: decrease calcium gluconate infusion by 10 mL/hr
	• 4.9–5.6 mg/dL: decrease calcium gluconate infusion by 15 mL/hr
	• >5.6 mg/dL: hold calcium infusion
	At very low or high levels, physician notification should be considered

Source: Burry LD, Tung DD, Hallett D, et al. Regional citrate anticoagulation for PrismaFlex continuous renal replacement therapy. *Ann Pharmacother.* 2009;43:1419–1425.

Appendix

Agents Implicated in Drug-Induced Thromboembolic Diseases

Agents Implicated in Drug-Induced Thromboembolic Diseases

Hemostatic Agents
Aminocaproic acid
Aprotinin
Cyanoacrylate
Desmopressin
Prothrombin complex concentrate
Recombinant factor VIIa
Tranexamic acid

Anticoagulants
Heparin
Low molecular weight heparin
Pentosan
Streptokinase
Urokinase
Warfarin

Hematopoietic Agents
Darbepoetin
G-CSF
GM-CSF

Estrogen-Containing Agents
Diethylstilbestrol
Hormone replacement
Oral contraceptives

Antiandrogenic Agents
Cyproterone
Flutamide
Goserelin
Leuprolide

Selective Estrogen-Receptor Modulators
Raloxifene
Tamoxifen
Toremifene

Aromatase Inhibitors
Anastrazole

Androgenic Agents
Danazol
Megestrol
Nandrolone

Follicle-Stimulating Hormone
Follitropin alfa

Antineoplastic Agents
Aldesleukin
Asparaginase
Basiliximab

(continued)

(continued)

Bevacizumab
Bleomycin
Carboplatin
Cisplatin
Dacarbazine
Denileukin
Docetaxel
Estramustine
Fluorouracil
Imatinib
Irinotecan
Lenalidomide
Paclitaxel
Thalidomide

Immunologic Agents
Cyclosporine
Dexamethasone
Foscarnet
Immunoglobulins
Infliximab
Interferon alfa-2a
Interferon alfa-2b
Interferon beta
Interferon gamma
Interleukin-3
Methylprednisolone
Muromonab
Prednisone
Sirolimus
Tacrolimus

Antipsycotic Agents
Chlorpromazine
Clozapine

Olanzapine
Quetiapine
Risperidone
Thioridazine

Other Psychotropic Agents
Clomipramine
Escitalopram
Lithium

Contrast Agents
Iohexol
Iomeprol
Iopamidol
Iothalamate
Ioxaglate

Cox-2 Inhibitors
Celecoxib

Miscellaneous
Acetohydroxamic acid
Botulinum toxin
Bromocriptine
Cocaine
Dihydroergotamine
Ectasy (3,4-methylenedioxymethamphetimine
   (MDMA)
Ergotamine
Metolazone
Papverine
Procainamide
Sildenafil
Topiramate
Tretinoin

Abbreviations: Cox-2 = cyclooxygenase-2; G-CSF = granulocyte colony-stimulating factor; GM-CSF = granulocyte/macrophage colony-stimulating factor; HIT = heparin-induced thrombocytopenia; HITT = heparin-induced thrombocytopenia and thrombosis; NK = not known.

Source: Garwood CL. Thromboembolic diseases. In: Tisdale JE and Miller DA, eds. *Drug-Induced Diseases: Prevention, Detection, and Management.* 2nd ed. Bethesda, MD: American Society of Health-System Pharmacists; 2010;941–961.

Appendix

Cancer-Related Thromboembolism

2-Year Cumulative Incidence (Chew HK, et al.)	Relative Risk (95% CI)[a] (Thodiyil PA, et al.)
Prostate	Noncancer in patients: (1.0) patients without cancer
• Localized (1.0%)	Head/neck: 0.29 (0.2–0.4)
• Regional (1.3%)	Bladder: 0.42 (0.36–0.49)
• Remote (1.2%)	Breast: 0.44 (0.40–0.48)
Breast	Esophagus: 0.76 (0.58–0.97)
• Localized (0.8%)	Cervix: 0.90 (0.68–1.18)
• Regional (1.3%)	Liver: 0.92 (0.076–1.10)
• Remote (2.6%)	Prostate: 0.98 (0.93–1.04)
Lung	
• Localized (1.3%)	Rectum: 1.11 (1.00–1.22)
• Regional (2.2%)	Lung: 1.13 (1.07–1.19)
• Remote (2.6%)	Colon: 1.36 (1.29–1.44)
Colon/rectum	Renal: 1.41 (1.25–1.59)
• Localized (1.0%)	Stomach: 1.49 (1.33–1.68)
• Regional (2.4%)	Lymphomas: 1.80 (1.65–1.96)
• Remote (2.9%)	Pancreas: 2.05 (1.87–2.4)
Melanoma	Ovary: 2.16 (1.93–2.41)
• Localized (0.3%)	Leukemia: 2.18 (2.01–2.37)
• Regional (0.9%)	Brain: 2.37 (2.04–2.74)
• Remote (2.9%)	Uterus: 3.4 (2.97–3.87)

(continued)

continued)

Non-Hodgkin's lymphoma
- Localized (1.5%)
- Regional (3.2%)
- Remote (2.1%)

Uterus
- Localized (1.2%)
- Regional (2.2%)
- Remote (4.8%)

Bladder
- Localized (0.9%)
- Regional (2.0%)
- Remote (4.3%)

Pancreas
- Localized (3.2%)
- Regional (3.0%)
- Remote (5.4%)

Stomach
- Localized (2.3%)
- Regional (3.4%)
- Remote (4.4%)

Ovary
- Localized (2.3%)
- Regional (3.4%)
- Remote (4.4%)

Kidney
- Localized (1.3%)
- Regional (3.8%)
- Remote (3.5%)

aPatients without cancers, but with other medical conditions were assumed to have a risk of 1.0 for VTE.

Sources: Chew HK, Wun T, Harvey D, et al. Incidence of venous thromboembolism and its effect on survival among patients with common cancers. *Arch Intern Med.* 2006;166(4):458–464; Thodiyil PA, Kakkar AK. Variation in relative risk of venious thromboembolism in different cancers. *Thromb Haemost.* 2002;87:1076–1077.

Appendix

Nondrug Causes of Thrombocytopenia

Nondrug Causes of Thrombocytopenia

Alcoholism

Anemia

Antiphospholipid syndrome

Blood transfusions/massive transfusion

Burns

Disseminated intravascular coagulation

Extracorporeal circulation

Hemolytic uremic syndrome/uremia

Human immunodeficiency virus (HIV)

Hyperthyroidism

Hypothermia

Idiopathic thrombocytopenic purpura

Intra-aortic balloon pump

Liver disease/hypersplenism

Myelodysplastic or metastatic disease

Nutritional deficiencies

Paroxysmal nocturnal hemoglobinuria

Pregnancy

Primary hematologic disorder

Pseudothrombocytopenia

Sepsis/infection

Systemic lupus erythematosus

Thrombotic thrombocytopenic purpura

Vasculitis

Drug-Related Causes of Thrombocytopenia

Agents Implicated in Drug-Induced Thrombocytopenia

Abciximab
Acetaminophen
Adefovir dipivoxil
Alprenolol
Aminoglutethimide
Amiodarone
Aminosalicylic acid
Amphotericin B
Ampicillin
Captopril
Carbamazepine
Chlordiazepoxide–clidinium bromide
Chlorothiazide
Chlorpromazine
Chlorpropamide
Cimetidine
Danazol
Deferoxamine
Diazepam
Diatrizoate meglumine
Diazoxide
Diclofenac

Digoxin
Efalizumab
Eptifibatide
Ethambutol
Etretinate
Famotidine
Fluconazole
Glyburide
Gold salts
Haloperidol
Heparin
Hydrochlorothiazide
Ibuprofen
Interferon alfa
Isoniazid
Levamisole
Linezolid
Lopinavir/ritonavir
Methyldopa
Minoxidil
Nalidixic acid
Naphazoline
Naproxen

Nitroglycerin
Octreotide
Oxprenolol
Phenytoin
Piperacillin
Procainamide
Quindine
Quinine
Ranitidine
Rifampin
Simvastatin
Sulfasalizine
Sulfvastatin
Sulindac
Tamoxifen
Terbinafine
Thiothixene
Tirofiban
Tolmentin
Trimethoprim–sulfamethoxazole
Sulfisoxazole
Valproate
Vancomycin

Source: Jones KL, Kiel PJ. Thrombocytopenia. In: Tisdale JE and Miller DA, eds. *Drug-Induced Diseases: Prevention, Detection, and Management.* 2nd ed. Bethesda, MD: American Society of Health-System Pharmacists; 2010;929–940.

Appendix

Disseminated Intravascular Coagulation (DIC)[a]

Causes	Sepsis/severe infection
	Malignancy
	Trauma
	Obstetrical (amniotic fluid embolism, Abruptio placentae)
	Severe toxic or immunologic reactions
	• Snake bites
	• Recreational drugs
	• Transfusion reactions
	• Transplant rejection
	• Vascular abnormalities
	• Severe hepatic failure
Diagnosis	Severe thrombocytopenia
	Elevated fibrin markers (D-Dimer, fibrin degradation products)
	Prolonged international normalized ratio or prothrombin time
	Fibrinogen level <1 g/L
Management Considerations	Treat underlying disorder
	Transfuse only for active bleeding
	Heparin in selected circumstances
	Exogenous antithrombin administration (laboratory indices improved, mortality benefit unclear)

[a]DIC is characterized as a systemic intravascular activation of coagulation that is triggered by a clinical situation leading to microvascular deposition of fibrin, which can lead to organ dysfunction. The activation of coagulation may deplete platelets and coagulation factors leading to bleeding.

Examples of Available Bleeding Definitions[a]

Bleeding Severity	TIMI	GUSTO-1	Landefeld Bleeding Index	ISTH (Nonsurgical)
Severe or Life-Threatening		ICH or bleeding with hemodynamic compromise requiring intervention	Fatal—death Life-threatening—producing MI, stroke, surgical intervention Potentially life-threatening (two of the following): • severe blood loss • hypotension ($>$20% drop in SBP to $<$90 mm Hg) • critical anemia ($\Downarrow$ Hct 20% to 25% or less)	
Major	**ICH** $\Downarrow$ Hct $\geq$15% $\Downarrow$ Hgb $\geq$5 g/dL Each transfused unit counts as 1 g/dL Hgb or 3% Hct		**Fatal** Severe $\geq$3 units of blood loss	**Fatal** Symptomatic bleeding in a critical area or organ $\Downarrow$ Hgb $\geq$ 2 g/dL leading to transfusion of $\geq$ 2 units of whole blood or red cells

(continued)

(continued)

Moderate		Bleeding that requires blood transfusion with hemodynamic compromise	≥2 units and <3 units	
Minor	GI or GU bleeding observed: ⇓ Hct ≥10% ⇓ Hgb ≥3 g/dL Not observed: ⇓ Hct ≥12% ⇓ Hgb ≥4 g/dL		Overt bleeding: GI, hemoptysis, hematuria Transfusion ≥1 unit and <2 units of blood Blood loss ≥1 unit/ week or ⇓ Hct >20% discharge Hct <30% + blood loss of ≥1 unit/week + drop of Hct of 20% or more	

[a]The definition of bleeding has varied between clinical trials. A universally accepted approach is not currently in place.

Sources: Landefeld CS, Anderson PA, Goodnough LT, et al. The bleeding severity index: validation and comparison to other methods for classifying bleeding complications of medical therapy. *J Clin Epidemiol*. 1989;42:711–18; Schulman S, Kearon C. Subcommittee on Control of Anticoagulation of the Scientific and Standardization Committee of the International Society on Thrombosis and Haemostasis. Definition of major bleeding in clinical investigations of antihemostatic medicinal products in non-surgical patients. *J Thromb Haemost*. 2005;3:692–694; Rao SV, O'Grady K, Pieper KS, et al. A comparison of the clinical impact of bleeding measured by two different classifications among patients with acute coronary syndromes. *J Am Coll Cardiol*. 2006;47:809–816.

Examples of Transfusion-Related Reactions

Noninfectious	Infectious	Immunologic
Transfusion reactions	Bacterial	Multisystem organ failure
• hemolytic	• Creutzfeldt-Jakob	Infections and sepsis
• disseminated intravascular coagulation (DIC)	Viral	T-cell dysfunction
• febrile nonhemolytic	• hepatitis (A,B,C,E,G)	Macrophage dysfunction
• anaphylaxis	• HIV, HTLV I, and II	Alloimmunization
• post-transfusion purpura	• Epstein-Barr	Graft-versus-host disease (GCHD) (immune compromised patients)
• acute lung injury	• parovirus	
• incompatibility reactions from blood typing errors	• cytomegaloviris	
Embolism	Parasitic	
• air of fat	• malaria	
Hypotension	• babesiosis	
Hypothermia	• Chagas' disease	
Metabolic disturbances		
• citrate-related anticoagulation (if calcium co-administration not included)		
• hypocalcemia		
• hyperkalemia		
• acidosis		
• hyperammonemia		

Appendix

Recommendations for Timing of Epidural Catheter Manipulation Relative to Use of Anticoagulants

Anticoagulant Agent[a]	Timing of Spinal Needle Insertion or Epidural Catheter Placement in a Patient Who Has Been Given an Anticoagulant	Catheter Manipulation in the Presence of Anticoagulation	Timing of Epidural Catheter Removal (if anticoagulant could not be avoided while catheter in place)	Minimum Time Between Epidural Catheter Removal and Administration of an Anticoagulant
Prophylaxis Dosing				
Unfractionated Heparin (5,000 units q 12hr or q 8 hr)		5,000 units SC q 12 hr—no time restrictions apply[b]		
		For doses over 10,000 units daily, assess on a patient to patient basis		
Low Molecular Weight Heparin	Delay needle placement for a minimum of 10–12 hr[c]	Caution: avoid any catheter manipulation while the patient is receiving an anticoagulant	Avoid removal during anticoagulant treatment	2–4 hr
Enoxaparin 30 mg SC q 12 hr			A minimum of 10–12 hr between the last dose and catheter removal is recommended; best if catheter removed just before the next dose, when the anticoagulant effect is at a minimum	
Enoxaparin 40 mg SC q 24 hr	Preoperative LMWH is not recommended with neuraxial procedures[d]			
Dalteparin 5,000 units SC q 24 hr				
Dalteparin 2,500 units SC q 24 hr				
Therapeutic Dosing				
Unfractionated Heparin (IV or SC)	Delay needle placement until the aPTT is <40 sec and/or ≥4 hr post-stopping IV infusion or >12 hr post-SC dose	Caution: avoid any catheter manipulation while the patient is receiving an anticoagulant	Avoid removal during anticoagulant treatment; hold infusion 4 hr prior to catheter removal; consider getting an aPTT (send priority one); target aPTT <40 sec and ≥4 hr post-stopping IV infusion or >12 hr post-SC dose	2–4 hr

(continued)

Anticoagulant Agent[a]	Timing of Spinal Needle Insertion or Epidural Catheter Placement in a Patient Who Has Been Given an Anticoagulant	Catheter Manipulation in the Presence of Anticoagulation	Timing of Epidural Catheter Removal (if anticoagulant could not be avoided while catheter in place)	Minimum Time Between Epidural Catheter Removal and Administration of an Anticoagulant
Low Molecular Weight Heparin Enoxaparin 1 mg/kg SC q 12 hr Enoxaparin 1.5 mg/kg SC q 24 hr Dalteparin 100 units/kg SC q 12 hr Dalteparin 150–200 units/kg SC q 24 hr Tinzaparin 175 units/kg SC q 24 hr	Delay needle placement for a minimum of 24 hr[c]	Caution: avoid any catheter manipulation while the patient is receiving an anticoagulant	Caution: avoid any catheter manipulation while the patient is receiving therapeutic anticoagulation; use of UFH is preferred over use of LMWH; if LMWH was started and an epidural is in place, hold LMWH and wait 24 hr to reach a low anticoagulant effect	2–4 hr
Therapeutic or Prophylaxis Dosing				
Fondaparinux Therapeutic or Prophylactic dosing	Delay needle placement for a minimum of 72 hr[c]	Avoid administration of fondaparinux if an epidural catheter is in place	Caution: avoid any catheter manipulation if the patient is receiving this drug; in the event fondaparinux was started and an epidural is in place, consider waiting 36–48 hr or longer before removing the catheter	2–4 hr
Warfarin	Stop warfarin 5 days prior to insertion; assess INR	Do not initiate until the catheter	If an epidural catheter is in place after warfarin started, the catheter	Can start any time after the catheter

(continued)

	the day prior to catheter placement; consider 2.5 mg PO vitamin K if INR >1.5	has been removed	should be removed before the INR exceeds 1.5; check the INR (send STAT or priority one) prior to removal	has been removed as long as no signs of bleeding are observed
Dabigatran[e]	Stop dabigatran 2–5 days prior to insertion; CrCl ≥ 50 mL/min: 2 days; CrCl <50 mL/min: 5 days	Caution: avoid any catheter manipulation while the patient is receiving an anticoagulant	Caution: avoid any catheter manipulation if the patient is receiving this drug; in the event dabigatran was started and an epidural is in place, consider waiting 36–48 hr or longer before removing the catheter	2–4 hr

Abbreviations: SC = subcutaneous; IV = intravenous; INR = international normalized ratio; aPTT = activated partial thromboplastin time; hr = hours; mg = milligrams; kg = kilograms.

[a] Additional details in the ASRA guidelines are provided in selected situations such as pregnancy, vascular, or cardiac surgery.

[b] Consider measuring the aPTT in individuals who may have a therapeutic effect when given 5,000 units of unfractionated heparin subcutaneously, such as individuals who are age 80 or older or who weigh below 50 kg. If the aPTT is above 40 seconds, consider removing the catheter at the time the next dose is due to be given and avoid administering the next dose for 2–4 hours before restarting.

[c] Longer hold periods may be required in patients with impaired renal function or who have a high risk of bleeding and who are at a low risk for thrombosis.

[d] A neuraxial technique is contraindicated in a patient who received LMWH/fondaparinux/direct thrombin inhibitor preoperatively. Indwelling catheters should be removed prior to starting but may be safely maintained if the patient is receiving prophylactic LMWH.

[e] Clot based assays such as the aPTT or thrombin time can be elevated in the presence of dabigatran and may suggest presence of a drug effect. Values in the normal range, however, can also occur and may not assure the absence of a effect. Checking these laboratory measures could be considered as a final safety check, but it should not supplant extreme vigilance to assure dabigatran is held for an appropriate time period prior to the procedure.

Sources: Horlocker TT, Wedel DJ, Rowlingson JC, et al. Regional anesthesia in the patient receiving antithrombotic or thrombolytic therapy. American Society of Regional Anesthesia and Pain Medicine Evidence-Based Guidelines. (3rd ed.). *Reg Anesth Pain Med.* 2010;35(1):64-101; Llau JV, Ferrandis R. New anticoagulants and regional anesthesia. *Curr Opin Anaesthesiol.* 2009;22(5):661–666.

INDEX

Note: *f* indicates figure; *t* indicates table